Investigation of Sudden Infant Death Syndrome

Diagnostic Pediatric Pathology

Series editors

Marta C. Cohen
Sheffield Children's Hospital
Irene Scheimberg
Royal London Hospital

Also available in the series

Placental and Gestational Pathology
Edited by Raymond W. Redline, Theonia K. Boyd, and Drucilla J. Roberts

Forthcoming

Pediatric Bone and Joint Pathology
Edited by Paul Dickman

Pediatric Dermatopathology
Edited by Isabel Colmenero, Antonio Torrelo, and Luis Requena

Pediatric Soft-Tissue Tumor Pathology
Edited by Rita Alaggio, Sheri Spunt, Erin Rudzinski, and Jennifer Black

Investigation of Sudden Infant Death Syndrome

Edited by

Marta C. Cohen
Sheffield Children's Hospital

Irene Scheimberg
Royal London Hospital

J. Bruce Beckwith
Loma Linda University School of Medicine

Fern R. Hauck
University of Virginia

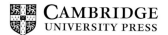
CAMBRIDGE
UNIVERSITY PRESS

CAMBRIDGE
UNIVERSITY PRESS

University Printing House, Cambridge CB2 8BS, United Kingdom

One Liberty Plaza, 20th Floor, New York, NY 10006, USA

477 Williamstown Road, Port Melbourne, VIC 3207, Australia

314–321, 3rd Floor, Plot 3, Splendor Forum, Jasola District Centre, New Delhi – 110025, India

79 Anson Road, #06–04/06, Singapore 079906

Cambridge University Press is part of the University of Cambridge.

It furthers the University's mission by disseminating knowledge in the pursuit of
education, learning, and research at the highest international levels of excellence.

www.cambridge.org
Information on this title: www.cambridge.org/9781108185981
DOI: 10.1017/9781108186001

© Cambridge University Press 2019

First published 2019

Printed and bound in Great Britain by Clays Ltd, Elcograf S.p.A.

A catalogue record for this publication is available from the British Library.

Library of Congress Cataloging-in-Publication Data
Names: Cohen, Marta C., 1961– editor.
Title: Investigation of sudden infant death syndrome / edited by Marta C. Cohen, Sheffield Children's Hospital, Irene Scheimberg,
Royal London Hospital, J. Bruce Beckwith, Loma Linda University School of Medicine, Fern R. Hauck, University of Virginia.
Description: New York, NY : Cambridge University Press, 2019. | Series: Diagnostic pediatric pathology | Includes bibliographical
references and index.
Identifiers: LCCN 2018049857 | ISBN 9781108185981 (alk. paper)
Subjects: LCSH: Sudden infant death syndrome. | Sudden infant death syndrome – Psychological aspects.
Classification: LCC RJ320.S93 I58 2019 | DDC 618.92/026–dc23
LC record available at https://lccn.loc.gov/2018049857

ISBN 978-1-108-18598-1 Print Online Bundle
ISBN 978-1-108-18600-1 Cambridge Core

Contents

Contributors

Srinivas Annavarapu, MD
Department of Cellular Pathology, Royal Victoria
Infirmary, Newcastle upon Tyne Hospitals, UK

Elijah Behr, Professor
MA Cantab Hons MBBS MD FRCP FESC
St George's Healthcare NHS Foundation Trust,
London, UK

**Peter S. Blair, Professor of Epidemiology and
Statistics**
Centre for Academic Child Health
Bristol Medical School, University of Bristol, UK

Marta C. Cohen, MD, FRCPath, DMJ (Pathol)
Histopathology Department, Sheffield
Children's Hospital NHS Foundation Trust,
Honorary Professor, Department of Oncology and
Metabolism, Sheffield, UK

Eve R. Colson, MD, MHPE
Yale School of Medicine, New Haven, CT, USA

Robert Coombs
Jessop Wing, Sheffield Teaching Hospital (retired),
Sheffield, UK

Theresa M. Covington, MPH
Within Our Reach, The Alliance for Strong Families
and Communities, and National Center for Fatality
Review and Prevention, Washington, DC, USA

Phillip Cox, MD
Birmingham Women's Healthcare NHS Trust,
Birmingham, UK

Robert A. Darnall, MD
Departments of Molecular and Systems Biology and
Pediatrics, Geisel School of Medicine at Dartmouth,
Hanover, NH, USA

Christopher Dorries, OBE
HM Senior Coroner, South Yorkshire (West) & The
Medico-Legal Centre, Sheffield, and Centre for
Contemporary Coronial Law, University of
Bolton, UK

Adèle C. Engelberts
Department of Pediatrics, Zuyderland Medical
Center, Sittard, The Netherlands

Juan Alberola Enguidanos, PhD
Department of Microbiology, Dr. Peset University
Hospital and Faculty of Medicine and Odontology,
University of Valencia, Spain

Phil Etheridge, BEng, MSt (Cantab)
Detective Chief Inspector and Sheffield Crime
Manager, Sheffield, UK

Andrew L. Falzon, MD, DABP (AP/CP/FP)
New Jersey State Medical Examiner, Office of the State
Medical Examiner, Trenton and Pathology and
Laboratory Medicine, Rutgers School of Medicine,
Newark, NJ, USA

Amparo Fernández-Rodríguez, PhD
Forensic Microbiology Laboratory, Biology Service,
Microbiology Laboratory, Biology Department,
Instituto Nacional de Toxicología y Ciencias
Forenses, Las Rozas de Madrid, Madrid, Spain

**Robert J. Flanagan, PhD, ERT, MCSFS, Chem, FRSC,
FRCPath, HFCMHP, FRCP Edin**
Toxicology Unit, Department of Pathology,
Sheffield Teaching Hospitals NHS Foundation Trust,
Northern General Hospital, Sheffield, and
Toxicology Unit, Department of Biochemistry,
King's College Hospital NHS Foundation Trust,
London, UK

Joanna Garstang MD, ChB, MRCPCH, MSc, PhD
Warwick Medical School, University of Warwick,
Coventry, UK

Michael Goodstein, MD, FAAP
York Hospital
WellSpan Health
York, PA, USA

Fern R. Hauck, MD, MS
Family Medicine and Public Health Sciences,
University of Virginia School of Medicine,
Charlottesville, VA, USA

Robin L. Haynes, PhD
Department of Pathology, Boston Children's
Hospital, and Harvard Medical School, Boston, MA,
USA

Barbara Himes, IBCLC
Director of Education and Bereavement Services,
First Candle/SIDS Alliance,
Indiana University–Purdue University Indianapolis,
Indianapolis, IN, USA

Monique L'Hoir, PhD
Wageningen University & Research (WUR), the GGD
North- and East-Gelderland, and TNO, Child Health,
Leiden, The Netherlands

Carl E. Hunt, MD
Department of Pediatrics, F. Edward Hébert School of
Medicine, Uniformed Services University of Health
Sciences, Bethesda, MD, and Department of
Pediatrics, George Washington University, Children's
National Medical Center, Washington, DC, USA

Alejandro Gustavo Jenik, MD
Neonatology Department, Hospital Italiano, Buenos
Aires, and Pediatrics Department, University
Hospital School of Medicine, Buenos Aires, and Task
Force on Sudden Infant Death Syndrome, Argentine
Pediatric Society, Argentina

Chris Miles, BSc, MB, ChB, MRCP
St George's, University of London, London, UK

Rachel Moon, MD
University of Virginia School of Medicine,
Charlottesville, VA, USA

Amaka Offiah, BSc, MBBS, MRCP, FRCR, PhD, FHEA
Reader in Paediatric Musculoskeletal Imaging and
Honorary Consultant Paediatric Radiologist
Department of Oncology and Metabolism, Academic
Unit of Child Health, Sheffield Children's Hospital,
Sheffield, UK

Simon E. Olpin, MSC, PhD, CSci, EuSpLM, FRCPath
Department of Clinical Chemistry, Sheffield
Children's Hospital, Sheffield, UK

Ashok Raghavan, MD, DNB
Radiology Department, Sheffield Children's Hospital,
Sheffield, UK

Jan-Marino Ramirez, PhD
Center for Integrative Brain Research, Seattle
Children's Research Institute. and Departments of
Neurological Surgery and Pediatrics, University of
Washington, Seattle, WA, USA

Sanja Ramirez
Center for Integrative Brain Research, Seattle
Children's Research Institute, Seattle, WA, USA

David A. Ramsay, MB, ChB, DPhil, FRCPC, FRCPath, MRCP (UK)
Department of Pathology and Laboratory Medicine,
London Health Sciences Centre, and Western
University, University Hospital, London, Ontario,
Canada

Deborah A. Robinson
Consultant, SUID Investigations,
Seattle, WA, USA

Daniel D. Rubens, MBBS, FANZCA
Department of Anesthesia, Seattle Children's
Hospital, and Center for Integrative Brain Research,
Seattle Children's Research Institute, Seattle, WA,
USA

Irene Scheimberg, LMS, MD, FRCPath
Department of Cellular Pathology, The Royal
London Hospital, Bart's Health NHS Trust,
London, UK

Micheal J. Shkrum, MD, FRCPC
Department of Pathology and Laboratory Medicine,
London Health Sciences Centre and Western
University, University Hospital, London, Ontario,
Canada

Peter Sidebotham, MB, ChB, PhD, FRCPCH
Warwick Medical School, University of Warwick,
Coventry, UK

Waney Squier, MBChB, FRCP, FRCPath
Neuropathology Department, Oxford University
John Radcliffe Hospital, Oxford, UK

James Steer, BSc
Sheffield Diagnostic Genetics Service, Sheffield
Children's Hospital NHS Foundation Trust, Sheffield,
UK

David Tipene-Leach, MBChB, NZCPHM
Faculty of Education, Humanities, and Health
Science, Eastern Institute of Technology, Hawke's
Bay, New Zealand

John M. D. Thompson, PhD
Department of Paediatrics: Child and Youth Health
and Obstetrics and Gynaecology, University of
Auckland, Auckland, New Zealand

**Alfredo E. Walker, MBBS, FRCPath, DMJ (Path),
MFFLM, MCSFS**
Eastern Ontario Regional Forensic Pathology Unit,
Ottawa Hospital General Campus, and Department of

Pathology and Laboratory Medicine, University of
Ottawa, Canada

**Elspeth Whitby, BSc (Hons), MB, ChB (Hons),
FFDRCSI, PhD**
Academic Unit of Reproductive and
Developmental Medicine, The University of
Sheffield, Sheffield, UK

Christopher G. Wilson, PhD
Lawrence D. Longo Center for Perinatal Biology,
Departments of Basic Sciences, and Pediatrics, Loma
Linda University, Loma Linda, CA, USA

Maarten Witlox, LLM
Cot Death Parent Association and Netherlands
Centre for Youth Health, The Netherlands

James R. Wright, Jr, MD, PhD
Professor, Departments of Pathology and Laboratory
Medicine, and Paediatrics, University of Calgary/
Calgary Laboratory Services, Alberta Children's
Hospital site, Alberta Children's Hospital, Calgary,
Canada

Foreword

J. Bruce Beckwith MD

Adjunct Professor, Pathology, and Human Anatomy Loma Linda University School of Medicine

The sudden and unexpected death of an infant is a tragic event that has occurred throughout human history. Until relatively recently, death at any age was so common an event that the sudden demise of a seemingly healthy infant was accepted as one of the risks of human existence. Only in the present era has the sudden unexpected death of an infant become recognised as a distinctive tragic event worthy of serious investigation.

An introduction to this problem occurred early in my career. I was attracted to the field of pathology in the first year of medical school. The birth of my first two daughters occurred during those student years, and watching their development proved so fascinating that it was a major factor determining my decision to become a paediatric pathologist. Graduating in 1958, a classmate planning a career in paediatric radiology and I were given the unique opportunity of being the first interns in clinical paediatrics at Children's Hospital in Seattle. We were ideal test pilots for a programme then being developed for future graduates aiming for a career in clinical paediatrics. That remarkable exposure to the field of disease in infants and children was followed by an opportunity to serve a first year of residency in Pathology at Children's Hospital of Los Angeles, prior to three years as resident in general pathology at Cedars of Lebanon Hospital in the same city. I returned to Children's Hospital for a final year of training in paediatric pathology.

The needs of a growing family necessitated supplementation of income during my resident training years. The Office of the Chief Medical Examiner of Los Angeles County served a huge metropolitan area including some ninety cities and towns. The central office was responsible for all coroners' cases in the downtown area and for suspected homicides from the entire county. Other cases for which the office was responsible were examined by deputy forensic pathologists in funeral homes in the area where death occurred. Most deputies were advanced residents in pathology. I served in this capacity three evenings a week and most Saturdays for three years.

A senior staff member in the central office was responsible for assigning cases to deputies. During my tenure this duty was in the hands of Phillip Schwartzberg. Because of my interest and training in paediatric pathology, Mr Schwartzberg made a point of assigning me to cases of infant and child death whenever possible, rather than the usual assignment of deputies to a particular area of the county. Though this required driving to disparate locations, it presented an unprecedented opportunity for me to investigate a substantial proportion of sudden and unexpected infant deaths occurring in a vast metropolitan region totalling some ten million inhabitants, exceeding the population of most states.

The tragedy now termed SIDS has undoubtedly existed throughout history, but escaped general recognition due to its low prevalence compared to the prevalence of infant mortality in past ages. Its subtle manifestations had also contributed to varying interpretations as to cause of death. The person responsible for deputy assignments made it possible for me to examine an average of one or two cases of sudden unexpected infant death each week. This unique experience made obvious the fact that a substantial majority of these tragedies manifested striking similarity in history and anatomic features.

A notable feature of those sudden and unexpected deaths for which no cause was apparent was an almost complete sparing of infants in the first month of life. Most deaths occurred during the 2nd through the 4th month, the victims having been unexpectedly found dead in their cribs without prior symptoms, and sounds of distress were never reported. Post-mortem examination revealed a stereotyped pattern of findings. Though none of these explained the cause, their consistent presence suggested a common mechanism for a majority of 'crib deaths'. The infants in question were consistently found dead, never being witnessed in the process of dying. An important finding in most cases was the presence of numerous petechial haemorrhages confined to serosal surfaces of the thorax. For example, while the entire intrathoracic surfaces of the thymus typically displayed numerous petechiae, the posterior aspect of the cervical lobes above the left innominate vein typically contained no petechiae, consistent with 'damping' of negative pressure by that vessel. The localised distribution of haemorrhages strongly suggested the presence of increased intrathoracic negative pressure during the dying process, with sudden end-expiratory airway occlusion as the presumptive mechanism of most of these deaths.

Among the proposed causes of these deaths was accidental suffocation in bedding. Vigorous struggle was implied by the consistent finding of tightly clenched fists, often clutching fibres of bedding materials, and disarrayed covers. However parents consistently reported hearing no sounds of struggle, and the face was often uncovered when found.

Prone sleep position was a frequently suggested contributory or causative factor. During the 1960s, prone sleep position for infants was virtually universal, as the result of numerous well-publicised studies that demonstrated significantly enhanced quality of sleep for infants placed in that position. Though some infants were found with the face straight down, head position alone seemed unlikely as the cause, as simply turning the head a few degrees would have created access to air passages, and many were found with face to the side. Though sleep position seemed a potential factor in the mechanism of death, this explanation was not consistent with the paucity of 'crib deaths' during the first month, the age when accidental suffocation would seem most likely to occur. Causation seemed to be linked to postnatal rather than developmental age, as prematurely born, and term infants presented similar postnatal age distribution curves.

Following five years of residency training in Los Angeles, three of which were spent at Los Angeles Children's Hospital, I returned in 1965 to Children's Hospital in Seattle as head of anatomical pathology and subsequently as Director of Laboratories. Prior to my return a combination of circumstances had created an ideal setting for serious research into this problem. The unexpected sudden death of an infant born to a member of a prominent and influential Seattle family had led to widespread community awareness of this problem, and of the need for

investigation of potential causes. Upon learning of my training, experience, and interest in this problem, the Director of Forensic Pathology was delighted to delegate responsibility to me for post-mortem studies of all infant deaths in King County, which included the city of Seattle and surrounding areas. This opportunity would soon lead to a research grant from the Eunice Kennedy Shriver National Institute of Child Health and Human Development (NICHD) to make possible extensive studies on all sudden and unexpected deaths of infants in King County, Washington. With the valuable co-leadership of Drs Abe Bergman and George Ray, and widespread community awareness, and support, our research team was able to carry out extensive studies of every potential case of the tragic phenomenon that would soon become generally designated as SIDS. This term was introduced at the NICHD-sponsored Second International Conference on Causes of Sudden Death in Infancy, held in Seattle in February, 1969, and was the title of a book containing proceedings of that conference, published by the University of Washington Press in 1970.[1] Despite early debates about precise definitions, this term soon became the favoured designation for this tragic event. Investigations by our group and many others, influenced, and supported by prior experience with this problem, led to presentations at national meetings, publications, and to general awareness of and interest in this problem.

Though sudden and unexpected death of infants obviously has many causes, a substantial subset of cases shared many circumstances and pathological findings in common, suggesting that a single cause or mechanism seemed likely for many such deaths. Shortly after beginning our studies in 1965, a preliminary publication alerted paediatricians to the existence and significance of this phenomenon.[2] This was soon followed by a more extensive illustrated report in a widely distributed medical periodical.[3] emphasising the narrow age range that spared the first several weeks of postnatal life, peaking in the second, and third months, with a rapid decline beginning in the fourth month, its consistently silent occurrence during sleep, and pathological findings indicating complete airway obstruction as the mechanism of death for a substantial majority of sudden and unexpected infant deaths.

The term SIDS and the concept it embodied were debated for a few years, but soon achieved widespread acceptance. A 37-page monograph published in 1973[4] was reprinted in 1975 by the US Government Printing Office by order of the Department of Health, Education and Welfare (DHEW) and sent to all practising physicians in the nation, leading to widespread awareness of the existence, nature, and importance of this entity.

While the concept of SIDS is widely accepted, it remains a topic of controversy. Clinical and pathological evidence indicating its association with sleep during a brief period of postnatal life is generally accepted. Its age distribution indicates a relatively narrow period of vulnerability, peaking in the second, and third postnatal months. Obstruction of the upper airway is widely accepted as the likely mechanism, but the exact nature of that obstruction is not revealed by the usual post-mortem dissection. In addition to intrinsic variability in structure, the laryngeal inlet is a dynamic area subject to alteration by the motility of adjacent structures. The most informative anatomical treatise on laryngeal anatomy in infancy and childhood that I have found is the chapter by Karl Peter in the two-volume treatise on paediatric anatomy edited by Peter, Wetzel, and Heiderich.[5] The larynx is situated high in the neck at birth, with the tip of the epiglottis at the level of the top of the first cervical vertebra. Throughout infancy and childhood the larynx descends in position. At six years of age it lies below that vertebra, later attaining its final position below the third vertebra. The configuration of the epiglottis and shape of the inlet manifests great individual variability, making it impossible to define specific shapes and dimensions for various age periods. Inlet configuration also changes in various positions of head and neck.

Pathologists typically examine the larynx after removal from the body. The larynges of SIDS victims that we and others have illustrated in publications may have provided a misleading impression of laryngeal inlet structure and patency in SIDS victims. Dissection in situ, including the influence of head and neck position in SIDS victims, could provide valuable information. Embalming of the body preserves anatomical relationships during manipulation, and it is possible that the well-justified emphasis of forensic pathologists upon performing dissections prior to embalming might have contributed to a lack of knowledge concerning the anatomy of this critical region in SIDS. In-situ study of this region in both unembalmed and embalmed bodies of apparent SIDS victims, with emphasis upon the effect of various head positions upon laryngeal inlet patency, could provide important information concerning the potential cause of death. Regrettably this consideration did not occur to me when I had ready access to abundant case material.

Even if this approach were to reveal insight into the cause and mechanism of SIDS, the rarity of this event indicates that the vast majority of infants have airways capable of remaining patent in any sleep position throughout the brief period of risk.

Though SIDS long remained unrecognised in the era when infant mortality was a common occurrence, the sudden and unexpected death of a seemingly thriving infant now constitutes a major concern for those confronted with this tragic event. The term SIDS will likely either undergo future refinement, with more rigorous limitation to a subset of cases comprising a majority of those currently included under that term, or replacement by terms for recognised causes of sudden unexpected death of an infant. But regardless of designation, there will always be a need for authoritative information on dealing with this tragedy. The present volume provides an impressive fulfilment of that need.

References

1. Bergman, AB, Beckwith JB, Ray CG (eds.). *Sudden Infant Death Syndrome. Proceedings of the Second International Conference on Causes of Sudden Death in Infants.* Seattle: University of Washington Press, 1970.

2. Bergman AB, Miller J, Beckwith JB. Sudden death syndrome: The physician's role. *Clin. Pediatr,* 1966; **5**:711–13.

3. Beckwith JB, Bergman AB. The sudden death syndrome of infancy. *Hospital Practice,* 1967; **2**:44–60.

4. Beckwith JB. The Sudden Infant Death Syndrome. *Curr Prob Ped,* 1973; **3**(8):3–36. Reprinted, Rockville, MD: US Department of Health, Education, and Welfare, 1975, DHEW Publication No. (HSA) 75–5137.

5. Peter K. Der Kehlkopf des Kindes. Band. In: Peter K, Wetzel G, Heiderich F, eds. *Handbuch der Anatomie des Kindes.* München, Verlag von J. F. Bergmann, 1938: 525–62.

Preface

On a beautiful early fall day in 2003, our lives turned upside down. Twice. In the early morning, our only son was born. He was greeted by his three sisters, his grandparents, and his parents, all of us who had been anticipating his arrival with so much excitement and love. A brother, a son, a grandson! The miracle of birth is life-changing, no matter how many times it is experienced.

Six hours later, our son stopped breathing. We went to the lowest of all possible lows in a matter of minutes. He was resuscitated, but his brain had been without oxygen for too long. He would never breathe on his own again. Two days later, he was removed from life support. We left the birthing floor of the hospital with an empty baby carrier, and empty hearts.

An autopsy was performed. We needed an answer. The result? SIDS. We buried our son and trudged forward. Most of what came next is a blur.

When parents lose a child, they are robbed of the hopes and dreams that are attached to that child. The wonder of what he would have become, how he would have changed the world. We'll never know.

When you lose an infant, you are also robbed of memories. Our son was with us for only six hours. There wasn't enough time to create memories. All of the memories of his short life can fit into a small hat box. And most of that box is filled with the bereavement cards we received. We have a few photos, a handprint, a snippet of his hair. But we can't remember the sound of his cry. The smell of his baby-ness. Mostly we remember the pain of his loss. Because instead of experiencing his life, we now endure a lifetime without him.

As if that isn't all difficult enough, imagine the result of an autopsy coming back as inconclusive. The experts have no idea why our son died. When cause of death is labelled as 'SIDS/or SUDI/SUID', you are also robbed of answers and of any chance of closure. The death of our infant was sudden. And it was unexplainable. The acronym fits. But there is no resolution in that. It is salt in the wound.

Our bereavement process started on that life-changing day and continues to this day. When we were able to come up for some air, and look a little more into SIDS, what we found was ever so frustrating. Any published work we could find focused on risk factors such as smoking, infant sleeping position, etc. None of that applied in our situation. But that seemed to be the end of the research story. Until about two years ago when we found some new research being conducted out of Seattle Children's Hospital that focused on physiological contributors to SIDS. We felt hope for the first time. From there, we dove in deep. And here is what we found.

For a first-world developed nation, it is inconceivable that so many infants die each year in the United States without warning and without explanation. SIDS is the leading cause of death in infants 1 month to 1 year of age in all developed nations. About 3500 infants die of sudden unexpected causes (SUDI or SUID) in the US each year alone! And that number has not improved since the mid-90s. There are pockets of research all over the world, but progress is slow. There are some data collected at the time of death, but the data are inconsistent, and difficult to access.

The answers to finding the causes of SIDS lie in research. And research needs accurate, consistent, accessible, and usable data. In 2017, in honour of our son, we formed the Aaron Matthew SIDS Research Guild of Seattle Children's Hospital, whose vision is a world where no parent ever experiences the loss of a child again to SIDS. The guild is focused on four key areas: 1) raising awareness of SIDS and SUDI/SUID with the aim of raising much needed research funding; 2) building a worldwide research collaboration to solve this terrible mystery; 3) working with government to enable researchers to access all available autopsy data in a responsible way; and 4) developing the first global infant genome database for medical professionals and researchers worldwide with a goal of reducing infant mortality.

We have never felt more hopeful about the future of infant health and survival rates. The collection of knowledge and research in this book is so critical to truly understanding the mechanisms and factors surrounding a SIDS diagnosis. We are blessed to have so many experts working on this topic, as we dedicate our lives to making a difference in the name and memory of our son Aaron. Through our collective work, we will be comforted in knowing that his short life changed the world for so many others.

John B. Kahan and Heather L. Kahan
Seattle, Washington

The History of SIDS – the Commonwealth's Contributions in its Formative Years

James R. Wright, Jr

The National Association of Medical Examiners (NAME) in the United States asked me recently to present the history of SIDS.[1] The context for this was an attempt to strike the term 'SIDS' from the medical lexicon, as proposed in the June 2017 theme issue of their journal *Academic Forensic Pathology* and replace this with 'undetermined'. The article[1] did not take sides on this thorny issue but was designed to provide historical context and help guide discussions within NAME. Since it was directed towards an American audience, it naturally had a somewhat American focus. My historical article caught the attention of the editors of this book, and they have asked me to write a brief historical entry highlighting important global contributions. While recognising that SIDS is not a single entity and that the use of this name, which dates back to only 1969, to classify deaths is controversial and may change in some jurisdictions, the term SIDS is used for simplicity's sake, even though the three 'SIDS investigators' I will discuss did much or all of their important work before 1969.

Prior to the 1940s and 1950s, SIDS was generally thought to be due to overlying, infanticide, thymic asthma, status thymicolymphaticus, smothering by bedclothes, and accidental suffocation[1] which will not be covered here. Fundamental work published in the 1940s suggested that SIDS is a natural entity with typical pathological and epidemiological findings. The first of these types of studies included the publications of New York City forensic pathologist Jacob Werne in 1942, Birmingham UK pathologist W. H. Davidson in 1945, and Werne, and his wife Irene Garrow from 1947 to 1953; these papers all suggested that many of these sudden, unexpected infant deaths had natural causes and that performing autopsies demonstrated explainable causes of death in some instances and provided histopathological findings demonstrating vague, mild respiratory disease processes in most of the rest.[1] These observations paved the way for the better understanding of SIDS

that took place in the latter half of the twentieth century and changed the way these deaths were classified.[1]

The next wave of investigators confirmed these preliminary findings and took epidemiological analyses much further, helping establish the entity that would be named SIDS by J. Bruce Beckwith in 1969.[1] These included Melbourne forensic pathologist Keith Macrae Bowden (1908–1999), *British Medical Journal* editor Douglas Swinscow (1917–1992), and Sheffield paediatric pathologist John Lewis Emery (1915–2000). By virtue of the fact that they were working on opposite sides of the world, the convergence of their findings, combined with those of American investigators,[1] were even more compelling.

Bowden published three important papers in the *Medical Journal of Australia* from January 1950 to November 1952.[2–4] He noted that about thirty babies per year were found dead in their cots in the Melbourne area. The first paper addressed the question 'do babies accidentally suffocate in the bedclothes or face downwards on the bedding?' It provides his intriguing analyses into babies' spontaneous choices of sleep position at 2–7 months vs. 7–18 months of age and it comes very close to outlining the full 'triple-risk model'[1] currently used to explain SIDS. Bowden reported his autopsy series and concluded that if complete autopsies were performed, pathological findings are usually present. He notes that: 'although in every case the question why sudden death occurred, and although the exact mechanism of death is obscure in some cases, in practically every case natural disease was present'.[2] In one of his cases, the cause of death was determined to be an inherited metabolic disease, predicting a fertile area of research that would begin several decades later.[1] In his second paper, he added bacterial cultures and in some instances influenza virus cultures into his analyses and concluded that in twenty of forty-three cases, 'histological evidence of respiratory tract infection can be found, but in which the aetiological agent was not isolated'.[3] He also observed that parents initially reported the infant to be 'quite well when last seen' before the death but, that when questioned later, 'a carefully taken history revealed evidence of several days or weeks of minor illness' in over two-thirds of cases.[3] Bowden's final study examined overlaying as a possible cause of death in 179 consecutive infants brought to the Melbourne City Morgue after dying suddenly and unexpectedly. In only 11 instances, was one or both parents actually sleeping with the infant and in 10 of these instances a complete autopsy established a natural cause of death. Bowden concludes that in all of Melbourne over the past four years, 'there has been one possible case of overlying'.[4] Bowden cited a forensic textbook claiming that accidental overlaying 'causes quite an appreciable annual loss of life' and that it is 'the most common form of accidental smothering', both of which he showed to be incorrect. All of Bowden's papers support his major premise: *'the more thorough the autopsy, the less the likelihood of a diagnosis of 'accidental suffocation''*.[3]

Swinscow wrote only one paper on SIDS, but it was influential.[5] 'So-called accidental mechanical suffocation of infants' was published in the *British Medical Journal* on October 1951; it called attention to the works of Davison, Werne and Garrow, and Bowden suggesting that many of these deaths had a natural cause. He then provided a detailed explanation of sex-ratio statistics and how they can be used to categorise deaths. Swinscow noted that: 'The two main factors concerned here are the sex distribution of the population exposed to risk and the differing susceptibility, characteristic of each sex, to death from a particular cause. When comparing the sex ratios of death from two or more causes in the same population, we find that the main effective reason for the difference between them is the fact that the deaths are caused by different agents'.[5] He then used England–Wales death statistics recorded by the Registrar-General for the years 1921–30, 1931–9, and 1940–9 to reveal that sex-ratio analyses showed a preponderance of male infants dying in cots and cradles when compared to infant deaths known to be accidental mechanical suffocation (eg., aspiration of food). He concluded 'many of the cot deaths are caused differently from (known accidental mechanical suffocation) deaths ... Yet all are alleged to be due to the same cause – accidental mechanical suffocation.'[5] He further stresses 'the effect that

such a diagnosis may have on the parents ... No infant's death should be attributed to accidental mechanical suffocation unless there is clear positive evidence of it.'[5]

John Emery's contributions to the understanding of SIDS began in 1956 and he published at least another seventy-five papers on the topic after that. In fact, studying SIDS became a lifelong passion. One of his own children died in infancy, which gave him compassionate insights allowing him to deal with grieving families. According to A. H. Cameron:

> He employed two methods as the basis of his work on cot deaths. First was the meticulous morphological post-mortem study, accompanied by statistically controlled comparisons with hospital deaths. Much of his published work studied one organ at a time, for example, the lymphoid aggregates in the lung or the progress of ossification at the costochondral junction. This led inevitably to a study of normal development, which he soon discovered was based on very scanty data at that time. Paradoxically in his early investigations, he planned to use cot-death material as normal controls for other projects, but he soon realized the error of his way. His second method was an investigation of the domestic environment, again with appropriate controls. By this means he identified certain risk factors which allowed the preventive community paediatric services to concentrate their attention on particular families. He always emphasised the dependence of team-work and, in particular, the close involvement of the Health Visitor service.[6]

Emery's first SIDS paper began by citing Swinscow's mortality statistics; next, he noted that Davidson 'thought that most of these deaths were due to natural causes, and that with skilled necropsy the cause of death would be found' but concluded, 'unfortunately this is not wholly true'.[7] He noted that others have found only non-specific chronic inflammation in lungs. He then presented his own Sheffield data showing the added value of better history-taking. He notes that 'in only five of 50 infants studied was the complete correct history available at the time of necropsy' and 'in 33 the history ... available to the pathologist was not only inadequate but misleading' (i.e., 'wrong enough to affect the diagnosis')[7] Emery also suggested that the autopsies be performed by a paediatric pathologist at the local children's hospital.

Emery published papers on the epidemiology of SIDS for forty years.[8–11] As a pathologist, he also published detailed papers on subtle pathologic findings suggestive of chronic hypoxia (fat-laden cells in the cerebro-spinal fluid (CSF), retention of periadrenal brown fat cells, histopathological changes in the trachea) seen in SIDS starting in the mid-1970s[12–14] as well as papers showing that some pathologic changes reported by others are not specific to SIDS.[15]

Emery performed retrospective case-control studies on SIDS and control infants examining obstetric and perinatal histories in order to identify prospective 'criteria for detecting children at increased risk of dying unexpectedly'.[16] He and his team then used this to develop a scoring system to identify infants at risk.[17] He established a programme of Sheffield 'health visitors', and Emery and colleagues reported that infants who were visited and weighed frequently and received safe-sleeping advice had fewer deaths than predicted.[18] Within the identified high-risk group, they found symptoms that further predisposed to death.[19] This work resulted in an interventional study which showed excellent results after seven years,[20] as well as the Care of Next Infant (CONI) programme funded by the Foundation for the Study of Infant Deaths (now The Lullaby Trust) to provide support to families with new babies after having experienced a cot death.[21] In the 1980s, Emery published controversial estimates that about 10% of 'SIDS' cases were actually filicide;[22] while it was important to acknowledge that some cases signed out as SIDS are really filicide and that forensic science cannot always identify these cases, current data suggests that his estimate was too high.[23] However, Emery did publish data proposing a much higher incidence in families in which two or more SIDS deaths have occurred,[24] a finding supported a decade later by the high-profile multiple infanticide convictions of Wanda Hoyt in New York and Marie Noe in Philadelphia,[1] as well as chilling publications from Sir Roy Meadows and David Southall showing parents deliberately harming their infants.[1,23] Emery's contributions to SIDS were many.

Keith Macrae Bowden, Douglas Swinscow, and John Lewis Emery made important pathological and/or epidemiological contributions to the establishment of SIDS as a diagnostic entity and helped advance its understanding. It is imperative that these be remembered, and their work has not been highlighted in a previous historical paper. For a more comprehensive history of SIDS and to see how the work of these three men fit into the overall picture, the readers are invited to read reference 1 below.

References

1. Wright JR Jr. A fresh look at the history of SIDS. *Acad Forensic Pathol*, 2017; 7(2):146–62.

2. Bowden K. Sudden death or alleged accidental suffocation in babies. *Med J Austral*, 1950; 1(3):65–72.

3. Bowden KM, French EL. Unexpected death in infants and young children: Second series. *Med J Austral*, 1951; 1(26):925–33.

4. Bowden KM. Overlaying of infants. *Med J Austral*, 1952; 2(18):609–11.

5. Swinscow D. So-called accidental mechanical suffocation of infants. *Br Med J*, 1951; 2:1004–7.

6. Cameron AH. Founders of Pediatric Pathology: John Emery (1915–). In: Garvin AJ, O'Leary TJ, Bernstein J, Rosenberg HS, eds. *Perspect Pediatr Pathol*, Basel: Springer-Verlag, 1992; 16:1–6.

7. Emery JL, Crowley EM. Clinical histories of infants reported to the coroner as cases of sudden unexpected death. *Br Med J*, 1956; 2:1518–21.

8. Emery JL. Epidemiology of 'sudden, unexpected, or rapid' deaths in children. *Br Med J*, 1959;2:925–8.

9. Emery JL. 'Sudden and unexpected' death in infancy. *Proc Roy Soc Med*, 1959; 52:890–2.

10. Sutton RNP, Emery JL. Sudden death in infancy: a microbiological and epidemiological study. *Arch Dis Child*, 1966; 41:674–7.

11. Emery JL. 'Cot death' rates on different days of the week. *Arch Dis Child*, 1998; 79:198–204.

12. Gadsdon DR, Emery JL. Fatty changes in the brain in perinatal and unexpected death. *Arch Dis Child*, 1976; 51:42–8.

13. Emery JL, Dinsdale F. Structure of periadrenal brown fat in childhood in both expected and cot deaths. *Arch Dis Child*, 1978; 53:154–8.

14. Wailoo M, Emery JL. The trachea in children with respiratory diseases including children presenting as cot deaths. *Arch Dis Child*, 1980; 55:199–203.

15. Cullity GJ, Emery JL. Ulceration and necrosis of vocal cords in hospital and unexpected child deaths. *J Pathol*, 1975; 115:27–31.

16. Protestos CD, Carpenter RG, McWeeny PM, Emery JL. Obstetric and perinatal histories of children who died unexpectedly (cot death). *Arch Dis Child*, 1973; 48: 835–41.

17. Carpenter RG, Gardner A, McWeeny PM, Emery JL. Multistage scoring system for identifying infants at risk of unexpected death. *Arch Dis Child*, 1977; 52:606–12.

18. Carpenter RG, Emery JL. Final results of study of infants at risk of sudden death. *Nature*, 1977; 268: 724–5.

19. Carpenter RG, Gardner A, Pursall E, McWeeny PM, Emery JL. Identification of some infants at immediate risk of dying unexpectedly and justifying intensive study. *Lancet*, 1979; **2**(8138): 343–6.

20. Carpenter RG, Gardner A, Jepson M, Taylor EM, Salvin A, Sunderland R, et al. The health visitors of Sheffield. Prevention of unexpected infant death: evaluation of the first seven years of the Sheffield Intervention Programme.*Lancet*, 1983; **1**(8327):723–7.

21. Emery JL, Waite AJ. These deaths must be prevented without victimizing parents. *Br Med J*, 2000; **320**:310.

22. Taylor EM, Emery JL. Two-year study of the causes of post-perinatal infant deaths classified in term of preventability. *Arch Dis Child*, 1982; **57**:668–73.

23. Milroy CM, Kepron C. Ten percent of SIDS cases are murder – or are they? *Acad Forensic Pathol*, 2017; **7**(2): 163–70.

24. Emery JL. Families in which two or more cot deaths have occurred. *Lancet*, 1986; **1**(8476):313–15.

Chapter

2

When a Baby Dies, a Community Cries – Family Perspective

Barbara Himes

In the early morning hours of Christmas Eve, our 2-month-old son starting fussing. It hadn't been long since he was last fed so I put a pacifier in his mouth and patted him gently until he went back to sleep. I rolled over in hopes for a little more rest myself. After several hours uninterrupted, I awoke to the light of day rather than a hungry little one. I tried to tell myself this was a milestone; Jake was starting to sleep for longer periods of time. I looked over at the crib just two steps away from my bed and could see his arm sticking out of the spindles of his crib. It had a purplish blue colour to it and I couldn't imagine what that was. That very moment changed our lives forever.

The range of emotions that come with expecting a child are different for every family and each pregnancy. Try to recall or imagine the moment that you learned you were expecting a baby. Excited? Scared? Anxious? Relieved? Just as each pregnancy is unique, so too are the feelings and circumstances surrounding each mother and father-to-be. Many are thrilled to become a parent. Some are depressed, sad, or worried after learning of an unplanned pregnancy. Often, being anxious about their ability to be a good parent. It is safe to assume many people are thrilled that their dream will become reality, while others might be weary of the situation or uncertain about the relationship with the other parent. No matter the circumstance, most parents wonder what their miracle will look like when they arrive and what life will be like with their new addition.

As dramatic as the uncertainty and anticipation can be, thoughts, and wonders become true reality when the baby is born. Emotions run high as parents are relieved the baby is okay, and they're often euphoric at the instant connection to the newborn. For many, the love is immediate, and intense. Let's remember, however, that for some new parents there may be deep fear of their ability to care for their newborn. This can be accompanied by embarrassment that they aren't overjoyed about their baby and a feeling of shame or guilt about feeling that way.

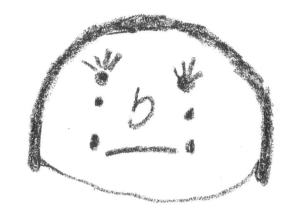

Figure 2.1

Then, in an instant, the incomprehensible happens for some families. It happened to me. A baby found lifeless, gone, never to wake again … What happened to this seemingly healthy baby?? Was it something I did or neglected to do? In the many years since my son's passing, I've heard some reoccurring comments and questions from other families. Those include the following: *What caused this? Am I being punished? Someone else was caring for my baby … what did they do? He was just at the doctor – why didn't the doctor catch it? How can a healthy baby die? Will this happen again? What does 'undetermined' mean and how does this explain my crisis?*

Through the years of learning from my own experience and involvement with siblings and peers, I've come to realise that how parents are treated, and an explanation for the family, is vital. It is imperative for healing and understanding. For my family and me, being presented with current evidence-based diagnosis and the available knowledge surrounding it in a way that we could understand proved very helpful in lessening the feelings of guilt, blame, and helplessness. My family was treated with compassion and my son with dignity and respect. The impact of an infant death involves so many emotions and challenges outside the intense desire to know why, but wanting to know why never goes away. This lingering quest for a 'reason why' has led many to wonder – what research is being done and how can I trust and believe in the information that I find?

I recently collaborated on a study entitled: 'The diagnostic shift to undetermined: are there unintended consequences?'[1] This study sought to describe the perceived effect(s) that a shift in cause of death has had among bereaved families. The survey collected information, through an online family forum for a two-week period, from bereaved parents who have suffered the death of an infant since 2002.

The number of family respondents was small and therefore findings may not be statistically significant, but offers a sense of the perceptions among families in this unenviable position. Fifty-five parents who had experienced the sudden unexpected death of their infant since 2002 answered the survey. All of these respondents had had a death investigation which ultimately was closed with a cause of death as SIDS (21.8%), Sudden Unexpected Infant Death in Infants (SUDI)/Sudden Unexpected Death in Infancy (SUID) (23.6%), undetermined (38.2%), and asphyxia (16.4%).

40% of the respondents stated that they did not clearly understand the final diagnosis assigned to their infant's death. This lack of understanding was predominantly among cases certified as SUDI/SUID (53.8%) and undetermined (66.7%). Deaths certified with asphyxia reported confusion (33.3%) specifically when parents perceived that evidence of asphyxia was speculative. Parents of SIDS cases reported the least amount of confusion with the diagnosis (16.7%). Individuals who assisted the parents with an improved understanding of the cause of death (COD) and its implications for their family differed by diagnosis. SIDS and SUDI/SUID cases more often reported the medical examiner (ME) or coroner assisted them with a better understanding of the diagnosis and the terminology used. However, parents of cases certified as undetermined reported they were more likely not to receive clarity from anyone.

Negative perceptions towards the medicolegal death investigation and public health were described by parents in our study. Distrust, frustration, and loss of respect were most significant for the SUDI/SUID group (38.5%), while parents of SIDS were spared. Dissatisfaction was most often related to their awareness of the inconsistency of death certification practices ('I know others in my same situation who were given SIDS-not undetermined' … 'the emergency room doctor told me it was SIDS and the medical examiner said it was asphyxia' … 'I don't think they tried hard enough, healthy babies don't just die!'). Legal implications and social stigma were also factors reported by parents.

These negative feelings could most likely be attributed to the gap between the medical community's definition of these unfortunate events and the very real emotions that the family is feeling. When a baby dies, it's a very definite end. They are gone. The first symptom is the last symptom. To wonder and labour over the reasons for the loss while being given vague reasoning from medical professionals can be a cause for added stress and torment. There is a definite need for help in understanding the events that transpire, and then there is also a need for direction in learning more about support and outreach.

The death of a child has a lifelong effect for both parents and siblings. Many stories of coping strategies, different sources of support, and the impact of engrained memories resonate with me. Our local parent support group hosted an annual memorial service where I met an elderly man who shared that he had lost his son to SIDS thirty-seven years previously. He often thought of him, but never spoke of him or felt he had an avenue to honour him. He was overcome with gratitude for this opportunity to acknowledge his son and for his spirit to live on through all of us.

A nurse who attended a 'Safe to Sleep' training programme that was designed to educate healthcare professionals on the risk-reduction messages shared her personal experience with infant death that spoke volumes. Her own mother had lost a baby to SIDS prior to her birth more than forty years ago. Her mother was now in a nursing home with Alzheimer's, and the nurse visited her daily for dinner. The elderly mother never recognised her nurse daughter or could remember her name these days, but always talked about the baby who died and called her by name.

I often wondered how our family survived the most devastating experience of our lives. Those questions were answered when I had the occasion to meet the owner of a local ambulance service at a support meeting. She introduced herself. She went on to say she remembered when our son passed away two years earlier. There were two runs that Christmas Eve for unresponsive infants; one that they were able to resuscitate, and one, ours, that they weren't. She went on to say the staff cried and prayed for us. I understood then the magnitude of a far-reaching support system. The death of an infant has a ripple effect on family, friends,

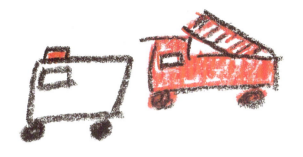

Figure 2.2

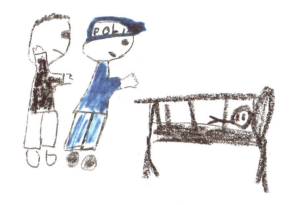

Figure 2.3

and community and leaves an indelible impression for all.

Siblings at home at the time of death experience emotional confusion, perhaps blocking out portions of their memories to protect themselves. A sibling who was three years of age at the time of his brother's death shared:

> The death of my brother to Sudden Infant Death Syndrome (SIDS) thirty-five years ago was traumatising to my family; the negative impact on the physical, spiritual, and psychological health of my family and I would last for many years. Despite being very young, I vividly remember the morning my brother died. I recall the police officers and first responders in my house speaking to my parents. I remember thinking the police were doing something nefarious; I thought they 'took' my brother away from our family. My mother and father were in a state of distress that I had never seen. There was crying and chaos everywhere. There were pleas from my mother to see her deceased baby one last time.

His four-year old sister expressed her feelings of confusion, wanting to keep her baby brother with her stuffed animals and not understanding why she couldn't, and being scared something would happen to the rest of her family too.

A 'Rainbow' baby is a baby born following a miscarriage, stillbirth, or infant loss. Rainbow children have similar and different experiences. They hear stories, often feel as if they knew the baby, maybe feel a missing piece and wonder how their parents were before the death. They might struggle to answer simple questions like, 'How many children are in the family?' For many children, it will go on to impact their view of themselves as parents and their relationships to others.

Another grown 'Rainbow' shares:

> As a kid, I don't think I realised the significance of being the first born after my brother's death. I was too young and naïve to understand that something very traumatic had affected and continued to affect my family and everyone close to them. Looking back on it, I was a little more coddled and protected by everyone. Before having any children of my own, I was always told that you will never understand the unconditional love that you will have for your kids. I now understand that the instant you see them, you immediately have a love for them that can't be described. The thought of losing a child makes me sick to my stomach. From time to time, I can't help but think about how cool having an older brother would be. I have to think that we would have done everything together, been best friends, had the same friends, been there for each other, and played sports together. It's odd that something that happened before I was born potentially changed the entire layout of my life.

Peer support groups played a powerful role in my own life as it provided a safe place to share feelings and provided an understanding of the facts. It truly helped me feel that we were not alone. Bereavement for many of us is a journey that doesn't end. It changes shape and purpose and morphs over time at different stages in a family life cycle. Some SIDS families are led to continue as advocates and as educators to help improve outcomes for everyone, providing another way to heal. These people help to provide a service that is so very necessary for new families, as evidenced in our experience.

We have been fortunate to make some incredible peer support connections with people who have have become lifelong friends. From the journey through the grieving process, to the birth of additional children, to the outreach of the community, to understanding the medical background of an infant death, to finding an avenue to help others down a similar path, I believe that there are so many ways to help those that experience these devastating losses. The responsibility of the medical community to help parents understand what has happened and the responsibility of the family and community to learn how to grieve and then grow are equal. The process is one that is lifelong. The death of a child is like a wound that heals, but the scar stays with you forever.

Acknowledgement

A special thanks and credit for illustrations goes to children involved in the sibling support meetings.

Reference

1. Crandall, L, Reno, L, Himes, B, The diagnostic shift of SIDS to undetermined: are there unintended consequences? *Acad Forens Path*, 2017 7(2):212–20; http://journals.sagepub.com/doi/abs/10.23907/2017.02 2?journalCode=afpa (accessed 30 October 2018).

Chapter 3

Care and Support of Parents After Sudden and Unexpected Loss of an Infant

Monique L'Hoir and Maarten Witlox

Introduction

The death of an infant is a major traumatic event for all family members, regardless if the death is explained or unexplained, expected, or unexpected. Children should not die earlier than their parents, but still it happens. Every death of a child is a shock for parents, siblings, grandparents, friends, and other involved people. The loss can cause anger and questions, 'why this child, why now, what could we have done to prevent it?' Parents, neighbours, bystanders, and healthcare workers all have these or similar emotions and questions.

Parents who have lost their infant suddenly and unexpectedly, without a clear explanation of death, almost all experience *post-traumatic stress reactions* and sometimes a *post-traumatic stress disorder* develops. The way parents are supported shortly after the loss of their child, the professional's attitude, their empathy can help parents immensely. Furthermore, everywhere in the world there are parent support groups, either on the web, or through meetings, that enable parents to meet fellow sufferers. If parents receive support that fits their needs by family members, friends, neighbours, professionals, and other cot death parents and have not experienced other traumatic events with which they have not come to terms, in general, they will be able to adapt eventually. But it takes much effort and quite some time.

In this article, suggestions are given how parents who suffer from the sudden unexplained death of their infant, can be supported. First, the organisation structure around sudden deaths is described. Next, attention is paid to the immediate care after the death and parental expectations, to involvement of healthcare workers, and the bereavement, and risks that may impede the grief process. Next, follow-up care, and care of subsequent infants is described and a conclusion is given. The perspective of parents, their needs, and expectations, their bereavement, which worldwide have more similarities than differences, are described in this chapter.

Definition

During the first international conference on sudden unexpected health in 1963, the definition of SIDS was introduced: 'the sudden death of any infant or young child, which is unexpected by history, and in which a thorough post-mortem examination fails to demonstrate an adequate cause of death'. [1] It has been recently proposed to replace these definitions into 'Sudden Unexpected Infant Death in Infants' (SUDI) or Sudden unexpected infant death (SUID).[2,3] 'Cot death' or 'crib death' is a definition parents understand, which Parent Associations use worldwide and because of its simplicity and clearance it gives support to all parents of all backgrounds and education levels.

For parents, if the conclusion after extensive protocolled investigation is a medical diagnosis, i.e. a lung disease or heart failure, this may facilitate their bereavement, especially when interventions to prevent a next sudden death is possible. But in most sudden and unexpected deaths, only a few risk factors are found, which together may not explain the cause of death entirely. Cot death/SIDS is a diagnosis of exclusion, which especially for Western, well-educated parents is very hard to understand and accept, because they feel they have, or should have, control over their life. Therefore, assessment and monitoring the need for practical and socio-emotional support is recommended for traumatic loss such as SUDIs.[4]

Cooperation Between Parents, Researchers, and Public Health

Worldwide, there are parent associations offering parents support. In the Netherlands, the Cot Death Parent Association was founded in 1981. Over the years much has changed. At first a possible

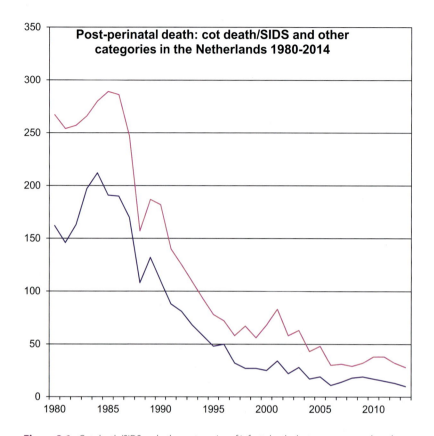

Figure 3.1 Cot death/SIDS and other categories of infant deaths between one week and one year registered at the Dutch Central Bureau of Statistics (2015). Other categories are: acute airway infections / pneumonia / unspecified symptoms / ill-defined condition / suffocation by food / accidental suffocation and strangulation in cot or bed (J00-J06, J20-J22, J10-J18, J40-J47, R00-R69, R95, R990, W79, W75).

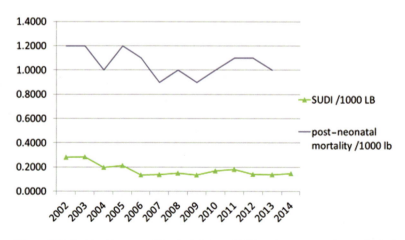

Figure 3.2 Sudden Unexpected Deaths in Infancy (SUDI) and post-neonatal mortality in the Netherlands 2002–14.

explanation for cot death was published almost weekly in the lay press and scientific journals. Then the high risk of prone sleeping was discovered and the cot-death incidence declined strongly (Figure 3.1,3.2).

In the Netherlands the cot-death incidence decreased from over 200 cases a year (1986) to less than 10–15 a year,[5] i.e. 0.06 per 1000 live births. In fact, Dutch parents of cot-death children aided this reduction by promoting and participating in epidemiological studies, which were initiated by Professor Dr G. A. de Jonge and Dr Adèle Engelberts.

Dutch Interdisciplinary Protocol

Since January 1, 2010, Dutch law states that in all deaths the attending physician must consult with the municipal coroner. In most cases the nature and cause of death are known. When after the death of a minor the cause of death is not (fully) clear and there is no evidence for a non-natural death, a protocol established by NODOK (Nader Onderzoek Doodsoorzaak van Kinderen) is followed.[6] This describes how further research into the cause of death should start, what information is collected and (additional) investigations shall be carried out, how the information will be reviewed, aggregated, and registered, and how parents are supported.

National Cot Death Study Group

Parallel to this procedure, but started earlier, namely in 1996, in-depth, standardised epidemiological information is collected by the National Cot Death Study Group (LWW in Dutch), which is a working group of the Dutch Association of Paediatrics (NVK in Dutch). This working group exists of mainly paediatricians, forensic paediatricians, pathologists, a cardiologist, a psychotherapist etc., and the paediatricians conduct home visits to the parents. In close cooperation with cot-death parents, epidemiological data are collected in a systematic way, about infant care practices, the previous medical situation of the child, etc. Together with data from ten nationwide surveys conducted between 1987 and 2017 into factors that might be associated with sudden death, this has contributed to a better understanding of the death of this group of infants and toddlers (0–2 years of age). In addition to the LWW, the Cot Death Foundation (whose work has been continued at the Netherlands Centre for Youth Health (NCJ in Dutch)) and the Cot Death Parent Association worked together intensively to turn these findings into preventive advice. This approach has been very effective and, together with the excellent preventive child healthcare system, has resulted in a large reduction of SUDIs. This is a real decrease and worldwide the most comprehensive.[2]

Child Death Reviews

In many countries so-called systematic 'child death reviews' are used to better understand the causes of death and to improve the care and support of parents.[7,8] It has recently been proposed to start reviewing only specific child deaths, such as theme-related deaths.[9] Death reviews conducted by the LWW are an example of a review which focuses on sudden unexpected deaths in infants and toddlers (0–2 years). The main difference with other, international 'death reviews' are the home visits by (retired) paediatricians, who generate important epidemiological information and are highly valued by the parents.

Initial Care of the Family is Crucial

The care, or the lack of care, that parents receive around the time of death has a great impact on the future adjustment and well-being of the parents. The initial care, and place of death (whether the child died at home, at the grandparents' home or, for instance, in a childcare centre) largely determines the course of bereavement.[10]

When parents dial the emergency number usually both ambulance and police arrive at the house. Parents will be in a panic, fearful, and overwhelmed. They can 'freeze', just sitting with their dead baby on their lap. Other parents may take the lead, start re-animation of their child, call the ambulance and family members, and are able to continue to think logically. Parents differ greatly when they first realise their child has died. For professionals it can be difficult to coordinate the situation. The family must wait for the forensic doctor to arrive and it helps the parents if the family doctor (i.e. the general practitioner) is involved shortly after the death of the child, as she/he is more likely to know the family well. He/she can start monitoring the family members, including siblings, offer emotional support, and can refer them to other professionals if necessary.

Not everything needs to be discussed in one interview. What is discussed during the first contact depends on the specific situation. Adequate care of the family immediately after the loss has positive effects on the mourning process and reduces the risk of developing a range of troublesome, sometimes long lasting reactions associated with bereavement, such as post-traumatic stress disorders, depression, and physical complaints.

All in all, 'support initiated by professionals should always include listening to parents and asking them at key moments after their child's death whether they need (extra) support and what kind of support they would like to receive'.[9]

Parental Expectations

Parents expect expertise, empathy, compassion, commitment, consolation, presence, normalising of what is normal, support and a proactive offer to help from healthcare workers.[11] Parents want to be acknowledged in their bereavement.[10] When healthcare workers and attending professionals (ambulance staff, forensic doctors, general practitioners, police officers etc.) give the impression that they are either incompetent, insensitive, cool, aloof, blasé, or uninterested, or generally respond insensitively, this harms the family's mourning process. It is important that the doctor who asks the parents' permission for autopsy (this is not mandatory in the Netherlands) explains to them what this encompasses and takes time to talk about this difficult subject. Because of the hectic situation, physicians cannot expect parents to immediately decide on an autopsy. A second talk, perhaps with the hospital doctor if the death occurred at home, should be offered. A brochure or website can be useful as a tool. Giving permission for autopsy may influence parental grieving process positively and may help exclude risks for future siblings. Parents will often say 'We did everything to find out why our child died'.

Involvement of Healthcare Workers

For parents it is important that healthcare workers show empathy, but it is just as important that they know what to do. As cot death is an infrequent occurrence this is not automatically taken for granted. Currently in the Netherlands forensic doctors and paediatricians are trained to guide parents through this sad situation and to facilitate the referral to the hospital.[6] The professionals who are initially involved inform the parents about the medical procedure, but also about the importance of saying goodbye to the baby. They will involve the family members in washing and dressing the baby themselves if they wish to, and encourage other rituals such as taking pictures.

There is an option to ask for pictures taken by a professional photographer attached to 'Make a Memory' (www.makeamemory.nl) and this can be offered by the paediatrician or nurse. Many parents embrace this concept. 'Make a Memory' is an organisation which makes pictures of the deceased baby in black and white and it is free of charge. The pictures are made by voluntary professional photographers. Parents may prefer to put the pictures away, unseen. At a later stage, they may decide to look at the pictures, and most parents are happy they have chosen to have them made. The pictures usually show the little hands and feet, and the family surrounding the infant.

The possibility to lay out the child at home instead of at a funeral home should also be discussed. It is important to follow the parents' own choices and rituals concerning their deceased baby in a sensitive way. The caregiver should always talk about the importance of arranging the funeral/cremation themselves.

Furthermore, the care, and support offered to the other children need special attention. If the parents are not able to offer this because of their own grief, aunts, uncles, or other people, such as caring neighbours, should be asked to give the children extra care and attention at that moment. The healthcare worker indicates that a difficult time lies ahead of the family, with a long and painful grieving process.

It is important that the healthcare worker talks about possible parents' stress reactions and how these are normal. Some parents feel that they are going crazy, they hear the voice of their baby or they experience physical pain in their (empty) arms. This is all part of extreme grief. Most important is that the caregiver listens to the parents, who at this time feel sad and shattered.

As other parents who have gone through the same experience can support and help cot-death parents enormously, the healthcare worker should always introduce the idea of the local parent associations. These groups welcome these parents as well as those who have lost their child due to accidental mechanical suffocation or an unknown cause or non-natural death.[12]

The healthcare worker will inform the parents about the possibly long-term supporting role of the preventive child health doctor and child health nurse and/or the social worker or psychologist.

Bereavement

Nowadays there is a greater understanding of the loss and pain parents experience after the death of their child, and bereavement care has changed.[7] In the post-war years parents were not always allowed to talk about their deceased child, to see their child after death or to show their grief.[11] In the meantime 'stage theories have made place for other, alternative approaches which may currently better represent grief and grieving processes'.[4,13] An example is the 'dual process model' of Stroebe & Schut.[14] This model indicates that both the confrontation with the loss and the attempt to avoid the loss are two effective ways of mourning. It is important to find a balance between 'loss orientation' and 'restoration orientation'. A parent who mourns will move back and forth between both extremes. An example is a father, who at the office seems to 'forget' the pain of the loss of his child by the distraction of 'business as usual'. But as soon as he gets on his bicycle to cycle back home, he may be in tears again, experiencing all the intense emotions and feelings. Moreover, those parents who get stuck in one of the extremes (either avoiding feelings or remaining in the loss orientation), have an increased risk of serious adverse effects on their physical and mental well-being.[14]

Grief

Grief is a combination of physical, emotional, cognitive, and behavioural reactions that occur after the loss of a person with whom a meaningful relationship existed. Mourning after the loss of a child is a normal process. The pain that parents feel is the price that they pay for the love they have for their child. Had they not loved their child, saying goodbye would not hurt. Every parent understands this explanation and it might help them to understand their emotional pain, which they feel precisely because they love their child. Differences in cause of death of an infant may affect bereavement. Parents and other relatives may react differently after a death due to a (traffic) accident, an illness, or violence.

Parents who lost their child suddenly and unexpectedly have had no time to prepare for, and adapt to, the death.[15] Also the age of the child, the age of the parents, the support parents give each other, work, level of education, and religious affiliations are all related. Complicated grief may be expected: a category in the reviewed International Classification of Diseases (ICD-11) of prolonged grief disorder, with a shorter bereavement duration (> 6 months) than persistent complex bereavement disorder (> 12 months). Only a minority of people have complicated grief, with

percentages around 10% depending on the bereaved subgroup, bereavement duration, and complicated grief criteria.[4]

Feelings of Guilt

Bereavement after the sudden and unexplained loss of a child will last for years in most cases. Of all emotions, feelings of guilt, even though there is no actual question of guilt, are very intense, and prolonged. The doctor should never deny those feelings, but encourage parents to talk about them and show that s/he is open to their deepest and most intense feelings. S/he can explain that adults have strong feelings of responsibility for their small and vulnerable babies which makes feelings of guilt normal. It is their absence, on the other hand, which is unusual.

Different Ways of Mourning

Family, friends, colleagues and employers may not understand that the grieving process after the loss of an infant takes so much time and therefore their support can fall short. In addition, the grieving process of mothers and fathers rarely develop in the same phase, the same way, and with the same intensity. They can lose each other during this process and it will feel as if they have to cope with the loss by themselves. Their own grief can be so intense that there is no room for someone else, not even their own partner. This is a normal part of grief and parents will be able to accept this better from each other when the caregiver informs them in advance about these possible differences of expression and experience of grief. Sometimes parents do nothing but try to 'prevent their partner to feel any pain' thus not expressing their own feelings, thus becoming blocked.[16]

Many damaging reactions are associated with bereavement, such as increased use of medication, psychosomatic complaints, nutritional, and sleep problems and economic problems. It has been affirmed that the most vulnerable people are the least inclined to seek help.[4] This is another reason why physicians, family doctors, and health nurses should be actively involved in outreach, and not merely tell parents: 'if you need me, just tell me and I'll be there'. This is a dysfunctional way of 'giving support'.

Constructive Mourning

Constructive mourning means that feelings can be expressed and that the social environment is accepting and supportive. Thoughts are shared, partners talk, and questions and memories are retrieved. Adaptive 'grief work' means that life makes sense again, an inner balance is found and the suffering and emptiness are built in the life after the loss. A grieving process can stagnate or become disturbed, or never stop. This can happen by prolonged denial and evading reality, which prevents recovery, acceptance, and adaptation. Effects of this ineffective way of coping can be depression, suicide ideas, and extreme passivity. Such reactions are definitely reasons for caregivers to refer parents to a psychologist or psychiatrist. But more is now known about the need for psychological treatments in general (i.e. counselling and therapy) and their impact. There is continued support for the view that bereaved people do not need routine referral to 'bereavement' interventions just because they have become bereaved.[4] Online interventions offer an alternative approach, which seems a useful form of support.

Post-traumatic Stress Reactions

Parents who experience the death of their infant, almost always experience post-traumatic stress reactions, especially if the death is unexpected and unexplained.[17] After traumatic events, such as cot death, these are normal reactions. Examples of post-traumatic stress reactions are repetitive nightmares, recurring images of the deceased child, avoidance of images of the child or other remembrances, diminished concentration, and increased irritability. Reliving occurs often by sudden and intrusive memories of the traumatic event, nightmares, or anxious dreams. These involuntary memories and the fear that they arouse, mainly cause physiological over-stimulation. Avoidance reactions aim to keep away reliving images of the traumatic event. These reactions are normal and will usually diminish gradually. Having a post-traumatic stress disorder is different. This psychiatric disorder can hinder bereavement or even block the start of the process, and should be resolved first. A diagnosis of 'post-traumatic stress disorder' (PTSD) means that significant complaints persist and suffering is prolonged. It is important that healthcare workers recognise signals and complaints and actively motivate parent(s) to seek help from experienced psychologists or psychiatrists. An option to treat post-traumatic stress successfully is a short-term treatment 'Eye Movement Desensitisation and Reprocessing' (EMDR). On a Dutch website www.EMDR.nl parents are able to find information about this form of help and where EMDR therapists are located. EMDR can also be used for siblings, especially if they have been witness to the extreme first reactions of their parents.

Siblings

Brothers and sisters of the deceased baby have just as much pain and sadness as the parents, but may express this differently. Sometimes it seems they are indifferent and the loss does not influence their feelings. It can help parents to inform them what reactions they can expect from their children and how they can cope with this. Healthcare workers can encourage parents to share their grief with their children. This may prevent fearful fantasies about the death of their little brother or sister. Open and honest conversations with their children increase the sense of security and avoid the development of feelings of guilt or rejection in children. It is often effective to explain things in simple, clear language; parents can talk with children about 'death' instead of 'sleeping forever'. Depending on which faith parents adhere to, specific words, and explanations can be given, such as 'in heaven' or 'one of the little stars above'. It may help parents to prepare them for ways children mourn, such as playing 'funerals' or drawing pictures of the deceased child. These are normal, valuable ways in which children express their feelings.

Continuation of Support

For most healthcare workers, offering guidance and support to parents whose child has died suddenly or to the siblings is not their daily work. The impact of the traumatic death on the family is important and for that reason there may be problems in the development of other children in the family or in the next infants. The parents' first support is a task for the doctors and other staff members in the hospital to which the deceased child is referred. Further support and assessment of the emotional balance within the family and possible reference to another healthcare worker – for example if an imminent disrupted grieving process develops – is primarily the task of the family doctor. In specific situations there may be a need for extra support after a period of apparent emotional balance.[18] Examples of situations or moments when extra care is appropriate or needed are the next appointment at the child healthcare clinic arranged before the baby's death to check or vaccinate the infant, the infant's next birthday, the appointment when the autopsy results are shared with parents, the anniversary of the child's death, or when parents have questions concerning future pregnancies. If healthcare workers are conscious of these important moments, they can anticipate, and take the initiative to contact the family. This can be a visit or a phone call. If this is offered one day before 'the special day' this is even more effective, because many parents plan special activities/rituals with their other children on special days, but on the day before, they often are in pain and sorrow.

Support by professionals should be offered repeatedly during the grief process. Of course parents decide whether they accept the offered support or not. Parents should be provided with information about the grieving process and options for support.

It has been demonstrated that 'parents appreciate contact with professionals six to twelve months after their child's death, to check whether the family needs any extra care or support. This contact should be initiated by the professional. Parents indicate that they would appreciate the provision of more support and follow-up appointments or contacts with a professional after the death of their child'.[11,19,20]

Risks That May Impede Bereavement

For all parents it is important to have a form of support after the loss of an infant. This is unrelated to the cause of death and the necessary procedures afterwards. After the loss of a child most parents have a strong need for an explanation based on a careful history and a thorough post-mortem examination. Healthcare workers must be able to give parents explanations about their deceased child, including when no clear cause of death is found.

If parents feel they are suspected of having contributed to the sudden, unexplained death of their child, this may influence the grieving process negatively and traumatise parents even more. Suspicion or the perception being 'suspected' evokes feelings of anger, powerlessness, and incomprehension. Explaining the conclusions of the findings of the post-mortem, death scene investigation and family history to parents requires tact, knowledge, and empathy. How the autopsy is offered to the parents, the way it is explained to them, how much time the parents get to consider it, and whether a second meeting is scheduled for example, are factors that influence the perception of the parents and influence their definitive choice.

The arrival of the police, after the parents have dialled the emergency number, can be cause for concern, depending on the police reaction. Naturally, the police also have a very positive function; they coordinate, reassure, explain, and support the parents, and assist them by warning other family members or other important acquaintances. Much depends on how the aid workers who are involved from the very beginning, including the police, behave. An overreaction from one of those involved (disrespectful behaviour and an attitude of suspicion) or passive and watchful waiting, is a complaint sometimes heard about the police action. Sometimes due to lack of knowledge concerning cot death, the police may suspect an unnatural death without any real evidence (for example because there is some pink froth in the baby's mouth, a common occurrence in cot death). Then a judicial autopsy is requested when an autopsy and investigation by a dedicated team would have been far more appropriate and more desirable for the parents.

Care of Next Infants

Dutch parents who are preparing themselves for a baby after having suffered a cot death, can get guidance comparable to the Care of Next Infant (CONI) programme developed in Great Britain[21] (www.nvk.nl; www.ncj/wiegendood.nl). For families who have experienced the sudden loss of a baby, it is very conceivable that during the next pregnancy, and often even more strongly in the first months after birth, feelings of happiness, and anxiety are entangled. In Great Britain as well as in the Netherlands, it is known that adequate professional support during this period helps parents dealing with their fears and uncertainties. By offering the CONI programme to parents, it helps parents to increase their feelings of control over the situation again.[22]

The purpose of the CONI programme is to include the entire chain of care (obstetrics, gynaecology, maternity care, youth healthcare [JGZ in Dutch], general practitioner and paediatricians) to offer parents the opportunity to get care that suits them best. By offering the CONI programme, which includes regular infant checkups, weekly weighing, and frequent home visits by a health nurse, parents feel less need to use expensive home monitors, which in fact offer a false sense of security. On the other hand, parents who still chose to use a home monitor should be informed in advance about the drawbacks of the equipment, and should be conscious that they use the monitor mainly to reduce their own anxiety. Open discussions about the limits of monitor care are a prerequisite in order to offer parents honest care. For this reason in the Netherlands a home monitor is not covered by insurance.

The CONI programme has been scientifically evaluated for usability and applicability and it has been used for many years by youth healthcare, general practitioners and paediatricians.[21,22]

Conclusion

The first care of parents after the loss of an infant is important and may offer support for the parents. For people who grow up in the Western world, where causal thinking is common, it seems difficult to accept that 'no apparent cause of death' is found. But it is possible, it does exist, and it should be in no case reason for hasty decisions or ill-conceived or unjust suspicions.

The Cot Death Parent Association urges doctors to always inform parents whose infant died suddenly and unexpectedly, about the existence of the Parent Association, independently of whether the death is categorised as SUDI, SIDS, cot death, asphyxia, or accidental suffocation.

Finally, we adhere to the opinion that central in the investigation after a sudden unexpected death is the care for the family, and not necessarily the (scientific) drive to explain the death. The immense decrease in cot death in the Netherlands proves that collecting epidemiological data about infants in close cooperation with parents, who (almost) always give their consent to use this information, has led to this unparalleled worldwide drop in sudden infant death.[2] We would like to finish with the following recommendations:

- It is important that the first doctor that puts forward to the parents the possibility of an autopsy explains it extensively and offers a second consultation on the subject, giving parents time to take this important decision. The perspective of future siblings should be taken into account.
- When the cause of death is unclear and there is no evidence of a non-natural death, the child will not be transferred to a forensic centre for autopsy, but will receive optimal and proper first care in the hospital the child and family are referred to. In the Netherlands there are six NODOK hospitals, where paediatricians, forensic doctors and pathologists work closely together and parents receive excellent support.

- Whether the working hypothesis is 'accidental suffocation', 'asphyxia', 'rebreathing', 'cot death', 'Sudden Infant Death Syndrome' or 'Sudden Unexpected Death in Infancy' (SUDI) or a similar category (see Figure 3.1); all parents should receive the same in-depth investigation, empathic, and careful treatment, follow-up care, and support.
- The family doctor is the one that supports the parents in the long term. For her/him to be able to do this adequately, s/he must be fully involved immediately after the death of the child and be kept well informed by the involved physicians.
- Parents whose infant or toddler died suddenly and unexpectedly should always be informed about the existence of the Cot Death Parent Association in that country.
- Physicians should be aware of problems that can arise during grief and possible effective treatments for trauma, such as (in the Netherlands) EMDR.[23]
- When parents expect a baby following this traumatic loss, they should be informed of the existence of the support programme 'Care Of Next Infants (CONI)'. Parents can get information about this programme through the Cot Death Parent Association, their paediatrician, or the preventive child health nurse.

References

1. Beckwith JB. Discussion of terminology and definition of Sudden Infant Death Syndrome. In: Bergman AB, Beckwith JB, Ray CG, eds. *Proceedings of the Seciond International Conference on Causes of Sudden Death in Infants*. Seattle, WA: University of Washington Press, 1970: 14–22.

2. Taylor BJ, Garstang J, Engelberts A, et al. International comparison of sudden unexpected death in infancy rates using a newly proposed set of cause-of-death codes. *Arch Dis Child*, 2015; **100**(11):1018–23.

3. Garstang J, Ellis C, Sidebotham P. An evidence-based guide to the investigation of sudden unexpected death in infancy. *Forensic Sci, Med Pathol*, 2015; **11**(3): 345–57.

4. Stroebe M, Stroebe W, Schut H, et al. Grief is not a disease but bereavement merits medical awareness. *Lancet*, 2017; **389**:347–9.

5. Dutch Central Bureau of Statistics: http://statline.cbs.nl/statweb/ (accessed 30 October 2018).

6. Further investigation in the cause of death in children. NODOK Protocol. https://www.nvk.nl/Nieuws/Dossiers/NODO.aspx (accessed 30 October 2018).

7. Gijzen S, Hilhorst M, L'Hoir MP, et al. Implementation of child death review in the Netherlands: results of a pilot study. *BMC Health Services Research* 2016; **16**:235.

8. Sidebotham P, Pearson G. Responding to and learning from childhood deaths. *BMJ*, 2009; **338**:b531.

9. Gijzen S. Child Mortality; Preventing Future Child Deaths and Optimizing Family Support. PhD Thesis: Twente University, Enschede, The Netherlands, 2017.

10. Gijzen S, L'Hoir MP, Boere-Boonekamp MM, Need A (2016). How do parents experience support after the death of their child? *BMC Pediatrics*, 2016; **204**:1–10.

11. Rudd R, D'Andrea LM. Professional support requirement and grief interventions for parents bereaved by an unexplained death at different time periods in the grief process. *Int J Emerg Ment Health*, 2013; **15**(1):5168.

12. Gijzen S, L'Hoir MP, Boere-Boonekamp MM, et al. Child mortality in the Netherlands in the past decades: an overview of natural causes. *J Public Health Policy*, 2013; **35**(1):43–59.

13. Doka K, Tucci A, eds. *Beyond Kübler-Ross. New Perspectives on Death, Dying, and Bereavement.* Washington, DC: Hospice Foundation of America, 2011.

14. Maes J, Dillen L, eds. *Je bent wat je hebt verloren. Een hedendaagse kijk op verlies en rouw. [You Are What you Have Lost. A Current View on Grief and Mourning].* Culemborg: Witsand Uitgevers bvba, Centraal Boekhuis, 2015.

15. Keyes KM, Pratt C, Galea S, et al. The burden of loss: unexpected death of a loved one and psychiatric disorders across the life course in a national study. *Am J Psychiatry*, 2014; **171**:864–71.

16. Dijkstra IC. Living with Loss. Parents Grieving for the Death of Their Child. PhD Thesis: Utrecht University, 2000.

17. L'Hoir, MP, Wolters WHG. Psychosocial aspects of cot-death; assessment of post-traumatic stress disorders. In: Walker AM, McMillen C (eds.), *Second SIDS Family International Conference, February 13–16, 1992.* Ithaca, NY: Perinatology Press, 1993:293–7.

18. Van den Akker A, Westmaas A. *Preventive Child Healthcare Guideline. Begeleiding gezin bij overlijden kind. [Counseling families in Child Death].* Bilthoven: RIVM, 2009.

19. Garstang J, Griffiths F, Sidebotham P. What do bereaved parents want from professionals after the sudden death of their child: a systematic review of the literature. *BMC Pediatrics*, 2014; **14**:269.

20. Aho AL, Tarkka MT, Astedt-Kurki P, et al. Fathers' experience of social support after the death of a child. *AJMH*, 2009; **3**(2):93–103.

21. Waite AJ, Coombs RC, McKenzie A, et al. Mortality of babies enrolled in a community-based support programme: CONI PLUS (Care of Next Infant Plus). *Arch Dis Child*, 2015; **100**:637–42.

22. Waite AJ, McKenzie A, Daman-Willems C. CONI: confirmation of continuing relevance after 20 years. *Community Practitioner*, 2011; **84**(1):26–30.

23. www.EMDR.nl. In the UK, see for e.g. Cruse (www.cruse.org.uk/); in the US www.bereavedparentsusa.org (all accessed 31 October 2018).

4

Chapter

Sudden Infant Death Investigation in the UK – the Coroner's Perspective

Christopher Dorries

Introduction

Under the law in England & Wales, the coroner has a central role in the investigation of deaths which:

- are of unknown cause
- give reason to suspect that the cause is unnatural
- have occurred in custody or otherwise in state detention.

This chapter examines the coroner's powers and duty to investigate such deaths, including the potential necessity for a post-mortem examination and in some cases an inquest. The reasons for the coroner's decisions at each stage will be considered, together with the nature of the enquiries made and the possible results. This basic law applies equally to child and adult deaths and the initial sections of this chapter will make little specific reference to children. The inquest and its possible conclusions will be considered, as will the potential complications of the 'right to life' under Article 2 of the European Convention on Human Rights (ECHR).[1]

A later section of this chapter considers the investigation of deaths in childhood from the perspective of an experienced and senior detective. Chapter 6 in this volume gives a view from the United States: in this regard it should be noted that use of the word 'coroner' in the US (and much of the rest of the world) means a pathologist or forensic pathologist rather than a coroner in the British sense who will almost always be legally rather than medically qualified.

The extent of the coroner's powers to gather evidence, and the fact that inquests are often held in the unremitting glare of publicity, may well give those involved cause for some unease, no matter how competent their actions surrounding the deceased were. It is hoped that this chapter will explain the realities (and counter some of the myths) surrounding the role of the coroner. Everyone has heard of the coroner – but in reality, very few people know what coroners actually do.

A Brief History of the Coroner's Role

To understand the modern role of the coroner it is useful to have a brief idea of the history of this ancient office. It is generally accepted that coroners came into being in 1194 when King Richard I created a counter to the corrupt and inefficient system of Sheriffs. Thus, the early coroners were often known as 'Crowners' because they were the King's men.[2] This has corrupted over the centuries to the modern word 'coroner'.

The early coroners had a number of fiscal duties for the King and were responsible for the maintenance of law and order although not the actual trial and sentencing of offenders – the latter point being referenced in the Magna Carta of 1215. Over time the fiscal responsibilities slipped and the coroner became more strictly involved in the investigation of death, although this had long been a good source of taxation for the Crown.[3]

The increasing complexity of society in the nineteenth century necessitated proper records of births and deaths. The Births and Death Registration Act 1836 rekindled the importance of the coroner's investigation, providing that there could be no burial without either a registrar's certificate or a coroner's order. At the same time, in the absence of any effective police force, it was often left to the coroner's jury to commit[4] those thought culpable of a homicide to the Assizes for trial, and it was only in 1926 that coroners were required to adjourn an inquest until the conclusion of indictable criminal proceedings.

Throughout the 1900s the coronial system became more regulated and an Act of 1988 consolidated earlier fragments of legislation. The system gained further importance following the Human Rights Act 1998 which gave effect in UK law to the ECHR, most particularly with regard to the investigation of deaths that might engage the provisions of Article 2 ECHR (as to which see later). The 2004 case of *Middleton*[5] in the House of Lords confirmed that the state's obligation to inquire into the circumstances of a death where Article 2 ECHR might apply would generally be met by the coroner's inquest.

Coronial law was brought up to date, in theory at least, by enactment of the Coroners and Justice Act 2009 ('the 2009 Act') which came into effect in July 2013. Supported by the Coroners (Investigations) Regulations 2013 ('the 2013 Regulations') and the Coroners (Inquests) Rules 2013 ('the 2013 Rules') the Act met much of the criticism surrounding the earlier legislation and gave a significant increase to the coroner's powers of investigation.

Note that the English/Welsh system of coroners and inquests is not replicated in Scotland. Northern Ireland and Eire have broadly similar (but different) legislation.

Who Does the Coroner Work For?

The coroner does not 'work' for anyone. He/she is an 'independent judicial officer' although the term 'judge' is used increasingly. While the facilities and (reasonable) expenditure of the coroner are provided by the local authority, with staff provided either by the authority or police, the coroner is not bound in any way to either organisation.

This unique level of independence is important. A coroner may be called upon to investigate a death which has occurred in a local authority setting, police custody, or in a government institution so this autonomy is a practical and effective safeguard for society.

The coroner's independence has an historical background. For very many years coroners were actually elected by the Freemen of a county but the County Councils Act of 1888 gave the task of appointing a coroner to the relevant local authority, sometimes termed an appointment by the people at one remove. This situation continues to the present day, the coroner is selected by a local authority after an open competition but from the moment of appointment holds complete independence and cannot be sacked or removed by the authority. The power to dismiss a coroner lies only with the Lord Chancellor in agreement with the Lord Chief Justice for incapacity or misbehaviour.

When Does the Coroner Deal with a Childhood Death?

At the time of writing, some coroners wish to hear about all deaths of children occurring within their areas. While the medical profession and others might agree that this brings benefits (not least of simplicity in understanding which cases need reporting) this is not the position in law.

It is expected that the introduction of 'medical examiners' (possibly by 2020) will bring a statutory duty on doctors to report certain deaths to the coroner for the first time; until then the sole responsibility to notify a coroner lies upon the Registrar of Births and Deaths. Children are not a specified category in the registrar's duty to report. Nor is it anticipated that the deaths of children will of itself form a reportable category in the new duty upon doctors.

It is appropriate at this stage to consider briefly the circumstances in which the doctor attending a patient can issue a Medical Certificate as to Cause of Death (MCCD) without reference to a coroner. Where the doctor has attended the patient for their last illness and has seen the patient within the last fourteen days they would be in a position to issue a certificate if:

- they were able to state the cause of death to the best of their knowledge and belief and
- the cause of death was wholly natural.

Such cases would not therefore be reported to a coroner. That said, it is common where a death is wholly natural and was expected by a doctor who has not seen the patient exactly within the fourteen days that reference to the coroner will elicit a certificate to the registrar (coroner's Form A) allowing the registration to proceed.

In simple terms, a death should be reported to the coroner where the patient (of whatever age) has died:

- of unknown cause
- of an unnatural cause
- in custody or otherwise in state detention (of whatever cause).

There are various lists which show circumstances where a death must be reported but the above is the basic premise of law. The complexity of a list is merely giving examples of an unnatural death, a subject dealt with in detail below.

Plainly, there are cases of infants dying unexpectedly. That would be reportable as a death of unknown cause but in reality, is going to be advised to the coroner anyway as there will almost inevitably have been a police attendance. The same will often apply where an unnatural death occurs because of trauma. There will be a police attendance and the coroner will be advised of the circumstances.

Note that the coroner does not presently have jurisdiction over babies who are stillborn. The definition of a stillbirth is a child born after the 24th week of pregnancy which did not at any time after being completely expelled from the mother breathe or show any other signs of life.[6] This brings a number of problems. Viability might now be regarded as 22 weeks rather than 24 and there can be difficult debate as to exactly what amounts to breathing or signs of life. However, in 2017 the High Court underlined that a coroner had jurisdiction where there were reasonable grounds for suspicion that a child had been born alive and then had the power to gain such further evidence as necessary to answer the question more fully, either by way of investigation or inquest as appropriate.[7]

Unnatural Deaths

Recognising an unnatural death is important. Not only must an unnatural death be reported to a coroner but it is also the prime legal requirement for the holding of an inquest.

Some examples of an unnatural death, such as drowning, entrapment, or motor vehicle impact are easily understood and recognisable as such. However, this can be a complex subject, commonly in connection with deaths related to medical treatment.

The basic premise is again simple, if a medical treatment or procedure has brought about, or contributed to, the death then the coroner must be informed. It matters not that the cause was a 'recognised complication' of the event, the fact is that the child would not have died at that time had the procedure not taken place. Nor does it affect the situation, that the patient would eventually have died anyway without the treatment.

In terms of 'faulty' medical treatment bringing about a death, the leading case remains *Touche*,[8] a 1999 death in London considered by the Court of Appeal. The court found that apart from the more obvious circumstance of a death from natural causes which had been contributed to by neglect (see below), a death was also to be regarded as unnatural where it was a wholly unexpected death, albeit from natural causes, resulting from some 'culpable human failure'. In a later part of the judgement the court described this as 'a death that should plainly never have happened'. It was made clear that omission was just as important as commission.

This is obviously far from saying that any death under medical treatment is unnatural and will thus result in the holding of an inquest; coroners recognise the complexities and balances involved in serious medical care. But the law is plain: where a death might be regarded as unnatural then there must be an investigation by the coroner and, if it thereafter continues to be viewed as unnatural, then an inquest must be held. The coroner holds no discretion to ignore an unnatural death on the basis that 'everyone was doing their best'.

The test in law for the coroner is whether there are 'reasonable grounds to suspect' that the death was unnatural. A mere unsupported allegation will not suffice, but the requirement only to have reasonable grounds to suspect is a low bar. It is, for example, lower than 'reason to believe' or a finding 'on the balance of probabilities'.

The Coroner's Initial Investigation

Once the coroner is informed of a death there will be an element of early inquiry which falls short of the formal stage of investigation that may develop later. For example, if the police have attended a child death at home but enquiries by the coroner's staff on the next working day confirm that this was a death expected by the medical team and is of a wholly natural nature then the matter is likely to go no further so far as the coroner is concerned. It is likely that this decision would only be made in close consultation with the police and attending doctor, and SUDI/SUID (Sudden Unexplained Death in Infancy/Sudden Unexplained Infant Death) or child death protocols will still be followed. It is probable that the coroner will issue a certificate for the registrar (Form A) confirming that s/he does not intend to make further enquiry.

However, in child deaths it is very common that some significant element of enquiry is necessary, often involving a post-mortem examination to ascertain the cause. Other enquiries will be made, usually by the police on behalf of the coroner. The coroner will also get an early indication of findings from the joint home visit by police and paediatrician (see below). In some cases, there may be a close examination of the scene of the death (commonly at home) by specialist officers. As much of this information as is available in time will be advised to the paediatric pathologist so that their examination can be made in light of the known facts. Wherever possible the autopsy should be conducted by a specialist in paediatric rather than general pathologist, although this may become less relevant with

21

young persons nearer the age of 18, particularly where the cause is traumatic rather than metabolic or from a complex disease. Police officers may well attend the autopsy to ensure that the pathologist is fully briefed even where the death is not overtly suspicious.

Paediatric post-mortem examinations rarely produce an immediate result, it is far more likely that the cause of death will not be given until the results of histology, bacteriology, and even toxicology are known. This can be some weeks and where the coroner is told that the result of the examination is 'pending' a more formal stage of 'investigation' will be announced. This allows, in suitable cases, for the coroner to release the body giving the family an authority for burial or cremation. Such an investigation can later be discontinued without the opening of an inquest where the autopsy eventually confirms a natural cause of death. The power to discontinue in these circumstances was probably the most useful change in the law contained in the 2009 Act.

Note that regulation 24 of the 2013 Regulations requires the coroner to notify the Local Safeguarding Children Board (LSCB) of the death of a person believed to be under the age of 18. In the UK, the LSCB is a multi-agency committee which must be established by the local authority to oversee the welfare of children and young people within its area. This must occur within three days of a decision to conduct an investigation or post-mortem examination. In practice the notification is unlikely to be delayed three days, nor would any distinction be made between an early informal investigation and a more formal investigation.

The Autopsy Decision and Tissue Retention

Ordering that an invasive post-mortem examination take place is a major step in the coroner's enquiries into any death, rarely welcomed by families. This is plainly all the more so in the case of a child death. The impact of such a decision will always be carefully considered by the coroner and his/her staff:

- objections raised by a family will be heard and the best possible explanation given.
- careful checks will be made to ensure that no medical practitioner is in a position to issue a Medical Certificate as to Cause of Death.
- consideration can also be given to the least invasive process compatible with a proper examination.

But ultimately, if the coroner's statutory duty to ascertain the cause of death requires an examination, then that is what must take place.

The coroner's decision on post-mortem examination (like many other coroner decisions) is open to an application for judicial review before the High Court. This is not an appeal, or an assessment of whether the High Court agrees with the decision: it is an application that the court review whether the coroner's decision is lawful and reasonable. Very few such applications are made.

Tissue retention at autopsy is very common, indeed almost invariable in paediatric cases. This is lawful only to ascertain the cause of death or (much more rarely) to assist in identifying the deceased. The coroner has no authority to permit retention for teaching or research. Of course, a family may be asked to give consent by a hospital for wider purposes but that is entirely separate to the coroner's authority.

The authority for such retention arises under Section 14(2) of the 2009 Act. Reg. 14 of the 2013 Regulations requires the pathologist to notify the coroner in writing of intended retention, whether of tissue samples or whole organs, and why this is necessary. Good practice is for the pathologist to specify the number of blocks. In turn the coroner will authorise the retention (if that be the case) and advise how long the material may be held. The coroner must also notify the next of kin (or personal representative of the deceased) that material is being retained and for how long. This will need to be carefully explained and the family will also be given a choice of the various options for disposal of the material once the period has expired. Curiously, there is no specific requirement in the coronial legislation for the coroner to pass on the family wishes to the pathologist (who bears the responsibility for disposal rather than the coroner) but no doubt this will inevitably be the case. The pathologist must maintain records of the disposal.

While coroners are not strictly bound by Human Tissue Act Codes[9] of Practice, these are generally accepted as good practice and followed. Coroners will also expect their pathologist to act in accordance with Royal College of Pathologist guidelines.[10]

Further Enquiries

At this stage the coroner is gradually building a picture of the circumstances surrounding the death of the child. The post-mortem examination report may confirm views that have been held about the death or it may send the whole enquiry in a different direction.

The coroner will be looking to gather information which is relevant to the death, remembering always the remit of the inquest (see below), from a range of sources. The police are likely to have obtained statements from witnesses as to the circumstances, the coroner officers will have obtained a report from the general practitioner with a copy of the surgery records. Reports will be obtained from treating clinicians where appropriate. If the death might be connected with an untoward event in a hospital or other place, the coroner will want sight of the relevant inquiry report. There may be information available from social services or perhaps even particular charities involved in the care of a child. There will usually be the report of a joint visit to the family (under an appropriate protocol) by police and a paediatrician (or a trained specialist nurse).

Formal enquiries by an LSCB[11] or Child Death Overview Panel[12] (CDOP) may or may not be completed before the inquest is held but again are likely to be a potential source of information. The LSCB is required to put in place procedures for a rapid response to individual unexpected child deaths and to review all childhood deaths in a systematic way. National guidance[13] underlines the importance of a clear working relationship between the LSCB, CDOP and the local coroner and all information on the circumstances of the death must be included in a report for the coroner within twenty-eight days, unless some of the crucial information is not yet available – which might often be the case because (inter alia) the cause of death may not be available four weeks after post-mortem.

However, to maintain visible independence it is important that neither the coroner nor a coroner's officer attend a LSCB or CDOP meeting about an individual case, the coroner should be at 'arm's length' from the panel deliberations and await the report. Being part of the review process could compromise the independence and public nature of the inquest.

In a limited number of cases the LSCB may hold a 'Serious Case Review' (SCR), or 'Child Practice Review' in Wales, with an independent lead reviewer in cases where neglect or suicide are suspected or the child has died in custody. Other than in exceptional cases the coroner would await a copy of the review report before proceeding to inquest. Where the death

was in custody there will also, in due course, be a report from the Prisons and Probation Ombudsman that the coroner will wish to see.

The coroner is entitled to sight of all and any of this material that might bear upon the death. Besides the common law power to summon a witness before the court, there are specific powers in Schedule 5 of the 2009 Act to require a person to produce a written statement, documents, or evidential objects within a reasonable period. Immunities from such production apply as before a civil court, otherwise the coroner has power to punish any failure to comply by a fine. Repeated failure to comply might be dealt with as a contempt of court.

The so-called 'Worcestershire Coroner case' of 2013[14] emphasised the importance and strength of the Schedule 5 procedures. The coroner sought access to management reviews and other information which the LSCB had gathered for an SCR. This was resisted on the grounds that it was in the greater public interest not to disclose, as such reports would have a higher degree of candour if report authors were assured that they would not become public. The High Court held that as the disclosure was to the coroner for the purpose of assessing the case rather than to the public (or even the 'interested persons' at the inquest), the public interest in the pursuit of a full and appropriately detailed inquest firmly outweighed the claim for immunity.

Notwithstanding the *Worcestershire Coroner* case, there is often a good working relationship between the coroner's office, LSCB, and CDOP with a recognition that the sharing of information is commonly to the benefit of all. For example, the coroner will often agree that the result of the post-mortem examination can be shared (on a confidential basis) with early meetings of the LSCB. However, if there are suspicions about the death such sharing may not be possible at an early stage.

The Inquest Decision

If, following autopsy and initial inquiries, the death remains of unknown cause, is unnatural, or occurred in custody or otherwise in state detention (regardless of cause), the coroner must hold an inquest. There is no discretion to hold an inquest if none of these criteria are met, nor is there discretion not to hold an inquest if one of the criteria is met. That said, the decision as to whether there is reason to suspect that a death is unnatural requires an element of judgement.

A coroner's decision not to hold an inquest is again susceptible to judicial review. There is no provision for the coroner to hold a form of court process allowing various 'interested persons' (see below) to make representations as to whether an inquest should be held but the author might express the personal view that this could be done, certainly with the agreement of all concerned. That said the author does not know of any case where this has occurred.

Those in the medical profession sometimes have the impression that the family or others can simply 'demand' that an inquest take place. That is not the case.

Suspicious Deaths

Cases where the coroner and the police fear that the death may be 'suspicious' will form an exception to some of the description given above. While there is a separate chapter in this volume (Chapter 5) written by a senior detective, some short explanation of the situation from a coroner's point of view may be useful.

Suspicions about a death may come to light in a number of ways. The police may report to the coroner that they have attended the scene of a death and that they have concerns. Alternatively, hospital staff may contact the coroner to advise that a child has just died (commonly in the Accident and Emergency (A&E) Department) and that they have concerns. On occasions the information being gathered by the coroner leads him/her to initiate further police inquiries, for example if the post-mortem examination reveals evidence of non-accidental injuries not initially apparent when the police attended.

In such cases the coroner will be in direct liaison with the police Senior Investigating Officer (SIO), generally someone of at least Detective Chief Inspector rank. The coroner will be asked to sanction a forensic autopsy. Often in the case of a younger child (dependent upon the circumstances) this may be a joint examination between a forensic pathologist and a paediatric pathologist, with the former taking the lead. Such examinations are still carried out on the instructions of the coroner notwithstanding what may be an intense police interest. The coroner will 'choose' the pathologist but must liaise with the police on this point – although in reality the forensic pathologist is likely simply to be the 'on-call' on a rota long agreed by police and coroner.

Where the suspicions persist beyond the autopsy, the police will lead the investigation and the coroner's direct role is likely to be no more than obtaining medical records etc. for the police.

There is often a delay in release of the body where there are suspicions. This may be because the results of tests must be obtained before it can be decided that no further examinations are necessary and the body can be released. Often, however, it is because the question of a second post-mortem examination arises. This is because where a homicide charge is anticipated it is normal to allow the potential defendant an opportunity to have a pathologist of their own choosing view the body. This may be particularly important in child deaths.

If homicide charges follow, the coroner must adjourn the inquest until the conclusion of the trial, sending a form to the registrar which allows the family to obtain a full death certificate. It is likely that the inquest will not resume but there can be exceptions, particularly if there are any issues involving Article 2 ECHR (see below).

The Remit of the Inquest

The inquest proceedings cannot just investigate whatever issues that the coroner or family feel might be interesting; there is a specific, and limited remit at law. Section 5(1) of the 2009 Act sets out the remit in a non-Article 2 engaged inquest as ascertaining:

- the identity of the deceased
- how, when and where the deceased came by her/his death
- registration particulars (for example, place of birth).

Importantly, s. 5(3) of the 2009 Act specifies that neither the coroner nor a jury shall express an opinion on anything other than these questions.

The evidence at an inquest will primarily be concerned with answering the question 'how'. This is generally interpreted as 'by what means' did the death occur, a narrower question than 'why' but it does not mean that the inquest must be limited to the last link in the chain of causation.[15] The High Court has recognised that such a limitation would defeat the purpose of holding an inquest at all.

Case law also makes very clear that the extent of the remit is a matter for the coroner in each individual case, but it is plain that the coroner should enquire into acts and omissions which are directly responsible for the death.[16] However, it is not the duty of the coroner to investigate every rumour or allegation brought to his/her attention.

See below as to the potentially extended remit of an inquest where Article 2 ECHR is said to be engaged.

The Nature of the Proceedings – What Actually Happens at an Inquest?

The inquest process is properly described as 'inquisitorial' rather than 'adversarial'. The inquest is the coroner's inquiry into the death, with the interested persons merely being present to assist in the task rather than trying to make their own case. Of course, the hearing is not always as straightforward as that.

Where an inquest is to be held, there will initially be a short hearing in court, often without the attendance of the family or others although they will always have the choice to attend, which simply takes formal evidence of identification and often notes the cause of death if known at that stage. Such proceedings, known as 'opening the inquest' must be recorded (as is the full inquest) and the press or public are entitled to attend.

At a later time, when all the information has been gathered and assessed, the coroner will list the case for hearing. In some cases there will be a pre-inquest review (PIR) at which those who the law recognises as 'interested persons' will attend while matters such as the list of witnesses to be called are discussed. 'Interested persons' will include the family of the deceased and organisations who had care of the deceased but whose conduct might be called into question at the inquest, for example an NHS Trust or a social services department. Interested persons have a statutory right to ask questions of the witnesses at an inquest and can make legal (but not factual) submissions about the proceedings.

When the inquest finally proceeds the coroner will generally start by outlining the role of the inquest and perhaps in particular that the hearing is to ascertain the facts of a death rather than attribute blame or guilt. The evidence of identification given at the opening is likely to be repeated and the coroner will then call the witnesses, commonly in chronological order save for the pathologist who is often called first.

It is the coroner who will first question the witnesses. Indeed, at an inquest all of the witnesses are called by the coroner for the benefit of the inquiry, they are not called by individuals seeking to prove one point or another.

The coroner will then allow the interested persons to ask their own questions of the witness, ensuring that only relevant, and proper questions are asked. With unrepresented families this means that the coroner often has to step in and help with the phrasing of a question that had started out as a long statement.

Where there is no disagreement upon a witness's evidence it is common that their statement or report is read out rather than them attending in person.

Once all the evidence has been heard the coroner will hear any submissions of law that those before the court wish to make. No-one is allowed to address the court upon the facts of the case, that is purely a matter for the coroner. Once submissions have been made the coroner will give a short summary as to her/his findings and set out the reasons behind the conclusion that is announced (see below).

It is not common, although not impossible, that an inquest into the death of a child would need to be heard before a jury, as this is only necessary where:

- the death occurred in custody or otherwise in state detention (which includes a Mental Health Act 'section') *and* was unnatural
- the death occurred from an act or omission of a police officer in the purported execution of the officer's duty
- the death occurred in circumstances making it notifiable to a government department or inspector. These are generally deaths reportable to the Health and Safety Executive so would include events such as the death of a child killed while playing on a building site.

The coroner's conclusion is dealt with separately below.

Article 2

The engagement of Article 2 ECHR at an inquest is a complex subject that has taken up many hours of argument before the High Court. What follows is only the briefest explanation.

The Human Rights Act 1998 gave effect in UK law to the ECHR for the first time, even though the UK had been a major contributor to the drafting and eventual ratification of the Convention in the late 1940s and early 1950s.

Article 2 ECHR is the 'right to life' and was originally drafted to forbid the wanton killing of citizens by their state. But the Convention is described as a 'living instrument' and over the decades the scope of Article 2 has expanded beyond recognition. Thus Article 2 is seen as requiring the state to safeguard life

25

by, for example, the proper planning, and control of the state's business. This includes:

- a negative duty – that the State refrain from taking life
- a positive duty that the state protect life in two ways:
  - putting in place a framework of laws, precautions, procedures, and means of enforcement to protect life or
  - taking appropriate steps to safeguard lives known to be at risk.

All of this impacts upon the coroner's investigation and inquest because the 2004 House of Lords case of *Middleton*[5] determined that the state's obligation to hold a thorough and independent examination of the circumstances of a death where there were grounds to suspect that Article 2 was engaged would be met by the inquest.

To recognise that a so-called 'Article 2' or '*Middleton*' inquest was different to the majority of inquests, the House of Lords set out that the remit, in appropriate cases, should be described as 'how and in what circumstances' rather than just 'how'. Although something of a play on words, the intended distinction is clear: an Article 2 inquest should have, where necessary, a widened remit over the chain of causation to ensure that all the requirements of a thorough and independent inquiry are properly met.

But the inquest has itself developed over the last decade and more modern case-law recognises that the wide discretion that a coroner has as to the remit of even a non-*Middleton* inquest now means that there is likely to be little distinction in the actual facts examined. Where, at least arguably, the Article 2 inquest differs maybe in more pejorative words that are available to the coroner or jury for the conclusion.

It is commonly believed that an Article 2 inquest must be heard before a jury. That is not in itself correct, but the requirement for Article 2 will sometimes mean that the requirement for a jury is also met.

The Conclusion

The word 'verdict' is no longer used for the process at the end of an inquest, and for good reason. The term 'conclusion' was introduced by the 2009 Act. Coroners spend much of their time in court trying to prevent inquests becoming adversarial (see above) yet 'verdict' is a very accusatory word suggestive of

a process in which people can be found guilty of an involvement in the death. It also infers that the finding of the inquest can be contained within a one- or two-word label, which is increasingly not the case.

Having heard all of the evidence, and any submissions on law that are to be made, the coroner will announce his/her decision as to the death. This theoretically comes in several parts but these are generally indistinguishable to the observer.

Depending upon the complexity and nature of the case, it is likely that the coroner will first briefly 'sum up' the evidence heard, perhaps indicating where particular evidence has been accepted or rejected. Possibly as part of the same process, or separately, the coroner will indicate the most important facts found. The coroner will then announce what is more properly called 'the conclusion', in part either by using a so-called 'short-form conclusion' or a 'narrative conclusion'. These are described more fully below.

In giving his/her conclusion and completing the Record of Inquest form (the legal record of the proceedings) the coroner must address the four statutory questions. S/he will first find the name of the deceased (who). The medical cause of death will be stated (part of 'how'). The coroner will then generally record a short statement as to the facts of how, when and where the deceased came by his death such as *John Smith died on 1/1/17 of injuries sustained on 31/12/16 when he fell off his bicycle in the path of a car on the High Street.*

The fourth question on the record form is referred to as the 'conclusion as to the death'. Here the coroner will either use one of the recognised 'short-form' conclusions (such as accidental death or natural causes) or use a 'narrative conclusion'. The latter is a brief, neutral and factual statement as to the circumstances of the death and are often used when the circumstances are more complex, or are uncertain, or fall between two of the traditional conclusions. For example, a coroner might record that the deceased *suspended himself on the staircase of his home, the question of intent remaining unclear*. Some coroners would use the word 'open' as a conclusion in these circumstances but it can be argued that the narrative makes the finding clearer without leaving any inference that there could have been foul play.

One notable conclusion open to a coroner is that the death has been 'contributed to by neglect'. In this context, 'neglect' is a much narrower concept than civil negligence and there are significant differences between the two. This means that it is shown on the balance of probabilities that there has been a gross failure to provide or procure for the deceased adequate nourishment, shelter, warmth or (more commonly) basic medical attention. The person must be in a dependent position by reason, for example, of youth, age, illness or incarceration and their physical condition will be such as to show (objectively) that they obviously need the care. Nonetheless, a mental health condition calling for medical attention will also suffice. There must be a clear and direct causal connection established between the failure and the cause of death.

Section 10(2) of the 2009 Act creates a significant restriction by forbidding a conclusion which appears to determine:

- criminal liability against a named person *or*
- civil liability.

Nonetheless, this restriction has to be put in context. The whole purpose of the inquest is to establish the facts of how a death came about, and that fact-finding is paramount. In the rare circumstances that there is a conflict between the restriction of s.10 and the requirement to find facts it is the latter which prevails. But in reality, a carefully drafted factual finding without emotional or adjectival wording can be very plain as to the (perhaps unhappy) facts found without even nearly breaching the restrictions of s.10. A finding that the death has been contributed to by neglect is not in breach of either s.5 or s.10.

Where the inquest has engaged Article 2 ECHR the wording can be more than merely factual. The case of *Middleton*[5] describes that the conclusion in an Article 2 case may be a 'judgemental conclusion of a factual nature [on the core factual issues], directly relating to the circumstances of death', without infringing either Section 5(3) or Section 10(2). The Chief Coroner's Guidance (number 17) on Conclusions[17] indicates that permitted judgemental words in an Article 2 case include 'inadequate', 'inappropriate', 'insufficient', 'lacking', 'unsuitable', 'unsatisfactory', and 'failure'.

References

1. See http://www.legislation.gov.uk/ukpga/1998/42/schedule/1 (acessed 31 October 2018).
2. Officially 'Custos Placitorum Coronae' or 'Keepers of the Pleas of the Crown'.
3. It was as late as 1846 that coroners lost the power to order forfeiture to the Crown of an object involved in a death, such as a railway locomotive.
4. A power that was not abolished until 1977.
5. *R (Middleton)* v. *West Somerset Coroner* [2004] United Kingdom House of Lords 10.
6. Section 41 Births and Deaths Registration Act 1953 as amended by the Still Birth Definition Act, 1992.
7. *R (T)* v. *HM Senior Coroner for West Yorkshire* [2017] England and Wales Court of Appeal (EWCA)Civ 318.
8. *R* v. *Inner N. London Coroner ex p Touche* [2001] EWCA Civ 383.
9. www.hta.gov.uk./ (accessed 4 October 2018).
10. www.rcpath.org/asset/874AE50E-C754-4933-995A80 4E0EF728A4/ (accessed 4 October 2018).
11. https://www.gov.uk/government/publications/working-together-to-safeguard-children–2 (accessed 30 October 2018).
12. www.gov.uk/government/publications/child-death-overview-panels-contacts (accessed 4 October 2018).
13. www.gov.uk/government/uploads/system/uploads/attachment_data/file/592101/Working_Together_to_Safeguard_Children_20170213.pdf (accessed 28 October 2018).
14. *Worcestershire CC* v. *Worcestershire LSCB and HM Coroner Worcestershire* [2013] England and Wales High Court 1711.
15. *R* v. *Inner West London Coroner ex p Dallaglio* (1994) 4 All ER 139.
16. *R* v. *HM Coroner for Western District of E. Sussex ex p Homberg* (1994) 158 JP 357.
17. www.judiciary.gov.uk/wp-content/uploads/2013/09/guidance-no-17-conclusions.pdf at para 52 (accessed 4 February 2018).

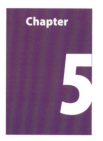

Chapter 5

Investigating Child Deaths in the UK – the Police Perspective

Phil Etheridge

Introduction

Every child who dies suddenly and unexpectedly has the right to have their death fully investigated, in order that homicides can be excluded and a cause of death identified.[1] With greater perceived understanding and the existence of prevention campaigns resulting in reductions in unexpected infancy deaths, the vast majority of remaining child deaths occur as a result of natural causes, such as disease or physical defects, or deaths caused by accidents.

A small proportion of deaths are, however, caused deliberately by violence, administered substances, or by careless use of drugs. Research has shown that up to 5–10% of sudden unexpected deaths in infancy (SUDI) might be covert homicides. In some child or infant deaths in which there is an identifiable natural cause of death, neglect and maltreatment by carers may have been a contributory factor.[2]

Additional to the Association of Chief Police Officers (ACPO) Murder Investigation Manual (2006), there are two principle guidance documents that assist the police in the investigation of death involving children. The first, commissioned by the ACPO, is the 2014 *A Guide to Investigating Child Deaths*.[3] The more recent is the Royal College of Pathologists' publication of 2016, *Sudden Unexpected Death in Infancy and Childhood*.[4]

Within the context of this paper, an unexpected child death is the death of an infant or child (less than 18 years old), which was not anticipated as a significant possibility (for example 24 hours before death), or where there was a similarly unexpected collapse or incident leading to or precipitating the events that resulted in death.

The investigation of child death is an extremely important, complex, and emotional area of police work. Children are not expected to die and the investigation into the sudden death of a child must be influenced by this basic fact.[3] When dealing with

sudden unexplained deaths in both infants and children all agencies, including the police, need to follow five common principles, especially when having contact with family members. These are:

- A balanced approach between sensitivity and the investigative mindset
- A multi-agency response
- Sharing of information
- An appropriate response to the circumstances
- Preservation of evidence.

Article 2 of the Human Rights Act (1998) states that everyone's life is protected by law. Public authorities are required to establish the cause of death, not only to provide explanations for grieving relatives, but also to understand the cause of death and, if necessary, create interventions to prevent future deaths of children.

In this, the police, and other agencies' prime responsibility is to the child, as well as other siblings and any future children who may be born into the family concerned. The police also have a key role in the investigation of child and infant deaths, whether criminal, or suspicious, for which they are the lead agency; the investigation conducted with, and on behalf of, the coroner.

The National Police Guidance describes three distinct strategic phases of investigations involving child death:

- Instigation and initial response
- The investigation
- Case management

Unlike traditional adult death investigation, with child death all three phases are conducted jointly with multi-agency partners.

Early Police Involvement in a Child's Death

The emergency services are often the first to hear of a sudden and unexplained child death occurring in the community. They get a phone call regarding an unresponsive child or infant at a given location (often, but not always, their home). The earliest priority of the first police officer attending should always be to preserve the child or infant's life. This could involve attempting first aid, often assisted by the family, until specialist medical care arrives.

There are also times when the call to attend is received initially by the ambulance service alone, but referred to the police for a number of reasons. First, ambulance referrals to the police will be primarily undertaken to see if the police are able to attend before the ambulance's arrival, to attempt to preserve the child or infant's life. Another reason for the referral from ambulance to police is that their arrival has revealed that the child or infant is already dead and unable to be resuscitated, the police then needing to be called to inquire on behalf of the coroner into unexplained child deaths. Lastly, there are times when the ambulance service discovers a dead child in circumstances which are suggestive to them, at this early stage, that a suspicious death may have occurred.

There are also occasions when the child or infant arrives at the A&E of a hospital or other medical location, and the police are notified that a child or infant has arrived and subsequently died, or that the child or infant has arrived dead with no obvious chance or opportunity to resuscitate her or him.

The coroner may contact the police directly when there is a child or infant death that the police may need to investigate. These referrals relate to child or infant deaths that have been notified to the coroner and the police in cases in which the child or infant was receiving medical care and their untimely death may involve some shortfall in medical care or medical or carer supervision.

By whatever means the child or infant death notification is reported to the police, ideally the first responder should have due considerations to the sensitivity of the situation and the effect that multiple uniformed police officers present at the location of the child's death may have on the family. Guidance[3] suggests that this first responder should be a plain-clothed detective officer using an unmarked vehicle, but practicalities of resourcing, and the primary concern of preserving life do not always make this possible.

When there are suspicious circumstances identified at the beginning of the investigation, a nationally qualified senior investigating officer will be appointed to take control of the investigation. For all cases involving a child or infant death, suspicious or not, a lead investigator should be tasked immediately with taking charge of the investigation. This will normally be an officer of at least detective inspector rank, who has been trained in child/infant death protocols. Either way, effective contact and cooperation between the police and the paediatrician is very important at this early stage, as an external examination and further tests including skeletal survey will begin to direct the investigation, and confirm or deny the existence of any suspicious circumstances.

First Actions by Uniformed Officers Attending

Following the arrival of the police to any child or infant death scene, it is important that the environment where the child or infant has died is sensitively and carefully secured, pending a joint scene assessment between the police lead investigator and the paediatrician.

Initial attending officers should always adopt an investigative mindset, using investigative evaluations, and developing hypotheses, when necessary, to begin to understand, and establish what has or may have happened, while at the same time being sensitive and discreet with the parents / carers who may be in shock and trying to deal with events.

Assuming that preservation of life is not possible, the police officers attending next actions should always be to identify and preserve scenes, secure evidence, identify victims and suspects (if applicable). These are known as the investigative building blocks and apply here as well as in a criminal homicide investigation.

If the body of the child is still at a location away from the hospital, the officers should make a visual check of the child and its surroundings, noting any factors that could make the death suspicious or, conversely, that takes suspicion away. After explaining the reason why the police presence is required in a child or infant death, the police should enquire, obtain, and record initial accounts make by parents, guardians, and/or witnesses. The police should also identify any potential scenes, taking sensitive steps to ensure that material or evidence is not removed, concealed, or destroyed. It is important that the death scene, and all items therein, is maintained as closely as possible to its original state pending a full scene assessment and future joint visit between the police appointed investigator and the paediatrician. The coroner should be notified of the death at this early stage.

In cases where there is no apparent suspicion, consideration should be given to ensuring that everything is done with sensitivity and, if possible, in collaboration with the parents and carers. A 'low-key' involvement approach will greatly assist the process, avoiding the presence of uniformed officers and marked police vehicles. Police jargon and parlance such as 'crime scene' and 'exhibit bags' should not be used.

Scene preservation and initial examination, using crime scene investigators should extend to recording room temperature, noting the position of the sun at the time of the arrival of officers as well as noting central heating settings and proximity of the child or infant to active heating sources within the home, and levels of clothing, and sleeping blankets.

At this stage it is crucial to reassure the grieving parents that the role of the police is mandatory for all unexplained child deaths, including their child's. The police have this role to assist and enquire with other key partners on behalf of the coroner, to understand why their child died, providing the parents, or carers with answers. It also allows an overall understanding of what may contribute to unexpected child death and to ensure, when possible, that the circumstances are not repeated within the family or in another family.

Circumstances That Might Govern the Level of the Follow-up Response

Whether the death is seen as suspicious or not will be one of the main factors that will dictate the level of a police and investigative response. Suspicious deaths involve the appointment of a senior investigating officer trained in homicide investigation and child death protocols. With this comes appropriately experienced police officers and staff trained in the necessary investigative areas such as crime scene management, child abuse investigators, family liaison officers, and specialist witness and suspect interviewing officers. This could also include, in consultation with the hospital staff, the referral of families to specialist bereavement services.

Should the suspicious child death be complex or have unknown offender(s) attached to it, then

additional resources may be sought and utilised by the senior investigating officer, including the recording, and coordinating of the many investigative actions that may be generated, by use of a either a paper-based or computerised action management system.

Based on research,[5] risk factors taken into consideration when making the assessment whether or not a death is suspicious include, taken in order of priority of suspicion, the following:

- History of violence to children
- Inconsistent account
- Mental health issues
- Previous atypical hospital visits
- History of alcohol abuse
- Child over one year old
- Child on protection plan
- Family known to social services
- History of drug abuse
- History of domestic violence
- Criminal record
- Previous sibling death.

Additionally, the following features found at post-mortem examination may be associated with suspicious deaths:

- Presence of features of rotational acceleration / deceleration impact injuries, sometimes referred to as the triad, which is subdural haemorrhages, brain swelling and retinal haemorrhages
- Toxicology detection of drugs of abuse
- Presence of fractures
- Bruising at unusual sites
- Post-mortem features indicating that the interval since death was significantly longer than that stated by parents.[3]

In essence, no two child deaths are the same and each child death and the circumstances, complications and complexities attached to it will need to be examined at an early stage and reviewed throughout the investigation, resourcing the investigation with the appropriate level of staff as needed.

Possible Tension Between Police Attending a Potentially Suspicious Death and Compassion for the Parents

There is a fine line to operate as an effective police officer in order to secure and preserve evidence for a potentially suspicious death and at the same time to show compassion for a family grieving for the death of their child, which will almost certainly turn out to be not suspicious. Police training has concentrated on this dilemma and staff attending a child death are now better able to deal sensitively with this situation. Given that a detective inspector has the initial responsibility for directing and coordinating resources, they are able to advise attending staff what they expect from them and what grieving families may wish to do, that would apparently be almost at odds with normal crime scene management and assessment.

Carers' Accounts and Their Importance to the Investigation

It is important that doctors and ambulance crew are clear about accounts that parents or carers have given, since these might be important to the investigation

Guidance[3] suggests that when dealing with a child or infant sudden death, all agencies should adopt the five common principles mentioned previously, especially when dealing with a grieving family. Local Safeguarding Children's Boards have developed protocols to ensure that child death investigations have that multi-agency approach which is very important, as later down the process the circumstances surrounding the child death may have to be reported as a Serious Case Review (SCR). An SCR takes place after a child dies or is seriously injured and abuse or neglect is thought to be involved. It looks at lessons that can help prevent similar incidents from happening in the future.

The lead investigator should direct attending officers and other investigators to identify and liaise at an early stage with ambulance crews and A&E medical staff to ensure that accounts provided by parents or carers of a child or infant who has died are accurately recorded. These accounts should particularly focus on the actions and words spoken by parents or carers present at the scene of the death, as well as the visual presentation of the child, any medical procedures, and the resuscitation techniques carried out. These should assist the forensic pathologist to explain any marks or bruises they may subsequently find on the child that can be eliminated since they occurred during medical intervention.

Any notes by this staff should be secured or at the very least copied. Depending on whether the death is deemed suspicious or not, the medical staff could be later interviewed as 'significant witnesses'; in that they might have been given versions of admissions or explanations from parents or carers early in the emergency response to the death, that may subsequently be missing or different from later accounts.

Valuable Physical Evidence

In addition to dynamics of the the scene, such as temperature and room orientation in relation to light and heating sources, physical evidence will include any material that will assist in providing a possible explanation that will allow paediatricians and pathologists to provide a potential cause of death. The child's position at death and where they have been subsequently moved to should also be noted, as well as any locations within the home where evidence appears to be missing or may have been moved. Photography and video are often used, as well as hand-drawn sketch plans.

Items that would also be of benefit and value to the investigation include material where there is forensic evidence such as blood, vomit, or other residues on bedding or clothing. Feeding, drinking, and medicinal implements would also be of value, as well as baby records (e.g. red book) undertaken and completed by visiting midwives.

Medical care records and social care records would also fall into the remit of physical evidence, although they are secured at a location away from the child's home.

The Police Presence at the Accident and Emergency Department

Unless there are signs of maltreatment that would deem the child death suspicious, a child who dies at home or in the community will be removed by the ambulance service to the A&E department of a hospital rather than to the mortuary. In some cases this may be the location where police have their first opportunity to speak with parents and carers who travelled with the child. Requests by parents to hold their dead child or be with their child should not be discouraged. The 'forensic link' between a parent and a child will always be present and would have little evidential value at any possible future crime scene evaluation or evidential recovery.

Accident and Emergency departments are never the easiest locations for the police to carry out their investigations, as hospital staff are primarily attempting to care for members of the public, including children. That said, many of the preliminary actions could only be completed at this location and the police's presence ensures that they have the maximum amount of information available to them in one place to allow them to make initial decisions around suspicious or non-suspicious child death and the level of complexity that the investigation may require, and resourcing it appropriately as identified.

A&E departments allow access to specialist paediatricians who will give an opinion as to nature and possible cause of injuries on the child, using external examination and other specialist skeletal or tissue survey methods available to them. Being present during the examination of the child with the paediatrician will allow police investigators the opportunity to see and record injuries and marks which may be of interest to their ongoing investigation.

Hospital records will provide a good indication of the child's underlying medical conditions prior to death, as well as a list of recent hospital visits and the reasons for them. Additionally, the hospital records will show which staff have actually seen the dead child and the parents while in the hospital, and what they have been told by parents, prior to police arrival, and involvement. Lastly, at the hospital police are also able to ascertain what medical samples have already been taken. These should be brought to the attention of the forensic pathologist as well as any medicines or substance (legal or illegal) found with the child at the time of its presentation at hospital.

Other medical professionals in the community, including general practitioners, and midwifery nurses can also be identified, as well as social care services from local authorities and any observations that they would have had during their interaction with parents and child.

The Police Perspective on the Home Visit and its Value

The home visit, undertaken jointly by the police and paediatrician, offers the investigation sufficient insight to the events leading up to and including the death of the child. The paediatrician, having examined the child, or infant, can contextualise injuries seen which may or not support the accounts made by parents and carers.

The paediatrician can also assist with the collation and interpretation of the child's medical records and, working with a forensic pathologist, can ask specific medical questions that they want answered at the post-mortem examination.

Experience from dealing with similar child death events and the participation of the same paediatrician, when possible, will ensure that the interviews of parents and carers by the police follow a consistent, sensitive approach. Information discovered from these accounts can be used to direct further investigative lines of enquiry, which will contribute to the overall understanding of the events that led up to the child's death and will assist the inquest process to ultimately decide upon a cause of death for the child.

A definitive cause of death may not always be found. A sudden death of an infant child under one year of age, which remains unexplained beyond post-mortem examination, review of the clinical history and following a thorough investigation is described as Sudden Infant Death Syndrome (SIDS).

Development of a Major Inquiry

Should the senior investigating officer feel that the death is suspicious, they have to consider who is suspected and how they should obtain from them investigative evidence, including an evidential account. Options such as voluntary attendance and whether to arrest need to be carefully considered, balancing the evidential requirements of the investigation of interviewing under caution with the sensitivity of family's requirements, allowing one, or both parents to grieve. Arrests would normally be considered in line with legislation when the 'prompt and effective' rationale allows investigators access to other legislative options such as searching and obtaining samples or impressions from the suspect. Should these ancillary powers not be required, then a voluntary, disc-recorded suspect interview conducted under caution would suffice.

In the absence of a clear suspect at time of a suspicious death, consideration should be given to interviewing the parents and carers as 'significant witnesses'. Their accounts (taken without need of caution), would be undertaken by specially trained interviewing officers, often by video recording, covering a range of subjects and topics relating to the child's history, including the events from forty-eight hours before the death and surrounding the discovery of the body, as well as actions taken thereafter.

Investigative strategies will then be devised and implemented by the senior investigating officer in order to secure and preserve evidence of what may have brought about the child's death, and exploring different hypotheses. These would include crime-scene assessment, forensic recovery, pathology, witness accounts, and family liaison as well as house search, house-to-house enquiries and victim/family enquiries, including material held on police and the databases of other statutory partners such as social services. Covert intelligence and evidential opportunities may also be explored, particularly when one parent may be responsible and one or both parents (or others) attempt to conceal events.

The use of specialist investigative support could also be called upon by the senior investigating officer to understand what had happened prior to and at the time of death. Scientific support could come from the request of a forensic biologist to assist with crime scene examination as well as other medical specialists to assist in the interpretation of injuries and fractures, including expert evidence regarding the degree of force used, to explain the sequence of events and contradict implausible accounts provided by parents and carers to explain the child's death.

Taking Statements from Witnesses

Consideration should be given to whether or not carers are interviewed together or separately, and in what capacity (i.e., suspect or significant witness). While grieving parents can find solace and support from each other when re-counting to the police events that led to their child or infant's death, care should be exercised to ensure that a dominant carer does not control the conversation. Separating carers will also allow each to account for their own actions and knowledge of their child or infant's death, which can be used later to corroborate with the medical evidence and history already known or being established.

Identification of witnesses is also crucial in order to establish key facts and corroborate the accounts of others. First accounts, which can include the initial telephone call to the emergency services, admissions made to first responders (including other relatives and other emergency service) and those accounts provided to the police upon their arrival should be recorded by the officers initially attending the scene. These accounts may be important to understand crucial facts at an early stage, such as the identification of scenes and the chronology of events leading to the child or infant's death. These accounts may also be vital when determining whether the death is suspicious or whether lack of parental or guardian care becomes an issue, since inconsistencies may emerge in the accounts as time after the child's death

progresses, which may, or may not be in direct contradiction of the medical evidence or history.

The identification of what type of event the ambulance and medical staff may have become witnesses to will depend on the incumbent circumstances that unfold. While they may not be witnesses to the child's death, other siblings living in the home may provide corroboration to parents' and carers' accounts, provide information that they may hold exclusively in their own right about their dead sibling (such as an accidental fall or injury known to them only) or, significantly, the interview of a sibling will provide information and an indication of the standards of care and welfare given by their parents to them and their dead sibling.

A 'Good' Statement

The key to any 'good' statement is that it is taken and produced by the police (often with the assistance of a paediatrician) in a standard format based in law that will allow the witness to explain what they have seen, done, or heard. This will allow the investigation to progress (in line with its strategic aims) and the witness to be called to criminal and/or coronial inquest at some later stage to provide their written or verbal evidence at that location.

The statement should be taken at a time when the person making it is best placed to give it, close to the event being recalled and sufficiently detailed and structured to achieve answers missing from, or needed by the investigation. This will allow others to understand what is being said by that witness in a complete, concise, and structured manner. There is no 'one-case-fits all' type for taking a statement in these circumstances, but guidance[3] suggests a number of key areas to be explored when taking a statement or account from a parent, carer, or material witness.

The child's welfare and health prior to death is always a good starting point. This may be followed by information about the parents (including employment status), other siblings, birth issues (including delivery and previous miscarriages/child-death history) and any medical conditions, diseases and injuries that the child (or other relevant children) have had to date. Visits to health practitioners should be explored as to frequency, reason, and outcomes, as well as contact or involvement with social work or other health, social care, and education specialists. The family setup and home could then be explored, with regard to who lives in the home, who sleeps where, who are the child's principal carers and what are the child's routines and behaviours, including school, and other activities, if applicable.

The chronology of events commencing 48 hours leading up to the death will then be explored. This includes the child's health condition, who was last with the child, who found the child dead, what was the child wearing, where s/he was sleeping, and what were the circumstances of that discovery, and finally, what the home condition is. The latter also includes food and drink consumed or refused by the child, any medicines the child was taking and the delivery routines around this; it will also extend to substances (legal or illegal) taken by or in the possession of parents, carers, or other relevant persons.

Finally the witness could conclude with what the parents or carers did after the discovery of the child, including contact with emergency services and who they contacted within their own family and friends' environment. In suspicious deaths, when the accounts of parents or carers may change, these first disclosures may prove important to establish who may be changing their accounts or who may have disclosed to others their maltreatment of the child that potentially caused the death.

The Decision on Criminal Process

The criminal investigation of suspects involved in the death of a child will involve a range of associated offences beyond the obvious ones of murder, manslaughter, and infanticide under common law. Legislation also extends to other offences surrounding the death of a child, including causing the death of a child, child destruction, child cruelty, abandonment of a child under two where life is endangered, and neglect of an infant under three caused by suffocation when the infant is in bed with adult carers who are under the influence of alcohol. This gives investigators a range of criminal offences to investigate and prove against parents, carers, or others depending upon their involvement and criminal responsibility.

Once a senior investigating officer feels that they have sufficient evidence to prosecute, they will present a summary of that evidence to the Crown Prosecution Service (CPS) for a decision to charge the identified offender with a criminal offence. A future criminal trial will hear the evidence and decide upon the facts of the evidence presented by the Crown and a decision will be made by a jury whether the offender is guilty or not guilty of the charges brought.

The CPS has a two-stage test: there has to be sufficient evidence for the prosecution to succeed and it is in the public interest for the prosecution case to take place.

Often the CPS will appoint a prosecutor to a child death case at an early stage, and liaison between CPS and the police will take place to advise on the evidence collated and what may be additionally required to support charges against the offender(s).

CPS will want and expect expert scientific and medical evidence, presented in a manner that will assist in supporting the offence charged and in a way that juries will understand, and offering expert opinion to provide for the robust rebuttal of any claims made by defendants to nullify or mitigate their involvement in the offences charged.

Working with the Coroner in both Criminal and Non-criminal Cases

While police are investigating the death of a child, there may be a number of additional proceedings being carried out at the same time. Family Court proceedings may be underway to protect other siblings within the family. A child homicide will also see the legislative commissioning of an SCR undertaken by Local Safeguarding Children's Boards, but additional to these is the fact that the coroner has the duty to enquire into all sudden unexpected deaths.

Coroners investigate deaths that have been reported to them if it appears that:

- the death was violent or unnatural
- the cause of death is unknown, or
- the person died in prison, police custody, or another type of state detention.

In these cases coroners must investigate to find out, for the benefit of bereaved people and for official records, who has died, and how, when, and where they died.

In all child deaths, the police will notify the coroner as soon as practicable. Early liaison with the coroner is vital in order to agree what factors are present that would lead the investigator to deem the death suspicious or not at that stage. The appointment of a paediatric forensic pathologist (or a joint appointment of a paediatric and a forensic pathologist) and the type of post-mortem examination will be agreed at this stage. Identification of the child will be agreed at this stage, and the method of identification may vary depending on the type of child death being investigated. Formal identification processes such as fingerprints, DNA and / or odontology could be considered when the child death is suspicious or arises from a dramatic disaster type of event.

In criminal cases, once a child death has been referred to the coroner, the inquest will be opened with basic facts and then adjourned pending the finalisation of criminal matters. In non-suspicious child deaths, the police will prepare a file of evidence obtained from a selection of witnesses' testimony, expert medical opinion, forensic and pathology findings, and other material aimed at allowing the coroner to answer the above questions. If it was not possible to find out the cause of death from the post-mortem examination, or the death is found to be unnatural, the coroner has to hold an inquest. An inquest is a public court hearing held by the coroner in order to establish who died and how, when, and where the death occurred. The inquest will be held as soon as possible and normally within six months of the death if at all possible.

Liaison with the coroner is also vital in the pre-inquest review, ensuring that the evidence collated will provide the coroner with sufficient information from which to make an informed decision as to the cause of death.

The coroner comes to a conclusion at the end of an inquest. This includes the legal 'determination', which states who died, and where, when, and how they died. The coroner or jury also makes 'findings' to allow the cause of death to be registered. When recording the cause the coroner may use one of the following terms:

- accident or misadventure
- alcohol/drug-related
- unlawful killing
- natural causes
- open
- road traffic collision
- stillbirth

The coroner or jury may also make a brief 'narrative' conclusion setting out the facts surrounding the death in more detail and explaining the reasons for the decision.

References

1. *Sudden Unexpected Death in Infancy; A Multi-agency Protocol for Care and Investigation.* London: Royal College of Pathologists, Royal College of Paediatrics and Child Health. 2004; https://www.rcpath.org and https://www.rcpch.ac.uk/ (accessed 30 October 2018).

2. Vaughan, J. *Infanticide: The Effects of Miscarriages of Justice.* Cambridge University Press, 2007.

3. ACPO. *A Guide to Investigating Child Deaths*, 2014; library.college.police.uk/docs/acpo/ACPO-guide-to-investigating-child-deaths-2014.doc (accessed 27 September 2018).

4. *Sudden Unexpected Death in Infancy and Childhood: Multi-agency Guidelines for Care and Investigation*, 2nd edn. London: The Royal College of Pathologists, 2016.

5. Mayes, A Brown, D Marshall, 'Risk Factors for inter-familial, unlawful, and suspicious child deaths'. *Journal of Homicide, and Major Incident Investigation*, 2010; **6**(1):77–96.

Chapter 6

Sudden Infant Death Investigation in the United States

Andrew L. Falzon

Introduction

Death investigation in the United States has undergone an arduous evolution over the years, with offices operating under various systems and with significant disparity in the level of competency. Although many offices are highly regarded for the high standards they maintain, in some jurisdictions within the country, this responsibility falls upon personnel with little or no medical training or any qualifications in medico-legal death investigation. Each state promulgates its own laws and regulations that govern death investigations, which will determine the types of cases that fall under the jurisdiction of the coroner/medical examiner, how each case is investigated, and the qualifications of the personnel responsible for the investigation. Deaths which are typically reportable to the coroner/ medical examiner include:[1]

- All violent deaths
- Deaths not caused by readily identifiable disease or disability
- Deaths under suspicious or unusual circumstances
- Deaths within 24 hours of admission to a hospital
- Deaths of inmates of prisons or law enforcement custody
- Deaths from causes that might constitute a threat to public health
- Deaths resulting from employment, or to accidents while employed
- Sudden and unexpected deaths in infants and children, and fetal deaths occurring without medical attendance

This does not necessarily mean that the medical examiner will assume jurisdiction of all these cases. Most natural deaths of patients who die outside of a medical facility but were under the care of a physician will be released to a funeral home, and the treating physician will be responsible for completing the death certificate in these cases. Accepted cases will undergo a post-mortem examination that may be limited to an external examination or an autopsy, depending on the circumstances surrounding the case and local laws and guidelines.

This chapter discusses the evolution of the death investigation process in the US, and the different investigation systems currently employed. As most state laws that deal with death investigation do not provide detailed guidelines as to when and how sudden unexpected deaths in infants and children should be handled, most forensic pathologists will rely on guidance provided by national government agencies, such as the Center for Disease Control and Prevention (CDC) and professional organisations such as the National Association of Medical Examiners (NAME). In addition, advocacy groups which have been instrumental in improving the standards of infant and child death investigations, and child fatality review boards that provide some degree of oversight of these cases will also be discussed.

The Evolution of Death Investigation in the United States

The early American settlers were instructed by the King of England to establish governments that mirrored those in the motherland, resulting in the appointment of coroners in Virginia and Maryland in the early part of the seventeenth century. Seventeenth- and eighteenth-century Colonial America saw little change in the setup of death investigation systems, which were conducted by local government officials (the justice of the peace, sheriff and coroner) and were based on English law. At this time, the main differences between coroners' offices in the different colonies were the method and term of their appointment and the number of coroners for each jurisdiction. The most recognised aspect of the coroner's role was the inquest, which typically started with the jury (consisting of adult white male property-owners) gathering to view the body as originally positioned at the site where the deceased was found. At the inquest, the coroner would chair the jury (the minimum number of which varied from one jurisdiction to another), playing little role in directing their conclusions. The investigation of childhood deaths was also considered part of the responsibilities of the coroner. Unfortunately, like many other investigations at the time, these relied heavily on the opinions and conclusions of lay witnesses that included midwives with little or no medical training, and rarely called on the expertise of physicians. In the early times following the formation of the new republic, the role of the coroner continued unchanged, eventually morphing into a more political position which often served as a platform for entering into the political arena.[2]

As the practice of medicine evolved and advanced, physicians in the US started to question the coroner's authority and approach to death investigation, advocating for a more scientifically based methodology. The issue of having non-medical trained coroners in charge of death investigation was raised repeatedly in the mid-nineteenth century, with numerous lectures, and articles written in medical journals advocating for a more scientific approach, with the performance of autopsies as practised in the British medicolegal system, and the utilisation of medical experts.[3] To this extent, a newly formed committee for forensic science formed within the American Medical Association (AMA) recommended that physicians be provided with training in medical jurisprudence in preparation for such expert testimony.[4] This AMA committee went as far as recommending the abolishment of the office of the coroner as it existed at the time, and that coroners be physicians appointed by the courts.

Following an outcry stemming from accusations of the incompetence and corruption of a Boston physician coroner by the name of A. W. K. Newton, the Boston Medical Association put forward a recommendation wherein they proposed the separation of the medical and judicial functions of the coroner.[5] The medical functions, including the identification of the body and the determination of cause and manner of death, would be performed by physicians that were appointed by the governor for a period of seven years.[6] A state law was enacted shortly thereafter, creating the Massachusetts Medical Examiner office, the first of its kind in the country,

which turned out to be a success. The push to eliminate lay-coroner systems spread to other states, including Michigan, Connecticut, and Rhode Island in the early part of the twentieth century; however, these efforts met with varying degrees of success stemming from the intense opposition and political pressure from the coroners. In January 1918, New York City appointed Dr Charles Norris as the first pathologist in the position of medical examiner, thus establishing the first true medical examiner system in the country.[7] Dr Norris was instrumental in the advancement of forensic medicine, having established the first forensic toxicology laboratory in the US. He also introduced the concept of medicolegal death scene examinations and encouraged training in forensic pathology for physicians, which led to the elevation of forensic pathology as a recognised subspecialty of pathology by the American Board of Pathology. The high standards he set for the office gave it a reputation as one of the best in the country, a reputation that continues to this day as exemplified by the highly regarded handling of the victims of the terrorist attacks of 11 September 2001.

At present, some medical examiner's offices are established within public health departments, some fall under law and public safety, while a few offices are established within a university setting. Since the medical examiner's office is a medicolegal agency rather than a strictly medical entity, and because public health departments are often underfunded, this arrangement can give rise to conflicts between these departments and increased bureaucracy. The major concern with offices that fall under law and public safety is the potential for lack of impartiality due to pressure on the pathologists to modify their diagnoses. In order to preserve the impartiality of the medical examiner's office, the National Association of Medical Examiners (NAME) strongly recommends that all offices be allowed to function independently and without political influence, and considers this independence an absolute necessity.[8] While none of the systems described above are perfect, the most important factors that guarantee a successful operation are adequate funding and freedom from outside political pressure. In part due to politics, and partly related to geographical factors, death investigation systems in the US lack uniformity across the country, and will typically consist of a coroner system, a medical examiner system, or some form of hybrid of the two. According to the CDC, the current

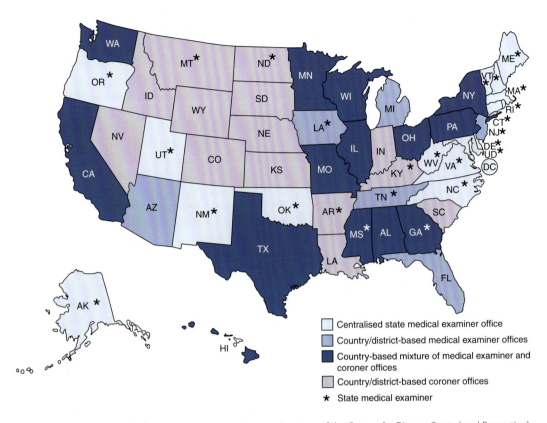

Figure 6.1 United States death investigation systems by state (courtesy of the Centers for Disease Control and Prevention)

situation with regard to the types of office setups is as follows (Figure 6.1):

- Centralised medical examiner system: sixteen states and Washington DC
- County or district-based medical examiner system: six states
- County-based system with a mixture of coroner and medical examiner offices: fourteen states
- County, district, or parish-based coroner system: fourteen states
- State medical examiner: twenty-five states[9]

A listing of the state-by-state distribution of the different forms of death investigation systems throughout the US, including the terms of office and references to the individual state laws can be found on the public health law section on the CDC website. The site also specifies the required training and qualifications of the physicians conducting post-mortem examination, since in some instances they are not required to be pathologists. The specific role of the coroner/medical examiners and the types of cases investigated in each jurisdiction are also outlined.

Deaths Investigated by the Coroner/ Medical Examiner

As outlined above, cases that fall under the jurisdiction of the coroner/medical examiner in the US are typically suspicious and unnatural deaths, deaths in custody (which would include all cases that involve interaction with law enforcement), unexplained paediatric deaths, on-the-job deaths, threats to public health, and cases where the cause of death is not clearly defined. The extent to which cases are accepted and the type of examination performed will vary from office to office depending on multiple factors that include local laws, caseload, and budgetary constraints. In many jurisdictions, the coroner/medical examiner will also be required to perform an autopsy if so ordered by a county prosecutor or a superior court judge. The laws and guidelines that specify when autopsies are required to be performed can be found on the CDC website.

The Investigation of Childhood Deaths

The CDC has played a major role in increasing the awareness and understanding of Sudden Infant Death Syndrome (SIDS), both within the medical community and the general public. Apart from providing important statistical information regarding sudden unexpected deaths in infants and children and identifying support groups for the benefit of the grieving parents, the CDC also provides guidelines and training related to the investigation of these cases. This training, which is intended for medicolegal death investigators, is in the form of multiple manuals that are easily accessible through the CDC website. These provide instructions for how to interact with parents and conduct interviews, conduct a thorough scene examination and perform the doll re-enactment of the scene. The latter is considered a critical part of the investigation, since in most cases the original scene findings are often disturbed and crucial information may be missed. A 'Sudden Unexplained Infant Death Investigation Form' which can be completed electronically is available online, and is intended to provide guidance for the collection of comprehensive information that includes investigative data, a witness interview, the infant's medical and dietary history, the pregnancy history, and an incident scene investigation.[10] Again, these are national guidelines which are recommended but not mandated by the CDC, and whether they are used will depend on individual state and/or local guidelines.

National Association of Medical Examiners Guidelines

NAME was founded in 1966, and serves as the national professional organisation for medical examiners. The organisation has grown over the years, and besides physician medical examiners, its members now include medicolegal death investigators and forensic administrators from across the US and beyond.

With the goal of setting standards and furthering excellence in death investigation, the NAME offers a voluntary and rigorous inspection and accreditation programme for medicolegal death investigation offices. This coveted certification is awarded for a four-year period, and serves as recognition of the achievement of a high level of competency with regard to office policies

and procedures. NAME members also work with other professional organisations such as the College of American Pathologists and the American Academy of Forensic Sciences in an effort to promote minimum standards of practice and the advancement of death investigations. Several position papers have been published by NAME, dealing with critical, and sometimes controversial topics that include autopsy performance standards, death certification, and the retention of post-mortem tissue samples for genetic testing. One position paper entitled: 'Recommendations for the Postmortem Assessment of Suspected Head Trauma in Infants and Young Children' provides guidelines relating to procedures that should be completed in the investigation of paediatric deaths resulting from abusive injuries, including a recommended list of photographs, a series of radiographs, and required histological sections.[11] Examination of the fixed brain by a neuropathologist is also encouraged in these cases, a concept that appears to be gaining popularity as cases become increasingly challenged in court. A complete listing of these position papers can be found on the NAME website.

A recent issue of the Academic Forensic Pathology, the official journal of NAME, was devoted entirely to SIDS. One of the articles in this issue, entitled 'Recommendations for the autopsy of an infant who has died suddenly and unexpectedly', discusses the paediatric autopsy, emphasising the fact that these cases represent a unique and distinct subspecialty interest within forensic pathology rather than a routine examination of a 'small adult'.[12] The article acknowledges the fact that although most forensic pathologists would agree that some form of invasive dissection is warranted in the examination of infants who die suddenly and unexpectedly, no current standard exists in the US detailing what should constitute a comprehensive paediatric autopsy. The article goes on to quote a survey conducted by the CDC among seven states which showed that whereas most of the pathologists agreed on the necessity of certain studies such as toxicology, viral, and bacterial cultures, histology, and radiography, there was less of a consensus regarding the use of vitreous chemistry studies and screening for metabolic disorders. Not surprisingly, genetic studies were the tests least likely to be conducted, although this is likely to change in the future as the role of genetic conditions becomes increasingly recognised and testing becomes more widely available and less expensive. This article does

39

not provide a step-by-step guide for how to perform a paediatric autopsy, but offers recommendations for ancillary studies and various autopsy dissection techniques. As in general forensic pathology, such investigations should be guided by history, findings of a thorough scene examination and evolving autopsy observations. The NAME is currently collaborating with other interested parties, with the goal of providing a joint position paper on best practices for the investigation, autopsy, and certification of sudden and unexpected deaths in infants and children.

The Impact of Advocacy Groups on the Investigation of Childhood Deaths

In the 1960s, parents who went through the experience of the sudden and unexpected death of their infants started coming together, driven by their frustration over the lack of progress in the understanding of the causation of these deaths. These parents formed organisations with the intent of promoting public awareness of the problem, while also advocating for research and support services for families. These efforts led to the passage of the Sudden Infant Death Syndrome Act (Public Law 93–270) of 1974, which among other things provided funding for SIDS research and the establishment of programmes that offered information and counselling to grieving families.[13] Multiple, non-profit SIDS support groups were formed, such as the American SIDS institute, CJ Foundation for SIDS, and the SIDS Alliance. The aim of these organisations was to promote and fund SIDS research and education, promote conferences, workshops, teaching programmes, and provide family support services through the use of brochures and direct contact with bereaved parents.

Grieving parents who dealt with the sudden loss of a child older than twelve months of age to SIDS-like deaths also started looking for answers. With the definition of SIDS as a sudden unexplained death in an infant one month to one year of age, these deaths could not be simply treated as an extrapolation of SIDS cases. Initially referred to as 'Post-Infancy SIDS', these cases were later referred to as Sudden Unexplained Death in Childhood (SUDC), which is the sudden and unexpected death of a child, twelve months or older, which remains unexplained after a thorough investigation that includes a death scene examination, history review, and a full autopsy with indicated ancillary testing. Like SIDS, SUDC is a diagnosis of exclusion, where the underlying cause of death remains unidentified.

Another programme that provides oversight of child fatalities is the child fatality review board. Almost all states have a well-established child death review programme, the majority of which are supported by state legislation. Team members typically consist of multidisciplinary and culturally competent professionals that include social workers, paediatricians, psychologists, and representatives from law enforcement agencies, the prosecutor's office, and the medical examiner's office. Multiple child fatality review boards may be established in any given state, as is the case in New Jersey, where the main board reviews all non-natural deaths, while subcommittees are established that limit their review to cases of SUDI/SUID and suicide. The purpose of the child death review boards is to review each paediatric death, identify any preventable issues or risk factors, and evaluate the investigation of the cases. In turn, this information is used to enhance governmental support systems, and to make recommendations to state and local agencies and legislators in order to establish policies that are intended to prevent similar deaths in the future.

Determining the Cause and Manner of Death

In the US, the mechanisms whereby conclusions are drawn following a death investigation differ from the inquests that are typically seen in England and Wales. The process generally starts with a death scene investigation that includes interviews of witnesses, which is most often conducted by a medicolegal death investigator. Once this preliminary investigation is completed, these investigators do not routinely engage in active ongoing investigations of the case, but will rely on law enforcement agencies for any updates. Identification is most often established by direct viewing of the deceased by relatives, or by showing the families post-mortem photographs which tend to be less emotionally traumatic. In some situations, for example when there is extensive facial disfigurement resulting from blunt-force injuries or fires, the pathologist will rely on scientific methods of identification including comparison of fingerprints and dental records, and less commonly DNA studies. In most jurisdictions, post-mortem examinations, whether external examinations, or full autopsies are conducted by pathologists, who will request any ancillary testing such as toxicology, radiography, and microbiology studies as indicated. Once all the information and test results are received, it is the responsibility of the pathologist to compile and review all the available information in order to formulate the cause and manner of death, a decision that lies solely with the coroner or medical examiner. Depending on the circumstances surrounding death and the autopsy findings, unnatural deaths are typically classified as accidents, suicides, or homicides. In cases where the manner of death cannot be ascertained, the manner of death will be classified as undetermined, with the proviso that if additional information becomes available at a later date, the case will be reviewed and amended accordingly. Unfortunately, some jurisdictions in the US have religious objection laws, which will permit the next of kin of deceased individuals to object to an autopsy based on the religious affiliation of the deceased. Such practice may compromise the investigation and prosecution of cases, especially cases of abuse, and neglect in infants and children. Other potential issues arising from this practice will include the failure to identify natural causes of death which may be of a genetic / hereditary nature and infectious diseases that may pose a threat to public health. A NAME position statement supports the repeal of such religious exemption laws.[14]

In the past, the deaths of infants between the ages of one month and one year where a thorough autopsy that included all recommended ancillary studies failed to reveal a definite cause of death, were typically certified as SIDS. In these cases, the manner of death was classified as 'natural'. The current preferred term in such cases is Sudden Unexpected Infant Death (SUID). When the history indicates the presence of risk factors that are typically associated with SIDS but lacks other remarkable findings, the manner of death is typically classified as 'natural'. When the history suggests the presence of unsafe sleep practices such as co-sleeping or the use of unsafe bedding items that may have contributed to death, the preferred manner of death is 'undetermined'. With the latter, it is strongly recommended that the pathologist include an opinion paragraph in the autopsy report in order to explain his/her findings and conclusions. This preferred designation is important from a public health point of view, as it highlights the potential role of these practices in the death of the child, and may help establish preventative guidelines and

policies. When definite findings of asphyxia such as suffocation by soft bedding with occlusion of airways or overlay by another person are clearly identified, the terms SIDS or SUID should be avoided, and the cause of death should clearly outline the events that resulted in the death. The manner of death in these cases should be classified as 'accident'.

One key lesson learned over time is that in the practice of forensic pathology, communication is crucial for the successful outcome of an investigation, and that the autopsy findings cannot be interpreted in a vacuum. This is even more important in the case of sudden unexpected deaths in infants and children, since many of the changes in these paediatric cases can be subtle and easily overlooked. Admittedly, completing the CDC-recommended questionnaire with grieving parents shortly after they have lost a child can be a challenge, and in some instances attempts to conduct a doll re-enactment of the scene have been met with aggressive responses from families. The role of advocacy support groups that can provide counselling and assistance should not be overlooked or underestimated, particularly when the person providing such assistance has experienced the loss of a child themselves, and are thus in a better position to relate to the parents. Obviously, the necessity of a thorough and detailed autopsy, with all indicated ancillary testing is crucial for the identification of any positive findings, with pertinent negative findings having an equally important significance. Once the autopsy report has been completed and the cause and manner of death determined, the pathologist should find the time to discuss the case findings with the parents, emphasising any need for follow-up in any other relatives. On a national level, guidelines for the investigation and autopsy of SUDI/SUID and SUDC cases, including the certification of the cause and manner of death will provide uniformity of the information obtained, which in turn will better guide future policies and recommendations for the prevention of these sudden unexpected deaths.

References

1. New Jersey State Medical Examiner Act, 2009. New Jersey Code Title 52 - State Government, Departments And Officers; 52:17B https://law.justia.com/codes/new-jersey/2009/title-52/52-17b (accessed 30 October 2018).

2. Jentzen JM. *Death Investigation in America: Coroners, Medical Examiners, and the Pursuit of Medical Certainty.* Boston: Harvard University Press, 2009: 10–11.

3. Editorial, *Boston Med Surg J*, 1846; **35**:350–5.

4. Mohr JC. *Doctors and the Law: Medical Jurisprudence in Nineteenth-Century America.* Baltimore: Johns Hopkins University Press, 1996: 226–36.

5. Tyndale TH. The law of coroners. *Boston Med Surg J*, 1877; **154**:246–7.

6. Editorial: The coroners must go. *Boston Med Surg J*, 1880; **109**:280.

7. *The Office of the Medical Examiner of the City of New York: Report by the Committee on Public Health, New York Academy of Medicine. Bull NY Acad Med*, 1967; **43**(3):241–9; https://www.ncbi.nlm.nih.gov/pmc/articles/PMC1806568/pdf/bullnyacadmed00252-0085.pdf (accessed 30 October 2018).

8. Melinek J et al. NAME position paper: medical examiner, coroner and forensic pathologist independence. *Acad Forensic Pathol*, 2013; **3**(1):93–8.

9. www.cdc.gov/phlp/publications/topic/coroner.html (accessed 30 October 2018).

10. www.cdc.gov/sids/index.htm (accessed 30 October 2018).

11. Gill JR, Andrew T, Gilliland, LJ, Matshes EW, Reichard R. NAME position paper: Recommendations for the postmortem assessment of suspected head trauma in children and young infants. *Acad Forensic Pathol*, 2013; **4**(2):206–13.

12. Pinneri K, Matshes EWl. Recommendations for the autopsy of an infant who has died suddenly and unexpectedly. *Acad Forensic Pathol*, 2017; **7**(2):171–81.

13. Govtrack. S.1745 – *An Act to Provide Financial Assistance for Research Activities for the Study of Sudden Infant Death Syndrome, and for Other Purposes.* 93rd Congress (1973–4) https://www.govtrack.us/congress/bills/93/s1745 (accessed 30 October 2018).

14. NAME Position statement in support of repealing certain religious exemption laws 2 March 2001; https://netforum.avectra.com/public/temp/ClientImages/NAME/8aa04f55-b815-4a3f-bfaa-236f571379d3.pdf (accessed 5 November 2018).

Chapter

7

Emergency Services: First Responders

Deborah A. Robinson

The definition of SIDS – the sudden death of a previously healthy infant in which no adequate cause of death is found after thorough scene investigation, complete autopsy, and review of case history – rests on the absence of an adequate cause of death. Conceptually the opposite of any other medical condition, this diagnosis is based on the lack of anatomic, biochemical, genetic, or physiological markers that distinguish disease. Despite years of medical research, no specific ante-mortem, or post-mortem markers exist for SIDS. While risk-reduction strategies have decreased the incidence of SIDS, it has not been eliminated. Without biological markers, SIDS has remained impossible to predict or prevent.

Furthermore, because no positive findings for SIDS exist, pathologists struggle with acceptable terminology for death certificates. Proposed guidelines suggest different labels and categories for SIDS, but they are no more satisfying and have the unfortunate consequence of creating confusion regarding the epidemiology of infant deaths.

Lacking compelling scientific explanations for SIDS, the 'triple-risk model' provides a useful conceptual framework for investigating infant deaths and recognising risk factors by organising various theories and risk factors into three categories: homeostatic development, intrinsic vulnerability, and environmental factors.

Regarding environmental factors, scene investigation is crucial for recognising modifiable environmental factors that increase the risk of SIDS and for revealing hazards that cause infant death.[1] Consequently, careful scene investigation is essential for competent death investigation and to prevent future infant deaths. Arguably, scene investigation, not medical research, is the basis for understanding hazards and risk factors and for promoting prevention strategies responsible for reducing infant mortality.[2]

Experienced death investigators understand that the infant death scene is the most challenging phase of investigation.[3] Unfortunately, the infant death scene is disrupted when a caregiver moves the body from exactly where death occurred. Furthermore, in many jurisdictions, emergency medical responders routinely remove a dead infant from the scene, effectively precluding meaningful scene analysis.

Death investigators also know that an infant death scene is typically one of confusion and emotional turmoil. Multiple family members, including children, along with police detectives, patrol officers, and chaplains often surround distraught parents. In this chaotic environment, a rigorous procedure is necessary: standardised protocols help provide a systematic methodology for collecting crucial scene investigation information, and a standardised form helps neutralise the investigation by focusing the caregiver's attention on a goal-oriented task. In the US and other countries, another useful investigative method utilises a stuffed, weighted no-descript doll, or similar prop, to recreate the conditions in which the dead infant was initially found. Since 1995, the King County Medical Examiner's Office (KCMEO) has used this technique to reconstruct the infant death scene. The objective of the KCMEO study is to assess the KCMEO's experience when doll reconstruction is employed in their investigations. From an investigator's perspective, doll re-enactment by trained investigators proves the most fruitful. When properly performed, a consistent, comprehensive, and compassionate doll re-enactment is not only critical for a complete death investigation, but it can engage grieving caregivers to be active participants in the process.

References

1. Byard RW, Jensen LL. How reliable is reported sleeping position in cases of unexpected infant death? *J Forensic Sci*, 2008; **53**:1169–71.

2. Centers for Disease Control and Prevention. *Guidelines for death scene investigation of sudden, unexplained infant deaths: recommendations of the Interagency Panel*

on Sudden Infant Death Syndrome. *Morb Mortal Wkly Rep*, 1996; **45**:1–22.

3. Shapiro-Mendoza CK. *Sudden Unexplained Infant Deaths in the Sudden, Unexplained Infant Death Investigation Training Manual: A Systematic Training Program for the Professional Infant Death Investigation Specialist. Centers for Disease Control and Prevention, Department of Health and Human Services*, 2007. https://www.cdc.gov/sids/pdf/suidmanual/Chapter1_ta g508.pdf (accessed 28 October 2018).

The Home Visit

Robert Coombs

The importance of the home visit in the UK can be traced back to the work of Carpenter and Emery in Sheffield via Fleming in Bristol and was mandated as a result of the Kennedy Report in 2004. It is part of a wider set of procedures and investigations of all these tragic deaths. There should be five objectives for this Child Death Review (CDR) process: to understand the cause of death, understand any contributing risk factors, support the family, learn lessons, and ensure that the statutory requirements in relation to death are met including criminal, civil, or child protection matters[1–4].

Who Should Do It?

In the UK it is usual practice for the home visit to be jointly undertaken by both healthcare and police. The latter is usually but not always a senior investigating officer with a child protection background but can also be a senior officer from the local division. Knowledge of who they are and their background is essential for a smooth joint-agency home visit. Ensuring that the Accident and Emergency (A&E) department obtains the appropriate contact details of the senior investigating officer clearly aids easy and rapid communication.

Often the first attendees at the house will be regular uniformed officers with little experience of these tragedies. It is important that they have access to appropriate help and protocols to avoid actions that may be regretted later. On review of cases one of the commonest criticisms is inappropriate actions by the front-line uniformed officers – designating a 'crime scene', inappropriate interactions with grieving parents and seizure of articles from the place of death. These should be left in situ for inspection at the home visit, though photography of the bedrooms before the home visit may avoid too many people in the house at the time of the visit.

The police will know the whereabouts of the family and are probably best placed to arrange the details of the home visit. They will also have done their background checks on the family and should freely share appropriate information.

The visit is a joint visit. The representative from health is often a trained paediatrician or specialist nurse working in the area of CDRs. There is no data yet to suggest that one model is better than another but interest and familiarity with the policies and procedures is critical, as is knowledge of normal child development and experience of normal infancy and its associated common illnesses.

There will be occasions when it may be appropriate to include other professionals who have known the family; these could include the health visitor or GP and in some cases the police will provide a Family Liaison Officer to support the family.

When Should It Occur?

Most agencies try to arrange the home visit within 24 hours of the death. There is little point in trying to organise one in the middle of the night and 2–3 hours should be pencilled in for the visit.

All the relevant information should have been collected before the visit including address and post code (for later use in applying postcode-related deprivation scores). Information from the A&E department where the child was taken and any issues raised by the initial medical review will help establish the circumstances of the death. Likewise it is important to know that searches have been made to establish if the child or family are known to social services. This helps with the communication with the parents who may be concerned the information may be misconstrued. There is no substitute for speaking to the A&E staff concerned or getting copies of the clinical record.

The need for the visit should have been introduced to the parents by the staff of the A&E department and should be seen as part of the normal protocol for trying to understand why these tragedies occur.

For centres where there is in-house pathology, discussion with the local mortuary technicians and pathologist gives you information about when the post-mortem may be taking place and if any contact has already been made between the mortuary staff, A&E and the parents. Introduction of the parents to the mortuary staff by A&E staff often alleviates many of the concerns the parents may have and lays the ground for possible ongoing bereavement support.

Liaison with the police is essential to establish when and where to meet the parents. It is usually in the parents' home, and death-scene review should always be with a parent present, but there are occasions when it seems inappropriate to force a parent to immediately return home and a relative's house is sometimes preferred for the initial discussions. On occasion a parent is in such shock that it is useful for a relative to be present to help obtain the important family histories. This can also be helpful in establishing the support the family will have available and ensuring that there are other members of the family who have heard what has been said.

The Home Visit

Obtaining the history is usually best done by the paediatrician with the police only asking supplementary questions where appropriate to clarify points. The police are best placed to look for evidence of risk factors such as alcohol ingestion and illicit drug use. The written record is taken by both the paediatrician and police.

Taking a family history often helps the family to relax a little and gives information as to any family history of SIDS or sudden deaths in children, adults, or stillbirths along with other familial conditions. Family background and education is often very informative as is the parents' physical and mental health history. The history should include all the children, starting with each pregnancy (whether planned and wanted, feelings concerning) progressing through birth to feeding and development along with any illnesses and/or hospital admissions.

In the UK families are issued with a 'Red Book' at the birth of each child. These are used as a hand-held record and contain entries made after each contact with a health professional. They should contain useful information on birth data, growth, development, and immunisations as well as evidence of hospital admissions.

While much of the initial interview is information-seeking, it is often best to let the parents tell their own story of the child over the last few days and night. This should include precise details of the last sleep and attempts at resuscitation.

As part of the investigators' review of their story it often clarifies the history to take them back to the death scene to clearly understand the circumstances of the death. Some have advocated use of a life-sized doll and either photographs or video of the death scene (see Chapter 7), actions which take great skill and experience to introduce appropriately to the family.

By the end of the interview information should have been collected on all the risk factors. These will include parental smoking habits, alcohol ingestion, illicit substance misuse as well as usual sleeping place and position, along with dress, sleep surface, and coverings.

Experienced investigators should at this stage be able to suggest to the parents the possible findings from the PM and explain the likely timescale for the PM report, multi-agency meeting and coroner's inquest (if there is likely to be one).

No visit would be complete without explaining possible avenues of support to the family from the voluntary sector (Lullaby Trust in England and Wales, Scottish Cot Death Trust in Scotland) and from local resources such as the health visitor, GP, or bereavement services. A planned visit after the multi-agency meeting is important, as is giving the parents a rough time line.

Leaving written information with the family is helpful. This should include a guide to the followup process, and contact details of people who will be involved in the ongoing investigations and multi-agency meeting that will conclude the information given to the coroner.

Following the home visit, a report should be prepared to be shared with all the relevant agencies, and in particular the pathologist who will be performing the post-mortem examination.

References

1. Carpenter RG, Gardner A, McWeeny PM, Emery JL. Multistage scoring system for identifying infants at risk of unexpected death. *Arch Dis Child*, 1977; **52**: 606–12.

2. Fleming P, Blair P, Bacon CJ, Berry P. *Sudden Unexpected Deaths in Infancy: the CESDI SUDI Studies 1993–1996*. London: The Stationery Office; 2000.

3. *Sudden Unexpected Death in Infancy; A Multi-agency Protocol for Care and Investigation*. London: Royal College of Pathologists, Royal College of Paediatrics, and Child Health. 2004; https://www.rcpath.org and https://www.rcpch.ac.uk/ (accessed 31 October 2018).

4. Garstang, J, Ellis, C, Sidebotham P. An evidence-based guide to the investigation of sudden unexpected death in infancy. *Forensic Sci Med Pathol*, 2015; **11**:345–57.

Autopsy: Current Methods and Ancillary Investigations

Irene Scheimberg and Marta C. Cohen

In cases of sudden unexpected death in infancy in the United Kingdom, a post-mortem is always ordered; in England and Wales by the Coroner and in Scotland by the Procurator Fiscal.[1,2] Depending on the jurisdiction, the coroner may request the post-mortem to be done by a paediatric pathologist alone (if there are no suspicious circumstances) or to be a joint procedure done by a paediatric and a forensic pathologist, even if there are no suspicious circumstances. Whenever there are any suspicious circumstances, there is a joint autopsy led by the forensic pathologist. The autopsy includes external and internal examination, infection screening, metabolic and genetic studies, and toxicology.[3–8] Some coroners will only allow toxicology in certain circumstances, including all suspicious cases.

The Autopsy

The autopsy should be done as soon as possible. However, as the availability of both paediatric and forensic pathologists may be limited, the body may have to be transported far from the place of death. At any point in the investigation, if something becomes suspicious the paediatric pathologist conducting a post-mortem alone should stop the examination and inform the coroner, who may then decide to call a forensic pathologist for a joint examination (see Section 3, Legal Framework, and Chapter 10, The Joint Forensic/Paediatric Post-mortem Examination).

Before commencing the autopsy procedure all cases are x-rayed. If available, MRI (Magnetic Resonance Imaging) and/or CT (Computerised Tomography) studies may be also carried out. The body is then photographed on its front, back, and side. Any abnormality noted at this stage should also be photographed.

After weighing the body, standard measurements are taken. Essential measurements include head circumference at the occipital-frontal level and body length (crown–heel). Other measurements that are

advised to be registered are chest and abdominal circumference, crown–rump, and feet length. Measurements are then compared with expected values for age and gender. If the baby is an ex-premature baby the comparison should be done using the baby's corrected age (premature baby's chronological age minus the number of weeks or months s/he was born early).[9]

External Examination

A careful external examination should record general nutritional status and hygiene, any abnormal findings in the skin or any evidence of disease, evidence of malformations, and evidence of medical intervention. All of these need to be carefully recorded in writing and/or with a diagram, and photographed if necessary. Distribution of post-mortem hypostasis adds to the information around the baby's death.

The external examination of the body starts with the head. Size and shape are important. The presence of a fontanelle and its measurements should be ascertained, although this should be measured again after reflecting the scalp. Any evidence of dysmorphism should be described.[10] Examination of the eyes should include the intercanthal distance compared to the palpebral fissure length; examination of the conjunctiva (looking for haemorrhages, jaundice, or pallor); and examination of the cornea, iris, and pupil to look for possible abnormalities. The position, shape, and rotation of the ears should be recorded. The nose and nostrils should be examined. Patency can be established with a swab for bacteriology studies. The philtrum, mouth, and palate are checked documenting clefts if present. In the mouth, the presence or absence of teeth should be documented, and the internal mucosa examined, as well as the state of the frenula and tongue.

The neck is examined for presence of oedema, injuries, or marks of intervention. The shape of the chest should be assessed as this may be abnormal in

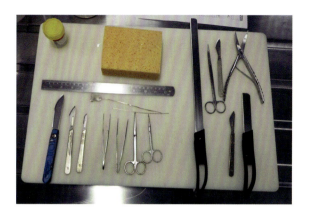

Figure 9.1 Set of instruments used in paediatric post-mortems.

Table 9.1 Minimum thoracic and abdominal histology samples and special stains if necessary

Heart: 1 LV, 1 RV, 1 septum	Septum: levels and EVG
Lungs: 1 from each lobe hilum to periphery	EVG, Perl's
Trachea with thyroid 1	
Larynx through epiglottis 1	
Gastro-oesophageal junction 1	
GI tract: rectum 1, Terminal ileum 1	
Liver: left lobe 1, right lobe 1	Reticulin, EVG, PAS, PAS-D
Spleen 1	
Pancreas 1 (consider longitudinal section)	
Kidneys: right 1, left 1	
Adrenals: left 1, right 1	
Gonads	
Bladder: 1	
Rib (5th or 6th) including costochondral junction	
Skeletal muscle: psoas 1; diaphragm 1	
Lymph nodes if relevant	
Any lesion	

certain syndromes. The shape and size of the abdomen are important as there may be general distention or masses. The baby should be rotated to examine the back. The limbs are then assessed to ascertain symmetry, size, and possible laxity. The genitalia including the perineum and the anus are examined and if the testes are descended this should be recorded. Presence or absence of nappy rash should be documented.

Before proceeding to the internal examination some bacteriology and virology studies should be undertaken. The nose and throat are swabbed routinely. A skin sample for fibroblast culture directed to metabolic investigations and genetic analysis (if the infant looks dysmorphic) is obtained using sterile instruments before the midline incision is made. A lumbar puncture may be also done at this stage (other technique would be direct puncture of the cisterna magna, see below).

Internal Examination

Most pathology departments have a special set of smaller instruments to be used in perinatal and infant autopsies (Figure 9.1). A standard set of samples is obtained during the internal examination of the neck, thorax and abdomen (Table 9.1)

The baby's neck and shoulders are placed on a block to provide better exposure of the chest for the initial incision. There are some variations of the initial incision but the aim is to offer maximal visualisation of the organs. The authors favour a T-shape incision as shown in Figure 9.2. The neck structures are removed through subcutaneous dissection, while lifting the skin with curved forceps in order to achieve better visualisation. The neck's skin is therefore preserved for viewing. If special visualisation of the genitourinary tract is required, an inverted Y may be the preferred incision. In any case, incisions are done in such a way that after reconstruction and dressing of the baby they will not be obvious to the parents.

Neck and thorax: The superficial neck muscles are examined for haemorrhages. If found. these should be correlated with the marks of intervention. The skin, subcutaneous tissues, and superficial muscles are reflected from the ribs. At this stage, if a pneumothorax is suspected a syringe with a needle and filled with water is inserted on the anterolateral chest wall between the ribs. If air is present in the chest cavity, bubbles will rise into the water in the syringe. The chest plate is removed by cutting along the chondro-costal junction from the sternoclavicular joint to the abdomen. The presence of fluid or other abnormalities is then noted in the pleural cavities. Pleural fluid may be collected for microbiology. After examining the pleural cavities, a sterile sample for bacteriology is obtained from each lung using a sterile forceps and scalpel. The size of the thymus should be noted and the presence of petechiae in the thymus,

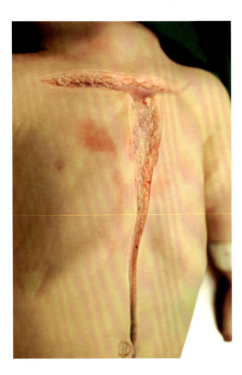

Figure 9.2 T-shape incision to access the thorax and abdomen and neck but preserving the appearances of the neck for viewing of the body

lungs, and pericardium assessed. After removing the thymus, the pericardium is incised, and the presence of fluid evaluated as for the pleural cavities. Any substantial amount of fluid should be measured. The heart is also examined for petechiae on the myocardium. Blood for ancillary studies (including bacteriology and measurement of vitamin D when available) may be obtained from the right jugular vein or the right side of the heart. Blood for toxicology (plain and preserved) is better obtained from the femoral vein, but if this is not possible, the site of origin should be stated (see Table 9.2).

The position of the heart, the great arteries, and the venous return is then assessed in situ. Some pathologists prefer to open the heart in situ and others after extraction of the cardiopulmonary block. In any case this is done following the blood flow,[1] usually accessing through the inferior vena cava.

After examining the thoracic organs, the tongue should be freed, the neck structures mobilised from the spine and the lungs, heart, and oesophagus extracted by cutting the aorta, inferior vena cava, and oesophagus at the level of the diaphragm. The oesophagus is opened, examined, and removed; the

heart is dissected, if it has not been done in situ, and separated from the lungs. The number of lobes and the position of the bronchi in relation to the pulmonary arteries can be ascertained, if it has not been done in situ; the trachea and bronchi opened and the larynx examined. The lungs are finally separated and weighed individually. Each lobe should be open and examined for the presence of focal lesions, oedema, haemorrhage, or secretions. Samples should be taken from each lobe and should include hilum and periphery. The right and left ventricles and the septum should be sampled. It is recommended that the left ventricle is sampled vertically to include the tip of one or both papillary muscles and the septum also vertically to include the AV (atrio-ventricular) node. The measurements of the valves and the ventricles should be recorded and the position of the coronary ostia noted. Any lesion such as an infarct must also be sampled. A section through the thyroid and the trachea and a section of the larynx should be taken as well as one from the thymus. The right fifth or sixth rib including the costochondral junction should be sampled to allow the histological examination of the growth plate, the bone marrow, and the bone. Any fracture, callus, or abnormality should also be sampled. A virology sample from the heart and lungs should be taken (see Table 9.2).

Abdomen and pelvis: Before introducing contamination in the abdomen, the spleen can be brought forward with sterile forceps and a microbiology swab taken after an incision with a sterile scalpel. The intestines are examined in situ and the rotation and fixation as well as distention, or any abnormality noted. Removal of the intestines exposes the retroperitoneal space and facilitates the examination of the liver, spleen, and pancreas. A sample of bowel content is sent to bacteriology and to virology, to rule out gastroenteritis.(see Table 9.2).

The abdominal block including liver, stomach, pancreas, and spleen is then removed for examination. The organs are separated and weighed and any external abnormality noted before serially sectioning them. The stomach is open and the gastric contents sent for toxicology. Some changes in the liver are obvious on macroscopic examination and should be recorded. The consistency of the spleen should be noted and recorded. Samples from the left and right lobe of the liver and the spleen are then taken.

Table 9.2 Recommended samples in the investigation of sudden unexpected death in infancy [Adapted from Sethuraman et al.[1]]

Sample	Send to	Handling	Test
Blood [#] cultures – aerobic and anaerobic 1 ml [****]	Microbiology	If insufficient blood, aerobic only	Culture and sensitivity
Blood [#] for Guthrie card	Clinical chemistry	Normal (fill in card; do not put into plastic bag)	Inherited metabolic diseases
Blood (serum) 1–2 ml	Clinical chemistry	Spin, store at -20 C	Toxicology (a chain-of-custody SOP should be adhered to)
Nasopharyngeal aspirate	Virology	Normal	Viral cultures, immuno-fluorescence and DNA amplification techniques[*]
Nasopharyngeal aspirate	Microbiology	Normal	Culture and sensitivity
Swabs from any identifiable lesions	Microbiology	Normal	Culture and sensitivity
Urine (if available)	Clinical chemistry	Spin, store supernatant at -20°C	Toxicology if indicated (a chain-of-custody SOP should be adhered to)
			Inherited metabolic diseases
Skin	Clinical chemistry	In Hams culture medium	Fibroblast culture for metabolic conditions and cytogenetics (if required)

\# when possible, blood should be taken from peripheral vein (i.e. femoral)

* Samples must be sent to an appropriate virologic laboratory.

**** Samples to be taken at bank holiday / weekend when baby arrives to Accident and Emergency. Additional samples to be considered after discussion with paediatrician.

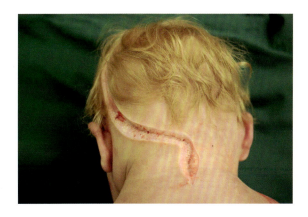

Figure 9.3 A 'question mark' incision of the scalp allows access to the base of the skull and the upper cervical spine.

Depending on the clinical history, it may be necessary to sample the pancreas extensively if there is a suspicion of persistent hypoglycaemic hyperinsulinism. A sample from the gastro-oesophageal junction, the small and large intestines, and sometimes the stomach are obtained.

Before extracting the bladder, a urine sample for bacteriology and metabolic studies may be obtained with a sterile needle and syringe. After in-situ examination, the adrenals, kidneys, ureters, and bladder are extracted. The adrenals are separated and are examined for evidence of haemorrhage. The adrenals may be weighed together or separately if there is a major discrepancy in the size. The kidneys are halved and the pelvicalyceal system and the patency of the ureters is ascertained. The kidneys are weighed separately. Finally the bladder is opened. The ovaries are examined and sampled and the uterus and vagina are opened. The location of the testes is ascertained and the testes are sampled.

Head and spine (see also Chapter 10): The body is turned and placed on its front. A semicircular incision is made on the back of the head from ear to ear just proximal from the occipital bone. This can be extended on one side like a 'question mark' to allow access to the base of the skull and the upper cervical spine (Figure 9.3). The scalp is reflected and examined. Haemosiderin deposits may be the result of birth-related haemorrhages. As the atlanto-occipital junction is exposed using the 'question mark'-shaped incision on the back of the scalp exposing the upper spine and occipital area, a sterile sample of cerebrospinal fluid can be obtained either with a pipette after incising the dura or by using a sterile needled syringe (Figure 9.4). The foramen magnum is exposed to look

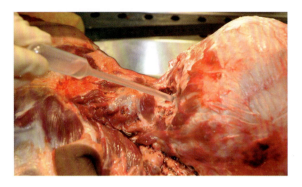

Figure 9.4 After removal of the atlas, a sterile pipette is used to obtain a cerebrospinal fluid sample for bacteriology and virology investigations.

Table 9.3 Central Nervous System samples

Brainstem	Medulla
	Pons
	Midbrain
Cerebellum	Vermis
	Dentate nuclei (right and left)
Cerebrum	Frontal cortex (right and left)
	Basal ganglia (right and left)
	Hippocampi (right and left)
	Occipital cortex (right and left)
	Insula
	Hypothalamus

for herniation of the brain. The upper cervical spinal cord is detached to facilitate subsequent removal of the brain. The skull bones are examined as there may be clear evidence of craniotabes, evidenced by patches of marked thinning in the skull bones. This can be better demonstrated after the brain extraction. The fontanelle is examined to see if it is bulging, sunken or normal, and measured before incision. The incision may be parallel to the superior sagittal sinus or in an angle following the lines of the fontanelle. The incisions are then continued along the sutures. It is important to be careful when cutting along the superior sagittal sinus, trying not to disturb it. As the bones are carefully reflected, the bridging veins may be assessed. The incisions along the sutures should result in five bony structures (two frontal, two parietals, and one occipital bone) that are reflected to expose the brain, which is examined in situ for oedema, subdural, and subarachnoid haemorrhages or any focal lesions. If the brain is very fragile, extracting it in water should be considered as a suitable option. Once the brain is removed, the duramater, especially the falx, and the tentorium should be examined and sampled if there is intradural haemorrhage. The venous sinuses are inspected and the pituitary removed. The basal dura should be removed to look for possible fractures. The middle ears are exposed and examined for the presence of infection. If pus is observed, swabs are obtained. The spinal cord can be exposed from the anterior aspect by cutting along all the vertebral pedicles and transecting the lowermost lumbar intervertebral discs. In-situ examination may reveal the presence of haemorrhage at this point. The cord is divided at the distal end and carefully lifted off the canal by dissecting the dura along the entire length.

The cord can also be removed from the posterior aspect by extending the scalp incision distally and exposing the cord. This method allows the brain and spinal cord to be removed as one unit, but is rarely used. In older babies with closed fontanelle and stronger bones, the brain may be removed as in an adult but cutting the superior calotte. If necessary a swab of the brain may be obtained after the incisions and before removal of the brain. The brain should not be sampled fresh and some formalin fixation is required for proper examination. The brain is placed in 20% buffered formalin for at least four days and preferably seven. In some institutions the brain is fixed at 37°C. Frequent changes in formalin during this period will increase fixation. Two hours before sectioning, the brain is placed in water at 4°C to facilitate cutting. The brain is carefully examined externally before slicing coronally, with detailed written, and photographic documentation of any observation. The brainstem and cerebellum are separated from the cerebrum; samples from the cerebellar vermis and dentate nuclei and from the medulla, pons, and midbrain are obtained. The cerebrum is sliced at the level of the mammillary bodies and subsequently cut using L-shape guides. The slices are oriented on a board to better assess the ventricles and any focal lesions. It is useful to photograph the slices to compare with histology if necessary. The brain is sampled for histology from standard locations.[11] Standard samples from the frontal cortex to include the watershed area (obtained from the frontal slice at the level of the mammillary bodies), the basal ganglia, the hippocampi, and the calcarine cortex are obtained. In ex-premature babies it is important to sample the white matter around the lateral ventricles (Table 9.3)

Microscopical Examination

The samples as detailed in Table 9.1 are fixed in formalin and embedded in paraffin. The sections are routinely stained with haematoxylin and eosin. We recommend standard Perls and elastic Van Giesson (EVG) (or trichrome) in at least two lung samples (one from the right and one from the left lung), levels and EVG on the heart septum, and some liver stains (reticulin, EVG, PAS-D) on the liver samples. Other special stains can be requested as necessary. Brain sections may be stained with βAPP and GFAP. If there are specific lesions it is better to obtain the opinion of a neuropathologist, preferably one with experience in paediatric neuropathology.

There are no specific histological findings in SIDS. Petechiae and small haemorrhages may be seen in the thymus, lungs, along coronary arteries, renal interstitium, and other organs. The lungs frequently show some degree of oedema and alveolar macrophages. Minor laryngeal and peribronchial inflammation with expansion of the mucosa-associated lymphoid tissue (MALT) may be seen with non-lethal viral infections. The presence of bronchopneumonia or other significant inflammation will point to a different cause of death.

Ancillary Investigations (see Table 9.2)

Skin samples for fibroblast cultures are important for inborn errors of metabolism and in cases of undiagnosed dysmorphism. These may be obtained at the hospital where the baby is taken if there will be a delay in performing the autopsy.

Blood and swabs for microbiology should also be taken at the hospital if there is a delay. These can also be repeated at the autopsy.

Bacteriology: CSF, blood, urine, bowel content, swabs from nose, throat, lungs, and spleen. Any lesion;

Virology: CSF, nasopharyngeal swab, lungs, heart, bowel content;

Frozen tissue for lipid stains and eventual molecular studies: heart, liver, kidney and skeletal muscle (stored frozen at -80ºC). Recent discoveries in the role of the brainstem in SIDS have led some institutions to also preserve a frozen sample from the medulla oblongata;

Frozen tissue for DNA: spleen or muscle;

Biochemistry: blood, vitreous humour;

Metabolic studies: skin sample, Guthrie card (newborn screening card), urine;

Toxicology: blood, stomach contents, urine, liver, vitreous.

Clinico-pathological Summary

This should include a careful review of the clinical history and autopsy findings including the ancillary investigations. A cause of death may have been found at the post-mortem examination (see Chapter 35) and an explanation of how this happened will help the coroner and the parents understand how the baby died.

If there is no cause of death found but there is a history of co-sleeping with more than one adult, and/or prone, and/or with misuse of drugs/alcohol and/or the baby is found under the blankets or there are some findings that do not explain the death but are abnormal (such as an old healed fracture) most pathologists will use the term *'unascertained'* or *'undetermined'* as the cause of death. In the instance of a sudden infant death while co-sleeping with an adult without the above detailed associated circumstances, most paediatric pathologists prefer to use the term SIDS, adding in the comment that there was co-sleeping.

When the sudden death of an infant under one year of age remains unexplained after a thorough case investigation, including performance of a complete autopsy, examination of the death scene and review of the clinical history,[12] a diagnosis of SIDS is made. As in the past most of these deaths occurred while the baby was sleeping in the cot, the term of *'cot death'* is still used by some physicians.

References

1. Sethuraman C, Coombs R, Cohen MC. Sudden unexpected death in infancy (SUDI). In: Cohen MC, Scheimberg I, eds. *The Pediatric and Perinatal Autopsy Manual.* Cambridge University Press, 2014: 319–29.

2. Dorries C. *Coroners' Courts: A Guide to Law and Practice.* Oxford University Press, 2014.

3. Byard RW. Sudden Infant Death Syndrome. In: Byard, *Sudden Death in the Young.* Cambridge University Press, 2010; 555–630.

4. Cohen MC. Fetal, perinatal, and infant autopsies. In: Burton J, Rutty G, eds. *The Hospital Autopsy. A Manual of Fundamental Autopsy Practice.* London: Hodder Arnold, 2010:184–202.

5. Cohen MC, Molina P, Scheimberg I. Paediatric and perinatal post-mortem techniques. In: Delgado S, Bandrés F, eds. *Legal Medicine*, vol. **3**. Barcelona: Bosch, 2011: 642–57.

6. Cohen MC. Sudden Infant Death Syndrome: post-mortem investigation and risk factors. In: Jamieson A, Moenssens A, eds. *Wiley Encyclopaedia in Forensic Sciences*. Published online, 15 December 2011; https://onlinelibrary.wiley.com/doi/abs/10.1002/978047006 1589.fsa1058 (accessed 30 October 2018).

7. Sidebotham P, Fleming P. *Unexpected Death in Childhood; A Handbook for Practitioners*. Chichester: John Wiley & Sons, 2007:347.

8. *Sudden Unexpected Death in Infancy and Childhood: Multi-agency Guidelines for Care and Investigation*, 2nd edn, London: The Royal College of Pathologists, 2016.

9. Scheimberg I, Ashal H, Kotiloglu-Karaa E, et al. Weight charts of infants dying of sudden infant death in England. *PDP*, 2014; **204**(17):271–7.

10. Gilbert-Barness E, Debich-Spicer DE. Pediatric autopsy. In: Gilbert-Barness, Debich-Spicer, *Handbook of Pediatric Autopsy Pathology*. New Jersey: Humana Press, 2005:7–74.

11. Squier W, Encha-Razavi F. Central nervous system. In: Cohen MC, Scheimberg I, eds. *The Pediatric and Perinatal Autopsy Manual*. Cambridge University Press, 2014:173–204.

12. Willinger M, James LS, Catz C. Defining the Sudden Infant Death Syndrome (SIDS): deliberations of an expert panel convened by the National Institute of Child Health and Human Development. *Pediatr Pathol*, 1991; **11**:677–84.

Chapter 10

The Joint Forensic/Paediatric Post-mortem Examination

Alfredo E. Walker

The Post-mortem Examination

In the United Kingdom, the approach to the performance of the post-mortem examination in sudden unexpected death in infancy (SUDI) is guided by the publication *Sudden Unexpected Death in Infancy and Childhood: Multi-agency Guidelines for Care and Investigation,* which was developed through collaboration between the Royal College of Pathologists (RCPath) and the Royal College of Paediatrics and Child Health (RCPCH). The reporting committee was chaired by Baroness Helena Kennedy QC, and the publication is more commonly referred to as the Kennedy Report.[1] First published in 2004, a revised edition was published in November 2016. The approach to the post-mortem examination is detailed in Appendix 6 of that publication which lays out the guidelines to be followed as a *minimum* standard by specialist paediatric pathologists asked to perform these investigations singularly in criminally non-suspicious deaths.

In cases which are deemed to be either frankly homicidal or criminally suspicious from the onset, the post-mortem examination should be conducted by either a forensic pathologist with significant expertise in paediatric pathology or jointly between a forensic pathologist and a paediatric pathologist as a 'double doctor' exercise. The latter practice is unique to the United Kingdom, as in other developed countries the post-mortem examinations in homicidal and criminally suspicious deaths in infancy are performed only by qualified forensic pathologists without the direct involvement of a paediatric pathologist. This is exemplified in jurisdictions that operate a US medical examiner's type of death investigation system as well as in Canada and Australia. It is advisable that paediatric pathologists embarking on post-mortem examination in cases of SUDI/SUID should be able to recognise atypical or suspicious findings that will precipitate abandonment of their

examination as a routine autopsy so that a forensic pathologist can be called in to take over or take charge of the examination. As such, upgrading a case to involve a forensic pathologist is best achieved when a systematised and standardised approach to the initial examination is adopted.

The post-mortem examination process involves a multiplicity of sequential steps as follows:

A. Obtaining information on the circumstances of death
B. Obtaining information from the examination of the death scene
C. Consideration of procurement of trace evidence from the external aspect of the body
D. Pre-autopsy radiography of the body
E. External examination
F. Evisceration of the organs +/- special dissection
G. Dissection of the organs +/- consideration of retention of whole organs for specialist examination in special circumstances (heart for cardiac pathology; brain, spinal cord, or cervical spine and for neuropathology, eyes for ophthalmic pathology, rib(s)/rib segments and long bones for bone pathology +/- assessment of metabolic bone disease)
H. Procurement of tissues and biological samples for ancillary investigations (routine histology, vitreous biochemistry, metabolic studies, cytogenetics, DNA extraction, and storage for targeted genetic testing if indicated)

A. Obtaining Information on the Circumstances of Death

Information on the circumstances of death is obtained from a variety of sources that should include the police and coroner's investigative reports, details of the decedent's medical, birth, and gestational history, the agonal illness and a description of the final sleep and sleep environment (if applicable) (see Chapters 7 and 8). In some jurisdictions, a standardised infant death pro forma questionnaire is completed by the investigating coroner, police investigator or SUDI/SUID paediatrician, which is then provided to the pathologist. In the United Kingdom it is called the SUDI/SUID questionnaire and in the province of Ontario, Canada it is called the *Investigation Questionnaire for Sudden Unexpected Deaths in Infants (Less Than One Year of Age)* which replaced its forerunner (the Death Under the Age of Five Years Questionnaire) as of 1 January 2013.[2]

B. Obtaining Information from Examination of the Death Scene

Information on the scene examination findings, especially for deaths that appear to be associated with an unsafe sleeping environment is very important. Such information can be gathered as part of the completed standardised sudden-death questionnaire pro forma, but must be purposefully sought out by the pathologist from the investigating authorities in jurisdictions where such questionnaires are not used. Ideally, pathologists should conduct their own examination of the scene of death, with, or without doll re-enactments, but this is not always possible or practical for non-forensic pathologists for a variety of reasons, the most common of which being the removal of the body from its in-situ position to facilitate resuscitation when it is discovered unresponsive. However, images of the scene must always be reviewed in the appropriate circumstances to assess for unsafe sleeping environments.

The goal of the infant death scene re-enactment is to accurately depict and replicate the environments into which the infant was placed to sleep and subsequently discovered. The re-enactment visually documents the body, head, and neck positions, materials found near, or next to the body, if the infant's airway was obstructed when discovered (nose and mouth) and the obstructing objects. Most death investigators agree that attempting to reintroduce and reposition a decedent's body into a scene for photographic reasons would not be a wise decision but doll re-enactments do just that with surprisingly positive results for both the investigator conducting the re-enactment and the family member or caregiver performing it. It is critical that the re-enactment be performed by the individual who discovered the body, either unresponsive, or dead, to ensure correct documentation of the infant death scene. A scene re-enactment doll is used to place the infant in the last position she/he was put to sleep as well as to place the infant in the position she/he was found (see Chapter 14). These two positions must be photographically documented and described descriptively.[3]

C. Consideration of Procurement of Trace Evidence

According to the circumstances, the forensic pathologist should consider the procurement of biological trace evidence samples from the body as evidential exhibits. This must be considered in all criminally suspicious deaths, not only for forensic analytical purposes but also to establish a clear chain of custody for these exhibits, should their handling be questioned in the future.

D. Pre-autopsy Autopsy Radiography

All cases must undergo a full skeletal survey using plain radiography prior to evisceration of the body as part of the post-mortem examination SUDI/SUID protocol, and the X-rays should be reported by an experienced paediatric radiologist (see Chapter 14). This will primarily allow for the evaluation of the possible presence of acute or healing bony injuries (acute fractures of the skull, ribs, or long bones, classic metaphyseal lesions, healing fractures with radiologically evident periosteal reaction and/or callus formation of the ribs and long bones), the degree of bone mineralisation (metabolic bone disease such as rickets etc.), other bone fragility disorders (i.e. osteogenesis imperfecta) and congenital anomalies including skeletal dysplasia. Where available, full-body CT scans and MRI of the body should be employed in addition to plain full skeletal radiography to provide additional information (see Chapter 11).

Any bony lesion which has been radiologically flagged (diagnosed or queried) must be excised for fixation, further specimen radiology, decalcification, and histological examination. As stated in the standard post-mortem procedures in SIDS, a fragment of non-lesional, non-decalcified bone (usually a small segment of rib) should be retained in formalin for the assessment for metabolic bone disease, should this be subsequently indicated in the case (see Chapter 9).

E. External Examination

A meticulous external examination of the body must be conducted in all cases with detailed documentation of the findings. The external examination is best conducted in a systematic manner of the different anatomical regions from 'head to toe' so that no cutaneous findings are missed. It is imperative that the findings are documented in triplicate in the form of (i) diagrammatic representations on completed body diagram templates (ii) narrative descriptions, and (iii) digital colour photography.

Apart from the basic physical characteristics of the identifying features and growth parameters which are normally documented at post-mortem examination, the following specific findings should be actively sought for and documented (see Chapter 36):

a. The pattern of hypostasis and inherent regions of contact blanching (i.e.: anterior hypostasis with a blanched area of the central face that includes the peri-nasal and perioral regions)

b. Boggy swellings or depressed regions of the scalp on palpation.

c. The nature of the anterior fontanelle on palpation if unfused (tense or depressed)

d. Congestion/cyanosis of the face (Figure 10.1)

e. Petechiae of the facial skin, eyes (palpebral and bulbar conjunctivae) and orogingival mucosa (Figures 10.2a and 10.2b).

f. Lacerations of the labial frenulum (fresh or healing) (Figures 10.3a and 10.3b)

g. Bruises/abrasions/lacerations of the inside of the lips

h. Injuries of the cheek and ears

i. Injuries on the lower jaw, submental region, and neck

j. Cutaneous blunt force injuries (bruises, abrasions, lacerations, and combinations thereof)

k. Burn injury (cigarette burns, scalds, electrical burns)

l. Patterned injuries (bite marks, tramline bruises, other patterned bruises/abrasions, patterned burns)

m. Sharp force injuries (superficial incised wounds, stab wounds)

n. Otherwise unexplained injuries of the ears, neck, torso, genitalia, and buttocks

o. Injuries inconsistent in their nature and location with having been sustained in an accidental

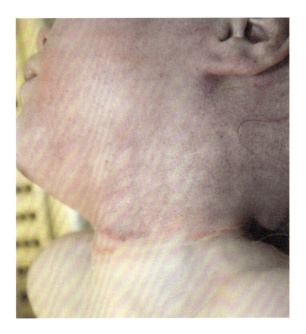

Figure 10.1 Congestion of the face and neck above a ligature mark

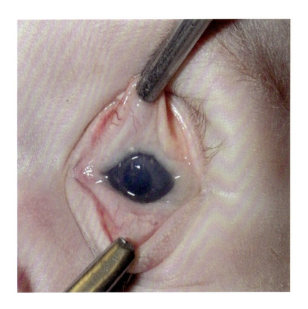

Figure 10.2a Assessment of the eyes for petechiae.

manner, considering the motor developmental stage of the child.

Caution is advised in the interpretation of apparent bruises and petechiae of the face, neck, and

57

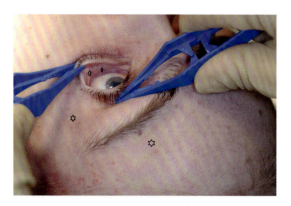

Figure 10.2b Assessment of the eyes for petechiae. Arrows point to the conjunctival petechiae and stars to the periorbital petechiae.

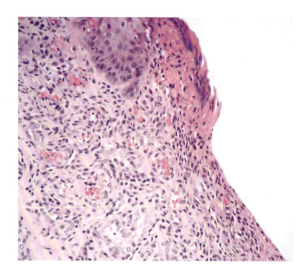

Figure10.3b Histology of healing laceration of the upper labial frenulum

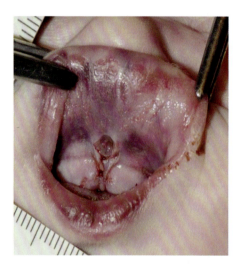

Figure 10.3a Healing laceration of the upper labial frenulum;

anterior chest when there is florid anterior hypostasis from the body having remained in the prone position for an extended period after death. Coarse hypostatic haemorrhages of the facial skin and anterior neck, and anterior cervical muscles may be post-mortem artefacts, which can be misinterpreted with disastrous medicolegal/judicial consequences.[4] Hypostatic haemorrhages of the palpebral and bulbar conjunctiva can also result and be misinterpreted for petechiae. Post-mortem hypostatic haemorrhages of the skin of the face, anterior neck, and eyes are only evident within the regions of skin that exhibit florid anterior hypostasis.

F-H. Evisceration and Special Dissections

To ensure that no subtle findings are missed, the evisceration of the body should either be performed by the forensic pathologist or paediatric pathologist or directly supervised by him/her if it is performed by an assistant. The standard cutaneous Y incision on the front of the torso can be used. Layered musculocutaneous dissection of the anterior torso to assess for subcutaneous bruising, and inspection of the anterior chest wall should be performed in all cases (Figure 10.4). The pectoralis muscles can be reflected off of the anterior chest wall. Any bruises detected on layered dissection can be sampled for histological examination from the internal aspect of the skin.

The chest and abdominal cavities can be opened in the standard manner. If the ribs are still cartilaginous, sharp scalpels can be used for incisional transection of their anterior aspects to facilitate removal of the anterior chest wall (Figure 10.5). The thoracic and abdominal organs are then inspected in situ prior to their removal and any abnormalities/injuries documented (Figure 10.6).

In order to assess the anterior cervical muscles for bruises and the larynx for injuries, in-situ layered dissection of the anterior neck structures to the level of the mandibular jaw line in a bloodless field, after removal of the brain and thoracic organs, is appropriate (Figures 10.7a and 10.7b). In cases of known or suspected compression of the neck, as well as in those cases

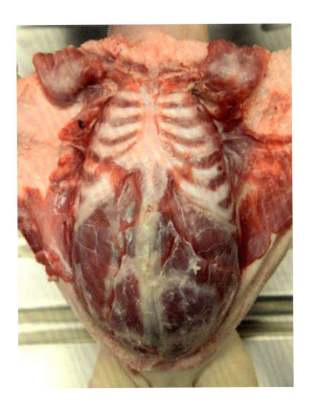

Figure 10.4 Musculocutaneous dissection of the anterior torso.

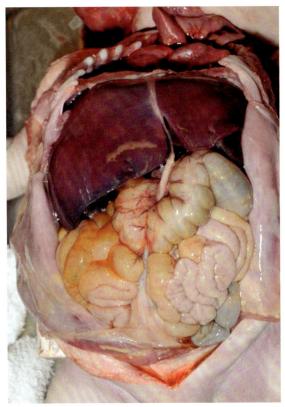

Figure 10.6 Opened chest and abdominal cavities.

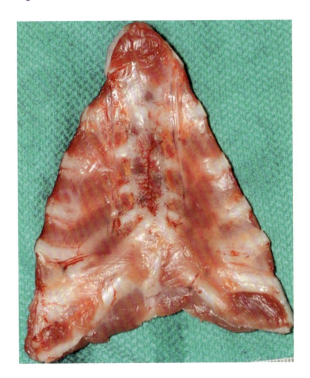

Figure 10.5 Excised anterior chest wall. Excision was facilitated through incisional transection through the still cartilaginous ribs.

in which both the cause and manner of death are undifferentiated, in-situ layered dissection of the anterior neck structures should be performed as a precaution.

Once the thoracic and abdominal organs are eviscerated, the thoracic, and abdominal cavities must be inspected in a bloodless state. The rib cage should be meticulously examined for evidence of healing or more recent rib fractures. An attempt must be made to correlate any findings on the skeletal survey report with abnormalities directly observed at post-mortem. Healing rib fractures will be apparent as nodular bony swelling above the background surface of the rib. Care must be taken not to miss/overlook paravertebral posterior rib fractures, which when bilateral and involve multiple sequential ribs, will be apparent as a vertical linear arrangement of nodular callosities along both sides of the vertebral column (Figure 10.8). The costo-chondral junctions of the ribs must also be specifically assessed for bulbous swellings and sampled for histological examination (Figures 10.9a and 10.9b). Haemorrhage of the

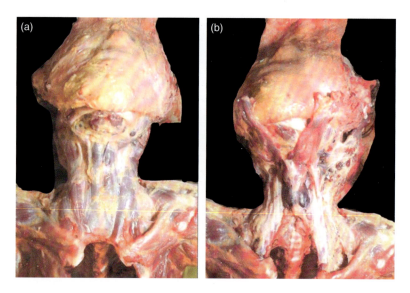

Figure 10.7a and b In-situ layered dissection of the anterior neck

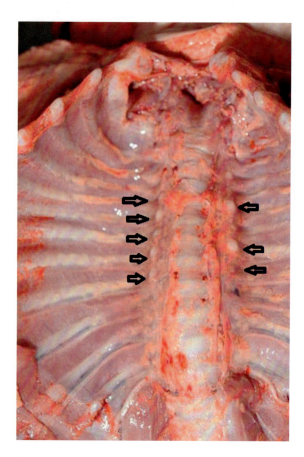

Figure 10.8 Appearance of the thoracic and abdominal cavities after removal of the thoracic, abdominal, and pelvic organs. Bilateral lines of fracture callus are evident on the posterior aspects of the ribs along the costovertebral junctions.

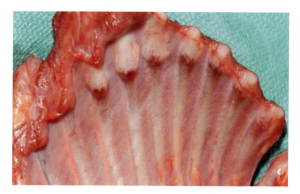

Figure 10.9a Bilateral bulbous swellings of the costochondral junctions of the ribs.

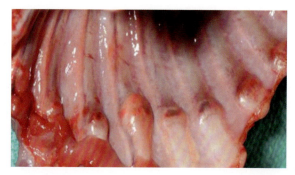

Figure 10.9b Bilateral bulbous swellings of the costochondral junctions of the ribs.

bulbous costochondral junctions may be a manifestation of recent fracture.

In certain situations, the following may need to be considered:

1. Layered dissection of the posterior torso and limbs (Figure 10.10) to permit assessment of subcutaneous and/or deeper bruising. Any bruises detected can be sampled for histological examination from the internal aspect.
2. Layered dissection of the posterior neck

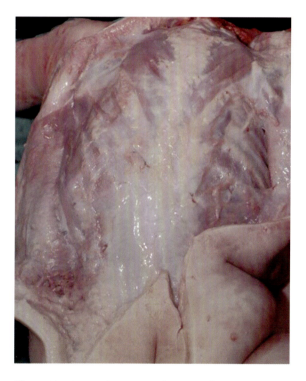

Figure 10.10 Musculocutaneous dissection of the posterior torso.

3. Removal of the eyes
4. Facial dissection
5. Excision of the cervical spine with the cervical segment of the spinal cord
6. Excision of the ano-genital organs (pelvic exenteration)

Removal of the Brain

The scalp can be incised in the traditional manner via an incision made across the mid-coronal plane of the crown that ends over the mastoid processes behind the ears and separates it into anterior and posterior segments. These two segments of the scalp are then reflected anteriorly and posteriorly respectively to expose the internal aspects of the scalp and the external aspect of the cranium which can then be inspected for bruising (subgaleal, intra-scalp and subperiosteal) and skull fractures, and documented accordingly. It may be necessary to strip away the periosteum from the outside of the skull to identify, fully appreciate, and document skull fractures (Figure 10.11 a–c).

Alternatively, the 'question mark' incision of the occipital scalp and back of the neck can be made to facilitate reflection of the scalp and exposure of the back of the cervical spine (see Chapter 9). The 'question mark' incision allows exposure of the posterior aspect of the cervical spine and musculature.

A sterile sample of cerebrospinal fluid (CSF) can be obtained by introducing a needle into the upper spinal canal through the membrane between C1 and C2 and aspirating into a sterile syringe. The sample can be divided and submitted for biochemical and microbiological analyses. This aspiration technique facilitates the early visualisation of blood within the subdural compartment. Another method is the

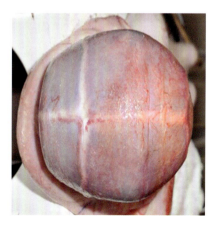

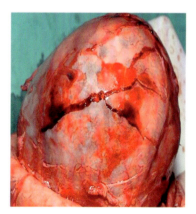

Figure 10.11 a) Normal crown view of the skull and internal aspect of the scalp on peeling back of the scalp; b) Y-shaped gaping fracture along the left frontotemporoparietal bone; c) linear fracture with gaping along the right parietooccipital bone on stripping away of the periosteum.

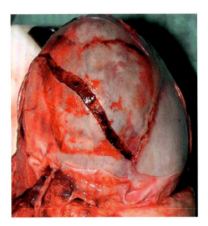

Figure 10.11 (cont.)

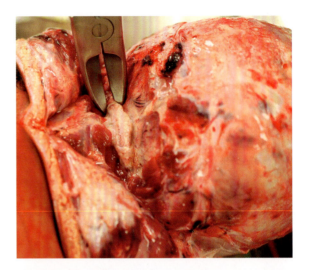

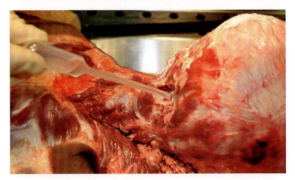

removal of the posterior segment of the atlas bone with bone cutters (Figure 10.12a), incision of the membrane, and aspiration of the CSF (Figure 10.12 b). This method also permits the identification of blood within the subdural space prior to opening of the skull (Figure 10.12c).

The technique used to open the skull differs depending on the age of the infant or child. In infants in whom the cranial sutures are not fused, the cranium can be opened by using a pair of scissors to cut through the fibrous suture lines, with backwards bending of the constituent skull bones to gain access to the cranial cavity. The final appearance of the opened skull bones using this method mimics the appearance of an opened flower with the brain being in the middle (Figure 10.13). In older infants and children in whom the sutures are fused, it will be necessary to use an oscillating electric saw to cut through the cranial vault in the conventional manner with manual removal of the skull cap to facilitate examination of the brain and the inside of the cranial cavity. After removing the skull cap, any epidural haemorrhage will be obvious. The dura mater is then incised around the periphery of the brain and reflected towards the midline so that the subdural space and surface of the brain can be examined and any findings documented. The identification of thin-film subdural haematoma (Figure 10.14) may indicate non-accidental head injury and should prompt the pathologist to consider examination of the optic nerves and removal of the eyes for opthalmic pathology assessment, and consideration of removal of the cervical spine for assessment, as recommended

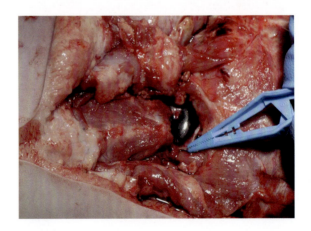

Figure 10.12 a) Excision of the posterior aspect of the atlas using bone cutters; b) using a sterile pipette to aspirate the subdural compartment clear cerebrospinal fluid has been obtained. c) Identification of blood within the subdural space of the cervical spine using the method described above.

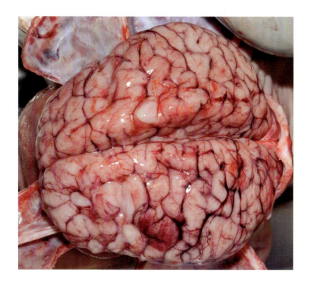

Figure 10.13 The skull is opened by cutting along its unfused fibrous sutures with backwards bending of its constituent bones to expose the brain.

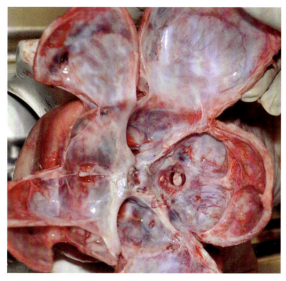

Figure 10.15 Opened skull (flower petals) appearance with in-situ dura mater.

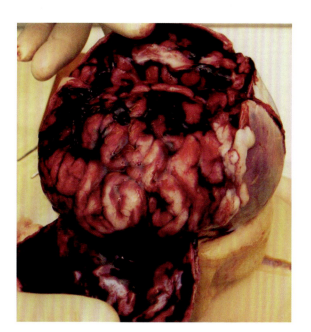

Figure 10.14 Patchy thin-film subdural haemorrhage in an infant.

by Matshes et al.[5] These considerations are especially indicated in the absence of external or internal evidence of blunt force impact injury to the face, scalp, and skull when violent shaking should be considered in the differential diagnosis.

Once the brain is removed from the cranial cavity, the base of the skull must be inspected before and after

the dura mater is stripped to permit the documentation of subdural haemorrhages and skull fractures (Figures 10.15). Pre-existent skull fractures are easily distinguised from post-mortem bending of the constituent bones.

Removal of the Spinal Cord

The spinal cord can be removed in its entirety by an anterior or a posterior approach. The posterior approach tends to be used when there are posterior rib fractures or other findings on the anterior aspect of the spine (i.e.: anterior cervical fracture) that need to be preserved for either second examination by another expert, or for histological sampling. Removal of the spinal cord by a posterior approach is easily achieved after subcutaneous dissection of the posterior aspect of the torso has been completed (Figure 10.16). Whether the anterior or posterior approaches are used, angled saw cuts through the rib arches into the spinal cavity will achieve the desired result of removing a narrow elongated window of bone to facilitate exposure of the spinal cord. The nerves can be divided along the entire length of the spinal cord and the cord can then be transversely divided in the upper cervical region at its proximal end and in the lumbrosacral region at its distal end, to facilitate removal. The excised spinal cord can then be inspected in the usual

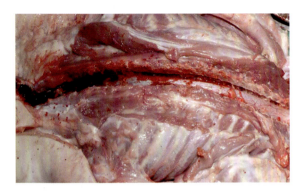

Figure 10.16 Appearance of the spinal cord within the spinal canal using the posterior approach. Clotted blood is evident in the extradural space in the lumbrosacral region (left side of the image).

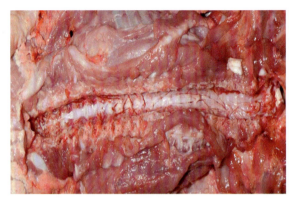

Figure 10.18 View on the spinal canal after the spinal cord had been removed (posterior approach).

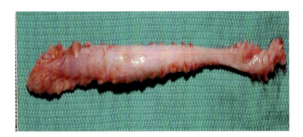

Figure 10.17 Excised spinal cord.

manner (Figure 10.17). Once the spinal cord has been removed, the internal aspect of the spinal canal can be inspected (Figure 10.18).

Facial Dissection

In some instances, a complete dissection of the soft tissues of the face away from the facial skeleton (facial dissection) may be indicated (Figure 10.19a and 10.19b). There are three reasons for the performance of a facial dissection:

First, it will allow for the identification, documentation, and histological sampling of the internal aspects of all facial bruises (subcutaneous component) which were evident on external examination of the body, without having to incise the skin itself, thereby preserving the cosmetic appearance of the face on reconstruction of the body. The histological examination of the bruise may assist in its histological dating but this is never accurate with respect to the actual age.[6]

Second, it will permit assessment of the facial skeleton so any bony injuries of the facial bones can be identified and documented.

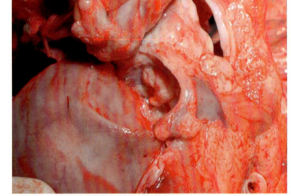

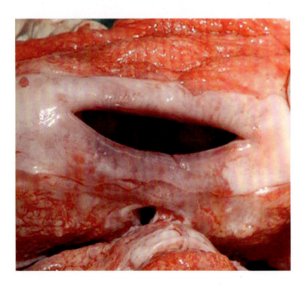

Figure 10.19 a) Facial dissection as seen from the right side of the face; b) view of the internal aspects of the lips after facial dissection.

Third, if indicated for other reasons, it will permit removal of the eyes with the optic nerves and periorbital fat at the end of the facial dissection, thereby removing the need to saw into the floor of the anterior cranial fossa (orbital roofs) as an alternative method of removal of the eyes.

The procedure to be followed for the performance of a facial dissection is well described and illustrated elsewhere[7] and involves the following sequential steps:

- Continuation of the standard rostral Y incision so that it joins the coronal scalp incision.
- Reflection of the skin of the neck to the jaw line.
- Incision of the oral mucosa.
- Continuation of the subcutaneous dissection of the facial tissues with transection of the external auditory meatii bilaterally.
- Reflection of the dissected skin towards the nose with extension of the dissection into the orbital cavities around the periorbital tissues with removal of the eyes from within the orbital cavities by transecting the optic nerves as far posteriorly as possible but keeping the eyes still attached to the facial skin by the conjunctivae.

Complete facial dissection will permit proper assessment of the internal aspects of the lips (Figure 10.19b) which may be useful in cases of suspected smothering.

Removal of the Eyes

In cases of clinically suspected non-accidental blunt force head injury (NAHI) with confirmed retinal haemorrhages on funduscopic examination, and for those cases in which thin-film subdural haemorrhages are detected as an unexpected finding during the post-mortem examination, it may be necessary to consider enucleation of the eyes with the optic nerves and periorbital tissues, for specialist examination specifically with respect to the identification, documentation and interpretation of optic nerve sheath and retinal haemorrhages (Figure 10.20). The significance of retinal haemorrhages is beyond the scope of this chapter; suffice to say that their identification and distribution may assist in the determination of the degree of energy transfer that the central nervous system had sustained.

There are three techniques that can be employed to remove the eyes: first, an external anterior approach (EAA), second, an internal anterior approach (IAA) and third, an internal posterior approach (IPA).

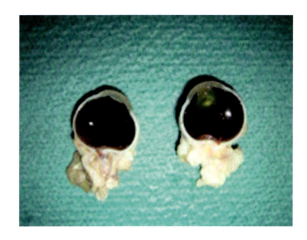

Figure 10.20 Excised right and left eyes with retinal haemorrhages.

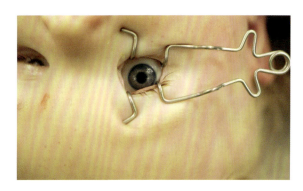

Figure 10.21 Use of a surgical eye retractor at autopsy to facilitate excision of the eye by the external anterior approach.

The EAA employs a surgical eye retractor and a pair of curved scissors that facilitates separation of the conjunctiva along the periphery of the globe through the junction of the bulbar and palpebral regions (Figure 10.21). The extra-ocular muscles and periorbital adipose tissues are then divided using the curved scissors held against the inside wall of the orbital cavity while applying gentle anterior traction of the globe to ensure that at least 1 cm of optic nerve remains attached to it before the optic nerve is cut as far posteriorly as possible.

When a facial dissection is performed for other reasons the IAA technique may be used. After cutting the optic nerve as part of the removal of the eye from the orbital cavity, but with it still attached to the facial skin by the conjunctiva, the conjunctiva is then incised around the periphery of the globe to release the eye from its attachment to the facial skin. Any haemorrhages of the periorbital tissues and optic nerve sheath can then be directly observed and documented.

The preferred method is the IPA, which involves removal of a window of the thin orbital roofs that constitutes the floor of the left and right anterior cranial fossae as depicted, to permit direct inspection and documentation of the periorbital tissues and optic nerve before removal of the eye by sectioning the optic nerve posteriorly as close to the optic chiasm as possible. This method can be routinely used (when removal of the eyes is indicated) after removal of the brain from the cranial cavity with documentation of the base of the skull and inside of the cranial vault (Figure 10.22).

Excision of the Cervical Spine

In 2011, Matshes et al. published their study on the investigation of thirty-five infants and young children.[5] They categorised the deaths into two broad groups: those cases with suspected hyperflexion/extension injuries of the neck (twelve cases) and those without such suspicion. They removed the entire cervical spinal column in each case (vertebrae, which contained spinal cord together with the neurovascular structures and adjacent soft tissues), decalcified them after formalin fixation, dissected them, and evaluated them microscopically. All the twelve cases with suspected or confirmed hyperflexion/extension injuries of the neck exhibited evidence of either bilateral or unilateral haemorrhage within or surrounding the C3-5 cervical spinal nerve roots. Based on this finding, they concluded that hyperflexion/extension forces experienced by the neck in shaken and impacted infants and young children is a more specific indicator of hyperflexion/extension injury than subdural haemorrhage alone and is also the mechanism of injury underlying the cause of the anoxic encephalopathy that occurs in this population as a result of injury to the cervical spinal nerve roots that innervate the diaphragm with subsequent apnoea. However, a baby that cannot use the diaphragm to breathe will use the intercostal muscles and will present with respiratory distress, therefore it is important to get a complete clinical picture before the collapse to interpret these post-mortem findings.[8] Since the publication of this paper, many practitioners (inclusive of this author) have resorted to removal and examination of the paediatric cervical spine as used in that

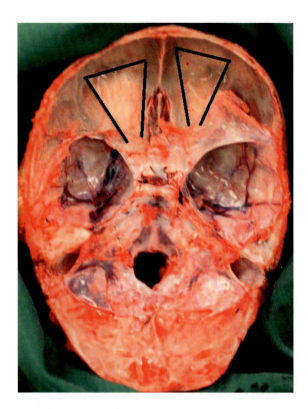

Figure 10.22 Image of the base of the skull with superimposed lines to indicate the linear saw cuts to be made over the anterior cranial fossa to facilitate removal of the eye by the internal posterior approach.

publication, which had been previously described by Vanezis for the post-mortem examination of the vertebral arteries in adults[9] and had been re-described more recently.[10] After removal of the brain and anterior cervical neck structures, the cervical spine is excised by making a square cut on the base of the skull around the foramen magnum and dissecting away the peri-cervical musculature anteriorly, laterally, and posteriorly. The excised cervical spine is then fixed in formalin for an adequate period of time before it is decalcified and serially sectioned for histological examination (Figures 10.23 a–d).

Removal of the Rib Cage

In cases with multiple, healing, rib fractures, excision of the entire rib cage or large sections of the rib cage may be indicated for further assessment. The excised rib cage (twelve pairs of ribs) or segments of rib cage can then be subjected to specimen radiography and fixation (prior to decalcification) so as to obtain better

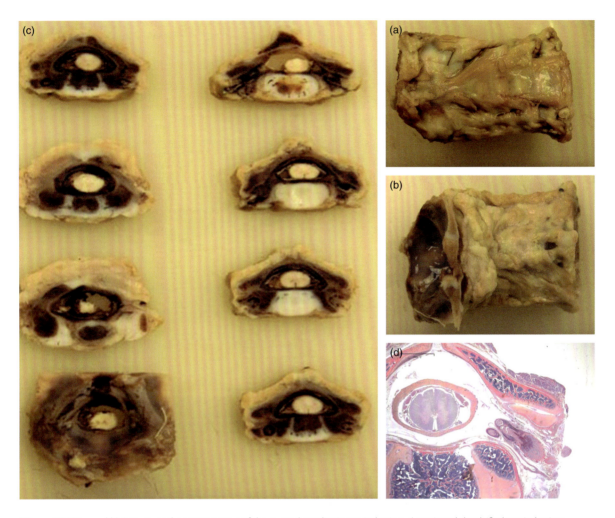

Figure 10.23 a and b) Anterior and posterior views of the excised paediatric cervical spine; c) sectioned decalcified cervical spine; d) histological section of cervical spine that depicts a crosssection of the the cervical spinal cord and one of its nerve roots.

radiographs with higher voltages that can impove on the radiological ageing of healing rib fractures, as there is less surrounding soft tissue to be penetrated. Specimen radiography can be obtained on the intact unit or on separated rib pairs and/or individual ribs.

Removal of the rib cage with minimal overlying soft tissue can be achieved by extending the subcutaneous dissection of the anterior torso laterally on both sides of the chest wall towards the midline of the back and dissecting the skin and subcutaneous fat away from the chest wall (Figure 10.24 a). The intervertebral discs of the C7/T1 and T12/L1 junctions can then be divided using a sharp scalpel to release the rib cage from above and below. This technique will permit the intact removal of posterior rib fractures, especially those located in the paravertebral and costovertebral regions. Alterations of this technique will allow the excision of rib-cage segments.

In cases with paravertebral/costovertebral rib fractures, in which removal of the spinal cord is also indicated for other reasons, the thoracolumbar segment of the spinal cord should be removed using the posterior approach (see removal of the spinal cord) so as to preserve the posterior costovertebral articulations for histological examination.

Once removed, the excised rib cage (or its separated rib pairs) are fixed in formalin and X-rayed again prior to decalcification and sampling for histological examination (Figure 10.24b, 25). The decalcified ribs can then be sectioned longitudinally for targeted histological sampling of fracture sites (Figure 10.26).

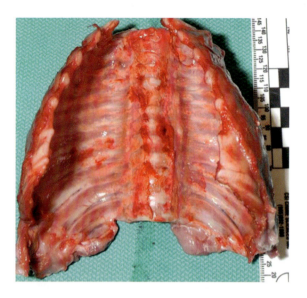

Figure 10.24 a) Removal of the rib cage

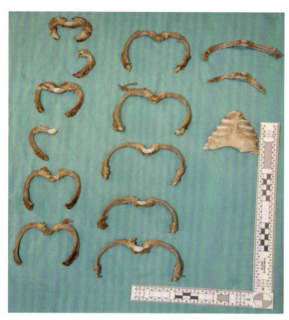

Figure 10.24 b) Individual examination of ribs.

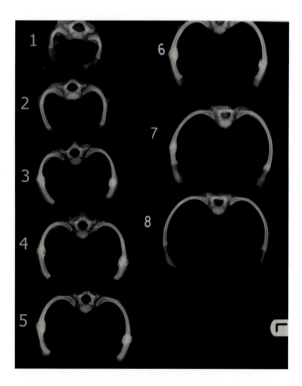

Figure 10.25 Specimen of the excised, numbered rib pairs that depict bilateral healing rib fractures of the lateral aspects of the 3rd, 4th, 5th, and 6th ribs, as well as the right 7th rib. The left-sided ribs are on the right side of the image.

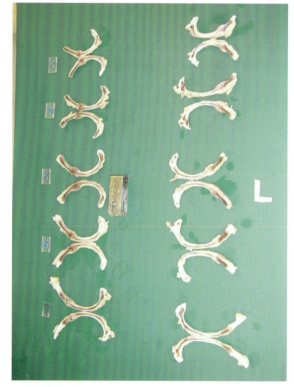

Figure 10.26 Longitudinal sections of decalcified ribs.

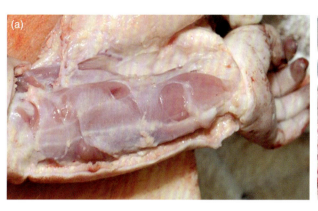
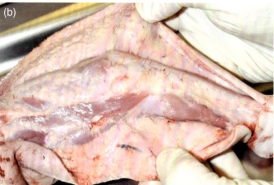

Figure 10.27 a) Rectangular skin flap incision of the left forearm to facilitate removal of the left radius and ulna; b) skin incisons of the medial aspects of the right and left lower limbs to facilitate removal of the femora, tibiae, and fibulae.

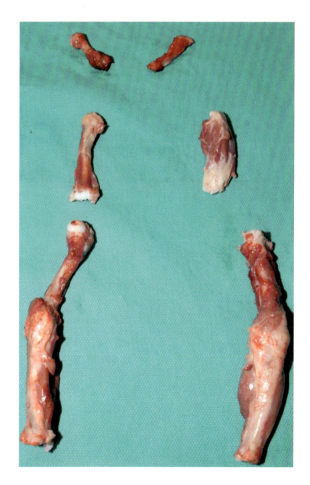

Figure 10.28 Excised individual long bones. Clockwise from top right: (i) left clavicle (ii) left radius and ulna (iii) left femur, tibia, and fibula in continuity (iv) right femur, tibia, and fibula in continuity (v) right humerus and (vi) right clavicle.

Removal of a Long Bone

When lesions of the long bones of the upper and lower limbs are detected or suspected radiologically, one or more of these bones should be excised for further examination. Irrespective of which long bone is to be excised, the principles of excision remain the same.

A longitudinal incision must be made along the medial aspect of the limb segment containing the bone to be excised, to facilitate the creation of a rectangular flap of skin and subcutaneous fat, which can be reflected laterally so as to expose the underlying long bone and its attached musculature (Figures 10.27a and b). The ends of the longitudinal incision must extend to the two joints between which the long bone articulates.The muscular attachments of the long bone being targeted must then be separated off; the long bone can then be isolated and removed from its anatomical position by releasing incisions made through its joint articulations. The excised long bone can be fixed in formalin, subjected to specimen radiography, decalcified, sampled, and examined histologically (Figure 10.28).

References

1. *Sudden Unexpected Death in Infancy and Childhood: Multi-agency Guidelines for Care and Investigation*, 2nd edn. London: The Royal College of Pathologists, 2016.

2. Office of the Chief Coroner for Ontario. *Paediatric Death Review Committee and Deaths Under Five Committee Annual Report*, 2013; www .mcscs.jus.gov.on.ca/sites/default/files/content/mcscs/d ocs/ec163306.pdf (accessed 30 October 2018).

3. Diebold K. Conducting the doll re-enactment in sudden unexplained infant death investigation. In: Centers for Disease Control and Prevention, *Sudden, Unexplained Infant Death Investigation*, 2007: 170–85. https://www.cdc.gov/sids/pdf/suidmanual/chapter7_tag508.pdf (accessed 30 October 2018).

4. Pollanen MS. Forensic pathology and the miscarriage of justice. *Forensic Sci Med Pathol*, 2012; **8**(3):285–9.

5. Matshes EW, Evans RM, Pinckard KJ, Joseph JT, Lew EO. Shaken infants die of neck trauma; not of brain trauma. *Acad For Path*, 2011; **1**(1):82–91.

6. Rossa CG, Langlois NEI, Heath K, Byard RW. Further evidence for a lack of reliability in the histologic ageing of bruises – an autopsy study. *Aust J Forensic Sci*, 2015; **47**(2):224–9,

7. Rutty GN, Burton JL. The evisceration. In: Burton J, Rutty G, eds. *The Hospital Autopsy: A Manual of Fundamental Autopsy Practice*, London: Hodder Arnold, 2010: 132–4,

8. Rouse C, Schmidt L, Brock L, Fagiana A. Congenital diaphragmatic hernia presenting in a 7-day-old infant. *Case Rep Emerg Med*, 2017 Article ID 9175710; https://www.hindawi.com/journals/criem/2017/9175710/ (accessed 30 October 2018).

9. Vanezis P. Techniques used in evaluation of vertebral artery trauma at postmortem. *Forensic Sci Int*, 1979; **13**: 159–65.

10. Matshes E, Joseph J. Pathological evaluation of the cervical spine following neurosurgical or chiropractic interventions. *J Forensic Sci*, 2010.**57**(1):113–19.

Minimally Invasive Autopsy

Elspeth Whitby, Ashok Raghavan, and Amaka Offiah

Minimally invasive autopsy is the 'new kid on the block' that has been researched and developed due to a decline in acceptance of the formal autopsy in cases where there has been parental choice. The decline is multifactorial but was initially blamed on the organs retention scandal that hit the UK in the 1990s. However, there has been an international decline in post-mortems, and parental views expressed through the media, social media, and social networking has contributed to this. There are numerous research proposals to obtain more data for the use of imaging as an alternative.[1]

Initial work in the UK centred on religious communities where speed of burial meant little or no time for the autopsy, and imaging was used to replace the formal autopsy.[2] This has expanded in the adult community with the establishment of facilities offering the service to anyone who can afford to access it. However, imaging alone lacks essential information that cannot be obtained without formal autopsy. Indeed, the autopsy process consists of far more than the dissection of the body. By replacing the dissection with imaging, while retaining the rest of the process, we arrive at the 'minimally invasive autopsy'. The additional components are an essential part of the process and vary depending on the circumstances. Additional investigations include a full external viewing, toxicology, genetic analysis, infection screens and (if consent is obtained) biopsy of any areas of concern.[3]

In our practice, to ensure the maximum amount of information is recorded in all cases, we use trained staff to obtain consent for the autopsy in a stepwise manner. The formal autopsy and its benefits are discussed first, and only if necessary do the staff suggest a limited autopsy and finally a full, minimally invasive autopsy. Ideally it would be beneficial to include biopsy of any abnormal area imaged and this can be performed under image guidance if required. In our institution, the service provision for minimally invasive autopsy is only available for fetal and neonatal cases.

Cases of Sudden Unexpected Death in Infancy (SUDI) are referred to HM Coroner (England, Wales and Northern Ireland) or the Procurator Fiscal (Scotland), who decide on the necessary investigations. Coroners may differ in their approach, depending on their experience, and on the local availability of the different investigative alternatives.

Information should be given to the parents about the medical aspects of the process, but also details on who looks after their baby when the parents are not there. Recent studies have shown that parents wish to know that their baby is cared for, dressed, and placed in a Moses basket, and is handled in the same way as a live newborn, with the same degree of care and attention, in a safe and secure environment.[4] These details provide them reassurance that the health professionals care and understand their stress and needs. As the minimally invasive autopsy service has evolved and research into imaging as an alternative to autopsy has expanded, it has become accepted by parents and professionals as a suitable form of investigation to try to establish a cause of death.[5]

Post-Mortem Radiography

Conventional radiography is the oldest radiological imaging method used in forensic medicine. Immediately after their discovery by Wilhelm Conrad Röntgen in 1895, X-rays were employed in post-mortem investigations, especially in anthropology. In this technique, the body is investigated via direct exposure to X-rays. Contrast is determined by the absorption properties of body structures, bone is associated with high absorption and soft tissues display less attenuation. Radiography is advantageous, as it is simple to perform, rapid, and cost-efficient.

Post-mortem radiographic protocols in neonates include depiction of both the axial and appendicular

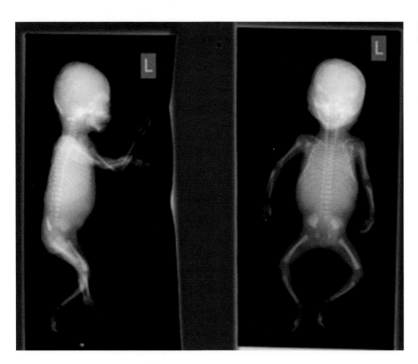

Figure 11.1 Lateral and AP radiographs of the whole skeleton of a fetus

skeleton. Two exposures are performed; one in the AP plane with the baby positioned as straight as possible, and the other in the lateral plane (Figure 11.1). It may be necessary to obtain separate views of the extremities. In infants and older children, however, particularly in the context of SUDI/SUID (when it is important to exclude fractures that might implicate inflicted injury as a cause of death), post-mortem radiographic imaging must be performed in the same way as an ante-mortem skeletal survey for suspected infant abuse, i.e. with separate projections of all anatomical sites and in accordance with national guidelines, such as those set out by the Royal College of Radiologists (RCR)/Royal College of Paediatrics and Child Health (RCPCH).[6] Because there are no radiation dose concerns for post-mortem radiography, image quality can be optimised for maximum spatial and contrast resolution.[7] All cases of SUDI/SUID should have post-mortem radiography performed as routine.

Post-Mortem Computed Tomography (PMCT)

Although PMCT is said to have almost complete concordance with autopsy for identifying cause of death in adults,[8,9] its role in children is more limited, due to the reduced inherent contrast in children (particularly in neonates and infants, compounded by their small size) compared to adults. As for post-mortem radiographs, there are no radiation dose concerns and therefore whole-body axial scans at 0.625 mm slice thickness can be performed, with subsequent coronal and sagittal reformats on soft tissue and bony windows, including 3D reconstruction (Figure 11.2).

PMCT is particularly beneficial for imaging the skeleton and excluding subtle rib and metaphyseal fractures. For this reason, PMCT is currently reserved for those cases where radiography shows equivocal skeletal abnormality, with post-mortem magnetic resonance imaging being the modality of choice in those infants for whom parental consent for autopsy has been withheld. PMCT is superior to PMMRI in infants only for imaging the bony skeleton and for detecting subtle calcification within organs.

Post-Mortem Magnetic Resonance Imaging (PMMRI)

This can provide structural details but not function. It provides good tissue definition (Fig. 11.3) and has been shown to detect as much, if not more than formal dissection for almost all body organs. The largest UK-based study in this age group was not specific for SIDS but included all causes of death across a large age range with over 90% concordance between minimally invasive techniques and formal autopsy in the fetal and stillbirth groups and over 75% concordance in the childhood group.[10–12] Very few of those included in the study were of the age group of SIDS cases and there were no age-based subgroup details, so it is difficult to ascertain the value of the PMMR in SIDS. In addition, the study used scans that took over two hours to complete and were interpreted by several different radiologists, making it an expensive way to perform MRI. Others have demonstrated that a clinical service can be provided by a small group of trained radiologists and that individual infants can be imaged in under forty-five minutes.[3] Their results demonstrate a high level of determination of the cause of death, but again this is in a diverse population, not just cases of SIDS.

To conclude: currently in those countries where consent for autopsy is required, if withheld, then radiography and PMMRI are the first-line radiological investigations of choice in cases of SIDS, with PMCT being an adjunct when there are equivocal skeletal abnormalities. As experience increases, PMCT may gradually replace radiographs, but in cases of SIDS, PMMRI is likely to play a key role in this investigation.

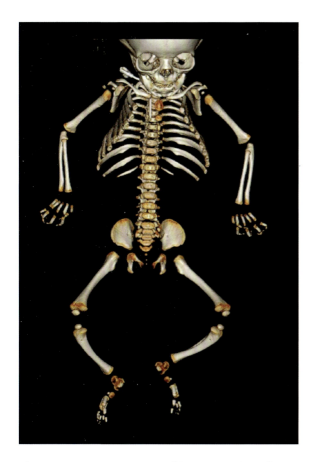

Figure 11.2 3D CT reconstruction of the normal skeleton of a male infant presenting with SUDI

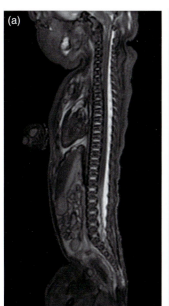

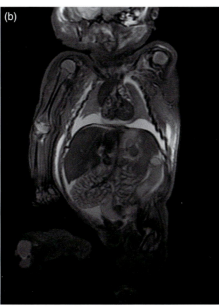

Figure 11.3 T2-weighted image of a structurally normal term baby
a. Sagittal section, note the pericardial effusion.
b. Coronal section, note the pleural effusions.

References

1. Ruegger CM, Bartsch C, Martinez RM et al. Minimally invasive, imaging guided virtual autopsy compared to conventional autopsy in foetal, newborn and infant cases: study protocol for the paediatric virtual autopsy trial. *BMC Pediatr*, 2014; **14**:15.

2. Roberts IS, Benbow EW, Bisset R, Jenkins JP, Lee SH, Reid H, Jackson A. Accuracy of magnetic resonance imaging in determining cause of sudden death in adults: comparison with conventional autopsy. *Histopathol*, 2003; **42**:424–30.

3. Whitby EH, Offiah AC, Cohen MC. Initial experience of a minimally invasive autopsy service. A report of the techniques and observations in the first 11 cases. *Pediatr Dev Pathol*, 2015; **18**:24–9.

4. Personal communication: K Reed and J Ellis, Faculty of Social Sciences, University of Sheffield, May 2017.

5. Kang X, Cos T, Guizani M, Cannie MM, Segers V, Jani JC. Parental acceptance of minimally invasive fetal and neonatal autopsy compared with conventional autopsy. *Prenat Diagn*, 2014; **34**:1106–10.

6. *Standards for Radiological Investigations of Suspected Non-Accidental Injury*. London: RCR/RCPCH, 2008; https://www.rcr.ac.uk/publication/standards-radiological-investigations-suspected-non-accidental-injury (accessed 31 October 2018).

7. Calder AD, Offiah AC. Fetal radiography for suspected skeletal dysplasia: technique, normal appearances, diagnostic approach. *Pediatr Radiol*, 2015; **45**:536–48.

8. Le Blanc-Louvry I, Thureau S, Duval C et al. Post-mortem computed tomography compared to forensic autopsy findings: a French experience. *Eur Radiol*, 2013; **23**:1829–35.

9. Roberts IS, Benamore RE, Benbow EW et al. Post-mortem imaging as an alternative to autopsy in the diagnosis of adult deaths: a validation study. *Lancet*, 2012; **379**:136–42.

10. Thayyil S, Sebire NJ, Chitty LS et al. Post-mortem MRI versus conventional autopsy in fetuses and children: a prospective validation study. *Lancet*, 2013; **382**:1980.

11. Shruthi M, Gupta N, Jana M et al. Comparative study of conventional and virtual autopsy using postmortem MRI in the phenotypic characterization of stillbirths and malformed foetuses. *Ultrasound Obstet Gynecol*, 2017; **51**(2): 236–45.

12. Vullo A, Panebianco V, Cannavale G et al. Post-mortem magnetic resonance foetal imaging: a study of morphological correlation with conventional autopsy and histopathological findings. *Radiol Med*, 2016; **121**: 847–56.

Chapter 12

Child Death Review: an Effective Approach for the Surveillance of Sudden and Unexplained Infant Deaths in the US

Theresa M. Covington

The Child Death Review Process

Multidisciplinary case reviews of infant deaths are an effective method to improve the surveillance of sudden and unexplained infant deaths (SUID, also known as Sudden Unexpected Death in Infancy, or SUDI) through improved identification, investigation, and classification. These reviews, known generally as child death reviews (CDRs) are also effective in catalysing local, state, and national action for improvements in agency systems of care and for risk-reduction and prevention actions. There are numerous interchangeable terms used to describe these reviews. These include CDR, child fatality review (CFR), infant and child death review (ICDR), child mortality review (CMR) and others. CDR is used throughout this chapter as representative of the different nomenclatures.

Originally developed in the early 1990s to improve the identification of, and children's justice response to, fatal child maltreatment, the CDR process has evolved into a public health model of child fatality and injury prevention.[1,2] In 1992 the United States Maternal and Child Health Bureau convened an ad hoc advisory group on CDRs. They acknowledged the important role of CDRs in addressing child abuse, but included a major departure from the norm: 'The primary purpose of the total (CDR) system should be prevention ... and state and local review teams should seek to implement the most expansive and comprehensive approach for identifying cases for review. Every fatality, birth to age 19, should be eligible for consideration at some level'.[3] A number of other countries were building CDR systems at the same time as the US. Comprehensive CDR systems are now in place throughout the United States, the United Kingdom, Canada, Australia, and New Zealand.[4] A number of other countries have more limited programmes and/or are developing expanded models.[5] In addition to reviewing child fatalities

related to maltreatment, many CDR teams throughout the United States review most SUDI/SUIDs, most fatal injuries, and many include reviews of natural infant deaths. The US also has a system of fetal and infant mortality review (FIMR). FIMR is similar to CDR but with significant differences: cases are de-identified, the purpose focuses on improving infant *and* maternal systems of care, and FIMR data is not typically aggregated and available for surveillance purposes. This chapter primarily focuses on CDR and the impact of CDR in the US on SUDI/SUID surveillance, risk-factor reduction, and prevention.

The US now has CDR programmes in all fifty states, the District of Columbia, and Guam. Reviews are also being conducted on military installations and in some American Indian nations. An annual report on the status of CDR finds that there are variations in the structure and process of CDR across states, yet in 2016 most states (37) utilised a model of local review teams with state advisory boards, and 12 states conducted only state-level reviews.[6] There are approximately 1,300 local CDR teams and 260 local FIMR teams in the US. The CDR process varies by state, even though most follow a similar model. State laws mandate or enable CDR in 44 states, including laws requiring local reviews in 34 states. State laws may mandate the type of process, membership, the types of deaths to be reviewed, and require an annual state report. Figure 12.1 describes the typical case review programme process.

Regardless of the programme structure, CDR is a process that supports an engaged, multidisciplinary community, telling a child's story, one child at a time, to understand the causal pathway that leads to a child's death and to identify pre-existing vulnerabilities and circumstances – in order to identify how to interrupt the pathway for other children. CDR generates a broad spectrum of data for an ecological understanding of the individual, community, and societal factors that interact at different levels to influence child health and safety. CDR leads to action to

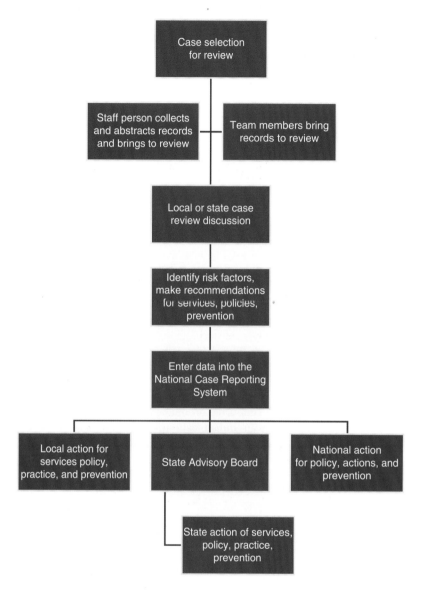

Figure 12.1 Steps in the case review process

improve systems and prevent deaths. Box 12.1 lists the primary objectives most common to the CDR process.

Most states review almost all of their SUDI/SUIDs. They also review a majority of their unintentional injuries, homicides, suicides, and death by child abuse and neglect of children ages 0–18. The US Department of Health and Human Services has a Healthy People (HP) 2020 objective specific to CDR and SUDI/SUID case reviews. HP 2020 objectives establish benchmarks and goals to improve the nation's health. HP 2020 objective *Injury and Violence*

Prevention 5.0 is to increase the number of states and the District of Columbia where 90% of SUDI/SUIDs are reviewed by a child fatality review team[7]. Thirty states met this standard in 2011 and twenty-five of those reviewed 100% of these deaths. Teams reviewed 69% of all US SUDI/SUID deaths in 2007, the benchmark year for measuring progress on this objective.[8]

Persons participating on a CDR team can be mandatorily assigned by legislation or policy, have jurisdictional responsibility to respond to child fatalities,

BOX 12.1 The objectives of child death review (CDR)

The objectives of CDR are to improve:

1. The accurate identification and uniform, consistent reporting of the cause and manner of every child death.
2. Communication and linkages among local and state agencies and enhance coordination of efforts.
3. Agency responses in the investigation of child deaths.
4. Agency response to protect siblings and other children in the homes of deceased children.
5. Delivery of services to children, families, providers, and community members.
6. Identification of specific barriers and system issues involved in the deaths of children.
7. Identification of significant risk factors and trends in child deaths.
8. Identification and action for changes in legislation, policy, and practices and expanded efforts in child health and safety to prevent child deaths.
9. Public awareness and advocacy for the issues that affect the health and safety of children.

or through a local identification process have the ability to obtain support for suggested recommendations. Team members are made up of professionals that are involved in the lives of children. Examples of team members participating on SUDI/SUID case reviews may include representatives from (but are not limited to): law enforcement, child protection services, attorneys, physicians, nurses, medical examiners, public health, emergency medical services, bereavement specialists, SUDI/SUID prevention specialists, political officials, educators, mental health professionals, maternal, and child health experts, home visitors, prevention partners, child-care licensing facilities, juvenile justice, housing authority, domestic violence experts, representatives of a particular culture within the community, and child abuse prevention. Teams can vary in size, depending on their jurisdiction, and population.

Information discussed in the review focuses on reports shared by agencies that responded to the child death. Information typically shared at a SUDI/SUID review includes:

- Autopsy reports
- Scene investigation reports and photos
- Interviews with family members
- Child-care licensing investigative reports
- Emergency medical services (EMS) run reports
- A&E department reports
- Prior child protection services and criminal background histories on child, caregivers, and supervisors
- Maternal and child health histories

BOX 12.2 Steps in the case discussion

1. Present case information: sharing the story of the child's life and circumstances of the death.
2. Discuss findings related to the investigation, services, agency systems.
3. Make recommendations to improve investigation, services, and systems.
4. Identify significant risk factors.
5. Discuss what is already happening to address risk factors.
6. Decide on what can be done to change behaviour, the environment, products policy, or laws?
7. Select the best recommendation(s) for action.
8. Decide on next steps and ensure persons/agencies take the lead to follow through.

- Criminal background checks on person supervising child at time of death
- Reports of home visits from public health or other services
- Any information on prior deaths of children in family
- Any information on prior reports that child had difficulty breathing
- Downloaded information from apnoea monitors, if applicable
- Information on product safety for materials found in sleep environment

A typical case review discussion includes a number of steps, see Box 12.2.

Although there is no national mandate in the US for SUDI/SUID case reviews, the National Center for Fatality Review and Prevention (NCFRP) is a federally funded resource centre that supports state and local CDRs and FIMRs in establishing and maintaining effective review systems. NCFRP has numerous resources available on CDRs, including a national programme manual, a guide to effective SUDI/SUID reviews, and the National CDR Case Reporting System. These are all available at www.childdeathreview.org.

The Role of CDR in Improving Outcomes

CDR can be effective in improving infant death investigations, services for families, and community members, agency policies, and practices in identifying risk and protective factors in SUDI/SUID deaths and ultimately and most importantly, in preventing deaths.

Improving the Investigation

Obtaining high quality and comprehensive information on SUDI/SUID deaths for surveillance purposes relies on information compiled from death investigations. The investigations include the autopsy, scene investigation, review of all pertinent records and histories, ancillary investigations (e.g. by day-care licensing or child protection services) and interviews. CDR has been found to improve the quality of investigations. Complete information on the investigation of a child's death is routinely shared at CDR meetings. When information is lacking or it is evident that investigations were incomplete or poorly conducted, reviews often lead to improvements. Key questions asked at a review related to improving investigations include:

1. Who is the lead agency?
2. Were the investigations coordinated?
3. Was there an autopsy? Was it comprehensive?
4. Was there a scene investigation?
5. Was there a scene recreation with photos?
6. Were there other investigations?
7. Was the family provided with information on bereavement services?
8. What were the key findings?
9. Was the investigation adequate?
10. Is the investigation complete?
11. What more do we need to know?
12. What can be done to help our investigators and the system?

The Scripps Howard News Service conducted an extensive study of SUDI/SUID and death investigation systems in 2007. The investigators reported that CDRs often led to investigation improvements. In an interview with a CDR state board team member in Mississippi they reported: 'What we have found in the child death review process is really troubling . . . About 85% of the time, information on each case is incomplete. By law, everyone is supposed to fill out a death scene investigation, especially in cases of sudden infant death. They just aren't doing it at all or they are doing it improperly.' Mississippi went on to adopt more rigorous guidelines for investigating and reporting SUDI/SUIDS deaths.[9] Anecdotally, numerous CDR teams report to NCFRP that their reviews led to significant improvements in the quality of death investigations, especially ensuring that SUDI/SUID deaths are referred to medical examiners or coroners instead of being certified by hospital physicians, that autopsies are conducted in all SUDI/SUID deaths, the place of death is considered the scene and an investigation is conducted there, doll re-enactments are conducted to help identify sleep-environment risk factors, and in improving investigator interactions with parents and caregivers to facilitate provision of bereavement services and healing. Numerous teams also report that their reviews led to local and state training for death investigators.

Improving the Diagnosis

It is widely believed that the influence of the CDR is in part responsible for the diagnostic shift from SIDS to undetermined or suffocation cause-of-death determinations.[10] The Scripps Howard study found that the more extensive the use of CDR is in a state, the more likely the cause of death in a SUDI/SUID will be other than SIDS. For example, they found that one in every six infant deaths were coded as suffocation in states with both local and state CDR compared with one in thirteen in states with only state reviews or no review programmes.[9] Quoting again from a Mississippi review board member, they report that in Mississippi, following the introduction of CDR, the state CDR team found that: 'about 20 percent of the SIDS deaths are not SIDS but suffocations and rollovers'.

Improving Services for Families and Agency Policies and Practices

CDR can be effective in improving services for families and community members, and agency policies, and practices and ultimately preventing deaths. Many CDR teams have ensured that referrals for services for SUDI/SUID families are made or that new services are put in place especially in the area of bereavement support. The multidisciplinary nature of CDR ensures that discussions related to different actions taken by agencies are often discussed and that improvements to policies and practices are recommended. One study in the State of Michigan found that the CDRs of maltreatment deaths led to a 35% decline in poor agency practices and a 9% decline in deaths associated with those practices. The study reported that the reviews were effective because the CDR process i) utilised a systematic process in the review discussions; ii) focused on identifying agency systems issues (findings); iii) developed specific recommendations to address those findings; and iv) assisted state agencies in implementing the recommendations.[11] The following set of discussion questions can help a team be effective in improving services and agency policies and practices:

Improving Services

1. Were there any services that the family was accessing prior to the death?
2. Were services provided to family members, other children, witnesses, first responders, or others as a result of the death?
3. Are there additional services that should be provided to anyone?
4. Who will take the lead in following up on these service provisions?
5. Does the team have suggestions to improve our service delivery systems?

Improving Agency Policies and Practices

1. Did agencies follow acceptable practice/policies in meeting the needs of the child and family before, at the time of, and after death?
2. Are there gaps in delivery of services to family and/or child?
3. Are there specific agency policies or practices that should be changed, improved on, implemented?
4. How can we best notify the agencies about our recommendations?

Examples of the way CDR has improved services, policies and practices include:

- Community mental health agency developing bereavement support programme.
- County EMS and police department requiring post-traumatic syndrome services for all first responders to a child death.
- County establishing a co-residential treatment programme for substance-using pregnant women that includes housing and support for their children.
- CDR data in one county leading directly to appointment by board of supervisors of Blue Ribbon Commission to examine racial disparity in SUDI/SUIDs.
- County moving from a coroner to a medical examiner system to improve quality of autopsies and other death investigation procedures.
- State child agency creating medical advisory committee to provide consultation to emergency departments across the state.
- State creating inter-agency task force to create risk assessment tools so providers can better identify and provide services to pregnant women with substance abuse problems.
- State requiring that all home visiting programmes through social services and public health include an assessment of infant sleep environments for families with infants.
- County conducting assessment and overhaul of EMS services after identifying delays in arrival times and transport.

Acting to Reduce Risk Factors and Prevent SUDI/SUIDs

The process of moving from a case discussion on a SUDI/SUID death to the identification of risk factors and actions that can be taken to reduce these risk factors is the most important task of CDR, and without which the CDR discussion becomes meaningless. Because CDR brings together multiple agencies and their case information, it allows the opportunity to systemically identify, report, and act to reduce significant SUDI/SUID risk factors. These factors include those intrinsic to the mother and baby; and behavioural, socio-economic, environmental, and product-safety factors known to be associated with SUDI/SUID.[12] Regardless of the diagnosis, e.g. SIDS, suffocation, or undetermined, a CDR team is able to describe the possible risk and protective factors in a SUDI/SUID death. Once identified, teams are able to identify specific actions that can be taken to reduce risks or strengthen protective factors. In their reviews of 15,657 SUDI/SUID deaths in 33 states, CDR teams reported that they recommended, were planning, or had implemented over 10,000 initiatives to reduce the risks of, or to prevent, SUDI/SUIDs between 2004 and 2016. These included parent education, media campaigns, provider education, and community or state safety projects.[13] Examples of these include:

- Provider training and education
- Home visiting
- Parent training and education
- Hospital-based safe-sleep education
- Community education
- Provision of safe cribs
- Child-care provider training and education
- Prenatal drug and alcohol treatment services
- Prenatal smoking cessation

Improving the Reporting of SUDI/SUID

One of the challenges of SUDI/SUID reporting and surveillance is the inconsistency of investigation and death certification, and the limited information available through death certificates to understand the circumstances in SUDI/SUID events. As has been extensively reported, the same set of circumstances in a SUDI/SUID event may be recorded as a SIDS, suffocation, undetermined, other natural, or even homicide. This is often dependent on the place of certification. Variations are found not only across states but within states, and even at times within the same medical examiner or coroner offices.[10,14-16] CDR affords a unique opportunity to enhance the limited information available in public health vital records surveillance systems.[14,16] Because CDR teams typically collect, discuss, and report on comprehensive SUDI/SUID information related to the infants, their caregivers, the investigations, the death event circumstances, agency factors, services, and risk factors, the findings from CDR can improve understanding of the medical, behavioural, and environmental risk factors in SUDI/SUID cases and help distinguish SUDI/SUID causes of deaths based on the quality of death investigations and other information provided at a case review.

The US National Child Death Review Case Reporting System

In 2005, the NCFRP created the National Child Death Review Case Reporting System (**CDR-CRS**).

This web-based reporting system is designed to allow review teams to input comprehensive data from their reviews into a database that allows for local team, state, and national-level analysis. The system is web-based, free to users, a confidential data entry platform, allows for local, state and national analysis, and is routinely updated with new or revised variables. By the end of 2016, 45 states were enrolled in the system with over 2,000 data enterers from local and state teams. Almost 200,000 reviewed deaths were in the database, including over 15,000 SUDI/SUID deaths from 33 states. Although the system is a rich source of data, there are limitations for its usefulness described in detail in a special supplement of the journal *Injury Prevention*, including:[17]

- Except in a few states that review 100% of all SUDI/SUIDs, there is no population data, and rates cannot usually be calculated using the data unless a state or jurisdiction is reviewing 100% of all deaths. Estimates can however be generalised in some cases.
- Standards vary across jurisdictions as to quality of scene investigations and case reviews, so the quality of data in the system also varies.
- There may be missing and/or incomplete information.
- Teams may classify deaths in a different way from the coroner or medical examiner, so one-to-one comparisons cannot be easily made between CDR-CRS data and vital records.

There are over 1,200 variables in the CDR-CRS. The system includes numerous variables related to SUDI/SUID. Many of these were incorporated into the case-reporting tool to enable reporting on variables related to the sleep environment consistent with the American Academy of Pediatrics Safe Sleep recommendations.[18] It is therefore a very rich source of information to help better understand these deaths. Table 12.2 is a partial listing of these variables. Figure 12.2 is an image of the section from the report form, Version 4.1, that allows teams to identify circumstances related to the sleeping environment.[19]

The nationally aggregated dataset is available to researchers through a formal application process. The first national reporting on the national-level SUDI/SUID data resulted from a secondary data analysis project conducted by NCFRP with funding from the US Maternal and Child Health Bureau. This was

o. Objects in child's sleep environment and relation to airway obstruction:

Objects:	Present? Yes	No	U/K	If **present**, describe position of object: On top of child	Under child	Next to child	Tangled around child	U/K	If **present**, did object obstruct airway? Yes	No	UK
Adult(s)	○	○	○	□	□	□	□	□	○	○	○
Other child(ren)	○	○	○	□	□	□	□	□	○	○	○
Animal(s)	○	○	○	□	□	□	□	□	○	○	○
Mattress	○	○	○	□	□	□	□	□	○	○	○
Comforter, quilt, or other	○	○	○	□	□	□	□	□	○	○	○
Fitted sheet	○	○	○	□	□	□	□	□	○	○	○
Thin blanket/flat sheet	○	○	○	□	□	□	□	□	○	○	○
Pillow(s)	○	○	○	□	□	□	□	□	○	○	○
Cushion	○	○	○	□	□	□	□	□	○	○	○
Boppy or U shaped pillow	○	○	○	□	□	□	□	□	○	○	○
Sleep positioner (wedge)	○	○	○	□	□	□	□	□	○	○	○
Bumper pads	○	○	○	□	□	□	□	□	○	○	○
Clothing	○	○	○	□	□	□	□	□	○	○	○
Crib railing/side	○	○	○	□	□	□	□	□	○	○	○
Wall	○	○	○	□	□	□	□	□	○	○	○
Toy(s)	○	○	○	□	□	□	□	□	○	○	○
Other(s), specify:											
____________	○			□	□	□	□	□	○	○	○
____________	○			□	□	□	□	□	○	○	○

→ If adult(s) obstructed airway, describe relationship of adult to child (for example, biological mother):

Figure 12.2 The CDR-CRS questions related to objects in the sleep environment
Form available from: National Center for Fatality Review and Prevention. National CDR Case Reporting System Case Report Form Version 5.0.

an early exploration of the limitations and possibilities of doing analysis on SUDI/SUID using the CDR-CRS data. The study described the characteristics and sleep circumstances of infants who died from SUDI/SUID and examined similarities and differences in risk factors among infants whose deaths are classified as resulting from SIDS, suffocation, or undetermined causes.[20] The study used data from deaths occurring between 2005 and 2008 from 9 US states to assess 3,136 SUDI/SUIDs. It found that only 25% of infants were sleeping in a crib or on their back when found; 70% were on a surface not intended for infant sleep (e.g., adult bed). Importantly, 64% of infants were sharing a sleep surface, and almost half of these infants were sleeping with an adult. Infants whose deaths were classified as suffocation or undetermined cause were significantly more likely than were infants whose deaths were classified as SIDS to be found on a surface not intended for infant sleep and to be sharing that sleep surface.

The first national reporting on local-level SUDI/SUID data was from a study conducted in Milwaukee, Wisconsin. The study demonstrates how CDR provides enhanced documentation of risk factors to help steer prevention efforts regarding SUDI/SUID deaths in a local urban community and reaffirms infants in an unsafe sleep environment have an increased risk of death. The study examined demographic characteristics, bed-sharing, incident sleep location, position of child when put to sleep, position of child when found, child's usual sleep place, crib in home, and other objects found in the sleep environment.[21]

Researchers reported on CDR data in which padded bumper pads were associated with suffocation deaths. The study authors reported that an additional 32 bumper-related fatalities from 37 states from 2008 to 2011 were reported in the CDR-CRS but not previously reported into the US Consumer Product Safety Commission (CPSC) database. This finding almost doubled the total number of deaths known throughout the US in which padded bumper pads were believed to be a significant risk.[22] This study and additional information from the CDR-CRS was provided to the CPSC in a public hearing on the potential risks of padded crib bumpers to the CPSC. Subsequently it was used in development of a joint

Table 12.1 Selected sample of data elements in the CDR-CRS related to SUDI/SUID

Information related to demographics, health histories, and socio-determinants of health	Investigation Information
Age at death	Autopsy performed
Race	Scene Investigation performed
Ethnicity	Scene re-enactments performed
Gender	Type of person certifying cause of death
Residence	Specific listing of autopsy tests
Type of Insurance	Agencies conducting scene investigations
Type of public services	Photo of scene uploaded
Birthweight	Official manner and cause of death
Child abuse history	
Breastfeeding	**Death in Sleep Environment Risk Factors**
Exposure to second-hand smoke	Place of sleep
Medical complications	Room of sleep
Metabolic screenings	Type of bed or object of sleep
Immunisation history	Position last placed
Injury history	Position found
Medications	Usual sleep place
Last meals	New sleep place
Mother's pregnancy history	Sleeping with a pacifier
Number of pregnancies	Temperature of room where found
Mother's smoking	Objects in sleep environment
Mother's drug/alcohol	Objects obstructing nose or mouth
Caregivers' ages	Persons or animals sleeping with infant
Family income	Room-sharing
Caregivers' education	Sleep positioners used
Caregivers' first language	
History of domestic violence	
History of child abuse	
Caregivers' police histories	
Mental health histories	
Caregivers' prior child deaths	

statement in November 2016 from four CPSC commissioners recommending that parents and caregivers not use padded crib bumpers.[23]

Researchers analysed the national CDR-CRS data in 2014 and found that risk factors for sleep-related infant deaths may be different for different age groups. Their analysis of CDR data found that the predominant risk factor for younger infants is bed-sharing, whereas rolling into objects in the sleep area is the predominant risk factor for older infants.[24]

Another analysis using CDR data in 2014 reviewed the risks associated with sofas and SUDI/SUID. Infant deaths on sofas were more likely than deaths in other locations to be classified as accidental suffocation or strangulation. They were also less likely to be Hispanic and to have objects in the environment; and more likely to be sharing the surface with another person, to be found on the side, to be found in a new sleep location, and to have had prenatal smoke exposure.[25]

A 2016 study of CDR data analysed how risks differed in in-home and out-of-home settings. The study found that sleep-related infant deaths in the out-of-home setting have higher odds of having certain risk factors, such as prone placement for sleep and location in a stroller/car seat, rather than in a crib/bassinet.[26]

Looking to the Future: Greater Surveillance and Prevention Possibilities with the US SUDI/SUID Case Registry

The US Centers for Disease Control and Prevention (CDC) had a mandate from the US Congress to improve infant death investigations, leading it to develop the National Sudden Infant Death Investigation Form. The CDC subsequently supported five training academies throughout the US, leading to thousands of persons attending ancillary trainings. In an effort to further improve reporting of information from SUDI/SUID investigations the CDC conducted a feasibility study in 2007–8 in seven states. This study led the CDC to conclude that CDR could be a suitable system for collecting data for the surveillance of SUDI/SUID at a national level.[27] A new programme, the Sudden Unexpected Infant Death Case Registry (SUID-CR) was implemented in 2009. The registry was designed to use the CDR process as the registry's reporting source and the

National CDR Case Reporting System as the reporting infrastructure for the registry. Working with the NCFRP at the Michigan Public Health Institute, refinements were made to the case reporting form and NCFRP was funded to provide technical support and management of the data. The purpose of the registry is to collect 'accurate and consistent population-based data about the circumstances and events surrounding SUDI/SUID cases, to improve the completeness and quality of SUDI/SUID case investigations, to categorise SUDI/SUID cases by the use of a decision-making algorithm with standardised definitions ... and to assist programme planners and policy makers with identifying targeted strategies to reduce potentially preventable infant deaths'.[27] Initially funding five states, the CDC expanded funding to nine states. Findings from this registry were used, in part, to establish an expanded registry, the Sudden Death in the Young Case Registry (SDY-CR).[28] This second registry is a joint project of the CDC, the National Institutes of Health (NIH) and the Michigan Public Health Institute. The CDC and NIH are funding eight additional jurisdictions to also identify, review, and report on all sudden and unexpected deaths of children to age 18. This registry also includes the collection and analysis of DNA. The NIH is also funding three research centres to study the case review report findings, medical data, and the DNA findings to improve understanding of SDY. All SDY-CR funded sites must review all of their SUDI/SUID cases. Thus, as of December 2017, thirteen states were doing state-wide SUDI/SUID surveillance and three states were doing the registry in limited jurisdictions.

Initial findings from the SUDI/SUID registry are encouraging. State grantees are meeting the requirement for population-based surveillance by identifying and reviewing all cases, data entry and data quality measures demonstrate states are obtaining comprehensive information from investigations and other sources, and are submitting accurate and timely data, and states are using their findings to implement improvements in practice and prevention.[27]

The registry is also allowing the CDC to classify all SUDI/SUID deaths in the registry in such a way as to capture the uncertainties that exist in current SUDI/SUID reporting. The classification being used in the registry categorises SUDI/SUID cases in terms of whether information was available on comprehensive scene and autopsy investigations, evidence on obstruction to breathing, and hazards in the sleep environment. It recognises the uncertainty about how suffocation or asphyxiation may contribute to death and that accounts for unknown and incomplete information about the death scene and autopsy. An initial study applied the classification system to 436 US SUDI/SUID cases that occurred in 2011 and were reported to the registry. This system helps the SUDI/SUID grantees and the CDC track SUDI/SUID subtypes, providing more information in identifying gaps in investigation and providing more information to inform SUDI/SUID risk reduction and prevention strategies.[29]

In summary, child death review is a robust multidisciplinary process that can be an effective approach to improving our understanding and response to sudden unexplained infant deaths. CDR has been shown to improve investigations, diagnosis, counting, agency policies, and practices, and services to families, and most importantly it has been shown to catalyse communities to act to reduce SUDI/SUID risks and implement prevention programmes. The efforts in the US to establish a nationwide SUDI/SUID case registry using CDR case reviews and reporting as a foundation show promise that a public health, population-based surveillance system can lead us to more accurate reporting on the true causes and circumstances of all types of sudden and unexplained infant deaths.

References

1. Durfee M, Gellert A, Tilton-Durfee D. Origins and clinical relevance of child death review teams. *JAMA*, 1992; **267**(23):3172–5.

2. Covington T, Wirtz S. The power of child death review to prevent maltreatment. In: Alexander A ed., *Research and Practices in Child Maltreatment Prevention*. St Louis: STM Learning, 2017:17–34.

3. *For All Our Children. Washington State Child Death Review Committee Recomendations: Preventing SIDS and Motor Vehicle Crashes*. Washington, DC, 2003; https://www.nwsids.org/documents/WashingtonStateChildDeathReview.pdf (accessed 30 October 2018).

4. Fraser J, Sidebotham P, Frederick J, et al. Learning from child death review in the USA, England, Australia, and New Zealand. *Lancet*, 2014; **384**:894–903.

5. Vincent S. *Preventing Child Deaths: Learning from Review*. Edinburgh: Dunedin Academic Press, 2013.

6. National Center for Fatality Review and Prevention. *Keeping Kids Alive: A Report on the Status of Child Death Review in the United States*, 2016; https://www.ncfrp.org/wp-content/uploads/NCRPCD-Docs/CDRinUS_2016.pdf (accessed 1 November 2018).

7. Office of Disease Prevention and Health Promotion. *Healthy People 2020*. US Department of Health and Human Services, n.d.: www.healthypeople.gov/2020/topics-objectives/topic/injury-and-violence-prevention/objectives (accessed 1 November 2018).

8. Office of Disease Prevention and Health Promotion. *Maternal, Infant and Child Health*, n.d. https://www.healthypeople.gov/2020/topics-objectives/topic/maternal-infant-and-child-health (accessed 30 October 2018).

9. Bowman L, Hargroves T, Hoffman L. Saving babies: exposing Sudden Infant Death. Scripps Howard News Service, 9 October 2007; http://www.editorandpublisher.com/news/scripps-wire-offers-saving-babies-investigative-report/ (accessed 30 October 2018).

10. Shapiro-Mendoza C, Kimball M, Tomashek K, et al. US infant mortality trends attributable to accidental suffocation and strangulation in bed from 1984 through 2004: are rates increasing? *J Pediatr*, 2009; **123**(2):533–9.

11. Palusci V, Yager S, Covington T. Effects of a citizen's review panel in preventing child maltreatment. *Child Abuse Negl*, 2010; **34**:324–31.

12. Carlin R, Moon R. Risk factors, protective factors and current recommendations to reduce Sudden Infant Death Syndrome: a review. *JAMA Pediatr*, 2017; **171** (2):175–80.

13. National Center for Fatality Review and Prevention. *Saving Lives Together! A Sampler of Prevention Outcomes from State and Community Child Death Review Teams*, 2016; https://www.ncfrp.org/wp-content/uploads/NCRPCD-Docs/OutcomesBrochure2016.pdf (accessed 1 November 2018).

14. Shapiro-Mendoza C, Tomashek K, Anderson R, et al. Recent national trends in sudden, unexpected infant deaths: more evidence supporting a change in classification or reporting. *Am J Epidemiol*, 2006; **163** (8):762–9.

15. Malloy M, MacDorman M. Changes in the classification of sudden unexpected infant deaths: United States, 1992–2001. *J Pediatr*, 2005; **115** (5):1247–53.

16. Shapiro-Mendoza C, Kim S, Chu S, et al. Using death certificates to characterize Sudden Infant Death Syndrome (SIDS): opportunities and limitations. *J Pediatr*, 2010; **156** (1):38–43.

17. Covington T. The US National Child Death Review Case Reporting System. *Inj Prev*, 2011; **17**(Supplement 1):34–7.

18. Moon, R. SIDS and other sleep-related deaths: updated 2016 recommendations for a safe infant sleeping environment. *J Pediatr*, 2016; **138**(5); http://pediatrics.aappublications.org/content/138/5/e20162938 (accessed 30 October 2018).

19. National Center for Fatality Review and Prevention. *National CDR Case Reporting System Case Report Form Version 4.1*; https://www.ncfrp.org/wp-content/uploads/NCRPCD-Docs/CDR_CRS_v5.pdf (accessed 30 October 2018).

20. Schnitzer P, Covington T, Dykstra H. Sudden Unexpected Infant Deaths: sleep environment and circumstances. *Am J Public Health*, 2012; **102** (6):1204–12.

21. Brixey B, Kopp L, Schlotthauer A, et al. Use of child death review to inform sudden unexplained infant deaths occurring in a large urban setting. *Inj Prev*, 2011; **17** (Supplement 1):23–7.

22. Scheers N, Woodard D, Thach B. Crib bumpers continue to cause infant deaths: a need for a new preventive approach. *J Pediatr*, 2016; **169**:93–7.

23. Consumer Product Safety Commission. *Joint Statement. . .Recommending Parents and Caregivers Not Use Padded Crib Bumpers*, 3 November 2016; www.cpsc.gov/s3fs-public/Joint%20Statement%20on%20Padded%20Crib%20Bumpers%20FINAL%2011.3.16.pdf (accessed 1 November 2018).

24. Colvin J, Collie-Akers V, Schunn C, et al. Sleep environment risks for younger and older Infants. *J Pediatr*, 2014; **134** (2): e406–e412; https://www.ncbi.nlm.nih.gov/pmc/articles/PMC4187235/ (accessed 30 October 2018).

25. Rechtman LR, Colvin JD, Blair PS, Moon RY. Sofas and infant mortality. *J Pediatr*, 2014; **134**: e1293–e1300; http://pediatrics.aappublications.org/content/pediatrics/early/2014/10/08/peds.2014-1543.full.pdf (accessed 30 October 2018).

26. Kassa H, Moon R, Colvin J. Risk factors for sleep-related infant deaths in in-home and out-of-home settings. *J Pediatr*, 2016; **138** (5): http://pediatrics.aappublications.org/content/138/5/e20161124 (accessed 30 October 2018).

27. Shapiro-Mendoza CK, Camperlengo L, Kim SY, Covington T. The Sudden Unexpected Infant Death case registry: a method to improve surveillance. *J Pediatr*, 2012; **129**(2)e486–93; http://aaspp.net/wp-content/uploads/2015/01/Shapiro-Mendoza-Camperlengo-Kim-Covington-2012-SUID-Case-Registry.pdf (accessed 30 October 2018).

28. Burns K, Bienemann L, Camperlengo L, et al. The sudden death in the young case registry: collaborating to understand and reduce mortality. *J Pediatr*, 2017; **139**(3); http://pediatrics .aappublications.org/content/139/3/e20162757 (accessed 30 October 2018).

29. Shapiro-Mendoza C, Camperlengo L, Ludvigsen R, et al. Classification system for the sudden unexpected infant death case registry and its application. *J Pediatr*, 2014; **134** (1):e210–e219; http://pediatrics .aappublications.org/content/134/1/e210.long (accessed 30 October 2018).

Chapter 13

Final Case Discussion and Child Death Overview Panels (CDOP) in the UK

Joanna Garstang and Peter Sidebotham

The Final Case Discussion

A final case discussion is held once all the investigations into the death are complete; this is typically four to six months after the death, but may be longer if more detailed pathological tests or other investigations are required. The aim of the discussion is to determine the complete cause for death, recognise any relevant contributory factors and address the needs of the family, including any child protection needs. In the UK, the final case discussion forms part of the statutory multi-agency response to unexpected child deaths; the Child Death Overview Panel (CDOP).[1] However, regardless of the jurisdiction, it is considered best practice that a diagnosis of SIDS is reached following a multi-professional discussion and that this conclusion should not be given by any individual professional alone.[2] There are many different models for investigating unexpected infant deaths internationally, but joint working by the different agencies of police, health, and social care is a key element for effective investigation and the case discussion is an integral part of this.[3,4] In this section we describe current English practice but the principles we use should hold true for other locations.

Practicalities of Arranging the Final Case Discussion

The final case discussion involves both professionals who were involved in the investigation into the death such as paediatricians and police officers, and those working with families on an ongoing basis, for example the primary care team. A suggested attendance list is shown in Box 13.1.

The meeting is usually led by the paediatrician; ideally the same paediatrician is involved throughout the SUDI/SUID investigative process. Meetings are often held at primary care centres to enable general practitioners to participate. If the pathologist is unable to attend it is vital that the paediatrician has obtained the post-mortem report prior to the meeting and discussed any queries with the pathologist. Although social care may not have had face-to-face contact with the family as part of the SUDI/SUID investigation it is important that they attend the discussion, particularly as child protection issues are often raised. In order to enable open conversation between professionals, families are not invited; however, part of the discussion should include a plan of which professional should visit the parents to explain the outcomes of the meeting.

If there are ongoing criminal investigations into the death, the case discussion will not be held until after these have concluded to ensure that police investigations are not jeopardised.

Reviewing the Case

The final case discussion involves reviewing all details of the case; infant and family medical histories, physical examination, post-mortem examination results, findings from the death scene analysis, police enquiries, and social care involvement. Having reviewed all information, the meeting should decide if a complete explanation for the death has been determined; this may be a medical or accidental cause of death. If the death remains unexplained after complete investigation the meeting should consider whether it is appropriate to label the death as SIDS. Possible contributory factors should be recorded for all deaths, not just SIDS, as many (for example missed immunisations, parental smoking, child protection concerns) are relevant for child mortality more generally.

The meeting should also discuss any potential safeguarding concerns that may have arisen as a result of the investigation; these may involve surviving siblings or those yet to be born. The presence of social care should enable these concerns to be addressed.

> **BOX 13.1** A list of professionals who may be invited to attend CDOP meetings
>
> Paediatrician, specialist nurse
> Child death team administrator
> Pathologist
> General practitioner (GP)
> Police officer
> Social worker
> Health visitor, midwife
> Early years or school staff (if older siblings)
> Coroner's officer

> **BOX 13.2** Potential membership of CDOP
>
> Hospital paediatrician   Community paediatrician
> Designated doctor for unexpected child deaths
> Midwife   Neonatologist
> Clinical governance representative   Health visitor
> General practitioner   Police officer   Youth offender services
> Social care   Education representatives   Public Health Local Government

Documenting the Discussion

The final case discussion should be documented, although there is no standard practice for doing so. A detailed narrative summary or a pro forma such as the Avon clinico-pathological classification[5] or the CDOP analysis form can be used for this purpose. Whichever method is used, the documentation should be shared with the coroner and the CDOP. It is good practice for a letter to be written for the parents, summarising the findings of the investigation and explaining the cause of death; this letter can be copied to the parents' GP.

Supporting Families

Parents will want to know the outcome of the discussion since understanding the cause of death is extremely important to them.[6,7] The case discussion should consider who is best placed to explain the findings of the investigation to the parents as well as to support their needs. Frequently the paediatrician visits the parents at home to share this information but it is helpful for a member of the primary care team, such as the GP or health visitor to accompany them, as they will be supporting the family in the longer term. Many coroners are keen that parents are able to discuss the cause of death with a paediatrician before the inquest, and parents certainly value being able to do so.[8] However, paediatricians should seek agreement from the coroner prior to discussing the cause of death with families.

The CDOP

Since 2008, all deaths of children from birth until they reach eighteen years of age are subject to review by the

CDOP.[1] The aim of this process is to improve the welfare and safety of all children in the locality and it is achieved by a multi-agency group of professionals categorising deaths and identifying relevant modifiable factors. As the CDOP reviews all child deaths in a locality, SUDI/SUID cases only account for a small proportion of their caseload.

Management of CDOP

CDOPs are geographically based on local government areas, as they are part of Local Safeguarding Children Boards (LSCBs); however, in some locations CDOPs may be combined between two or three local government areas. Until recently CDOPs were managed by the Department for Education, but following a review[9] they are now managed by the Department for Health, in recognition that deaths are predominantly due to medical causes. In the future CDOPs may also be regionally rather than locally based, covering much larger populations.

The CDOP chair should be from an agency that does not provide direct services to children, to avoid any conflict of interest; frequently they are chaired by public health physicians. The membership is from agencies with responsibility for children, such as health services, education, police, social care, and local government. Within health services, representatives include paediatricians, midwives, obstetricians, and primary care. Membership is flexible and can be varied according to the cases under review; for instance when considering deaths in a house fire, representatives from the fire service may be invited to contribute. Potential membership of CDOP is shown in Box 13.2.

Analysis of Deaths

CDOPs are notified of all child deaths, which then request information about deceased children from each service (i.e. primary care, hospital, police, social care, education) that these children were known to. All documentation from the joint agency SUDI/SUID investigation and final case discussion should be forwarded to the CDOP. All relevant information for each case is then anonymised for review.

Cases are discussed at CDOP meetings and reviewed using a standard template, the CDOP Form analysis. Possible contributory factors are analysed in four domains: those intrinsic to the child, factors in the social environment including family and parenting capacity, factors in the physical environment, and service provision. Panel members also determine whether the death is considered preventable; this is defined in the child death review statutory guidance as 'those in which modifiable factors may have contributed to the death. These are factors defined as those, where, if actions could be taken through national or local interventions, the risk of future child deaths could be reduced'.[1]

There are difficulties with CDOP analysis in that there are no clear guidelines as what constitutes a contributory factor in parenting capacity or service provision, leading to inconsistencies between different CDOPs.[10]

Learning from Deaths

CDOPs can make recommendations based on the deaths they review. These recommendations can be agency specific, local, regional, or national. Learning from CDOPs has led to local public health initiatives such as safe-sleeping campaigns and recommendations for health visitors to ask to see where infants sleep rather than just discuss safe-sleeping practices with parents.

CDOPs may identify deaths where abuse or neglect may have been a factor; these cases should be referred to the LSCB or Safeguarding Partners for consideration of a Serious Case Review if this need has not been already recognised.

Currently, CDOP data are only analysed at a local level, although there are plans for a national database to be established in the near future. This project has huge potential for understanding why children die and reducing child mortality.

References

1. HM Government. *Working Together to Safeguard Children: A Guide to Inter-Agency Working to Safeguard and Promote the Welfare of Children*. 2015, London: Department for Education.

2. Bajanowski T, Vege A, Byard RW, Krous HF, Arnestad M et al. Sudden Infant Death Syndrome (SIDS) – standardised investigations and classification: recommendations. *Forensic Sci Int*, 2007: **165**:129–43.

3. *Sudden Unexpected Death in Infancy and Childhood: Multi-agency Guidelines for Care and Investigation*, 2nd edn. London: The Royal College of Pathologists, 2016,

4. Garstang J, Ellis C, Sidebotham P. An evidence-based guide to the investigation of sudden unexpected death in infancy. *Forensic Sci Med Pathol*, 2015: **11**:345–57.

5. Platt MW. Learning lessons: reviewing child deaths. In: Sidebotham P, Fleming P. *Unexpected Death in Childhood: A* Handbook *for Practitioners*, Chichester, John Wiley & Sons Ltd. 2007: 205–31.

6. Garstang J, Griffiths F, Sidebotham P. What do bereaved parents want from professionals after the sudden death of their child? A systematic review of the literature. BMC Pediatr, 2014; 14:269; https://bmcpe diatr.biomedcentral.com/articles/10.1186/1471-2431-14-269 (accessed 30 October 2018).

7. Garstang J, Griffiths F, Sidebotham P. Parental understanding and self-blame following sudden infant death: a mixed-methods study of bereaved parents' and professionals' experiences. *BMJ Open*, 2016: **6**:e011323.

8. Garstang J, Griffiths F, Sidebotham P. Rigour and rapport: a qualitative study of parents' and professionals' experiences of joint agency infant death investigation. *BMC Pediatr*, 2017: **17**:48.

9. Wood A. *Wood Report: Review of the Role and Functions of Local Safeguarding Children Boards*. Department for Education, 2016; https://assets.pub lishing.service.gov.uk/government/uploads/system/ uploads/attachment_data/file/526329/Alan_Wood_re view.pdf (accessed 31 October 2018).

10. Garstang J, Ellis C, Griffiths F, Sidebotham P. Unintentional asphyxia, SIDS, and medically explained deaths: a descriptive study of outcomes of child death review (CDR) investigations following sudden unexpected death in infancy. *Forensic Sci Med Pathol*, 2016: **12**:407–15.

Imaging Findings on Autopsy

Elspeth Whitby, Ashok Raghavan, and Amaka Offiah

Post-mortem Skeletal Radiography

Diagnostic Accuracy of Post-mortem Radiography

The published usefulness of radiography in post-mortem imaging in the perinatal period varies between authors. The yield is dependent on the population studied and selection criteria used. Olsen et al. suggested that the success of radiographs in providing pathologically relevant information is around 10%,[1] while a more recent paper by Arthurs et al. has suggested that routine post-mortem radiography in fetuses and neonates is not diagnostically useful and that a more selective protocol would be more cost-effective.[2]

Radiographic Findings

Fractures

In cases of Sudden Unexpected Death in Infancy (SUDI), radiology plays an important first line role in identification of unsuspected fractures and is compulsory in all cases. If present, fractures raise the suspicion that death was inflicted.

As mentioned in Chapter 11, radiographs of all anatomical sites should be obtained individually and carefully assessed for fractures. Where there is any doubt, repeat radiographs, Computed Tomography (CT) and specimen radiographs (or high quality fax-itron images) should be performed (Figure 14.1).

Some radiographic findings can be more difficult to appreciate at autopsy, such as fractures from birth trauma or resuscitation and deformities of the foot or chest. These findings need to be considered within the clinical context.

Post-mortem Computed Tomography (PMCT)

There is growing evidence to suggest that PMCT may be a preferable option to the radiographic skeletal survey and the use of PMCT for skeletal imaging (particularly where abuse is suspected) is increasing. PMCT provides clearer imaging and allows for 3D reconstruction, which can be useful in legal cases.[3] Other researchers have found that CT is more sensitive than radiography in the detection of rib fractures (Figure 14.2) and that near perfect concordance between PMCT and autopsy can be achieved in the identification of fractures in general[4–6]. It has been reported that interpretation of images by those with little experience of PMCT may result in many false positive fractures, and therefore the experience of the radiologist is important.[4] Proisy et al. identified two 'healing metacarpal metaphyseal fractures' on PMCT, but reported that these bones were undoubtedly normal on radiography.[7] Conversely, false negative CT findings have also been reported, for example, skull fractures were missed in one study, which error the authors explained as being due to the large slice thickness (5 mm) used.[8]

Although PMCT may not always identify the specific cause of death and has less resolution than MRI, it can sometimes be helpful in detecting non-skeletal abnormality.[9] Pathology that has been identified includes (but is not limited to) brain haemorrhage/oedema, volvulus, pneumonia, pneumothorax, pulmonary hypoplasia, and fractures.

Perhaps of more relevance, given that this is a relatively new field of imaging, is an understanding of normal and iatrogenic findings on PMCT, a brief discussion of which follows.

Post-mortem Change

These changes are part of the decomposition process and have no pathological significance, but may result in diagnostic confusion. They include intravascular gas bubbles, gas in bowel/stomach distension, intra-articular gas (Figure 14.3) and pulmonary changes (e.g. atelectasis, lobar collapse/consolidation).[7,10]

Normal Variants

These are non-pathological changes in anatomy that occur because of genetic or epigenetic factors. There is a wide range of normal variants that can occur and

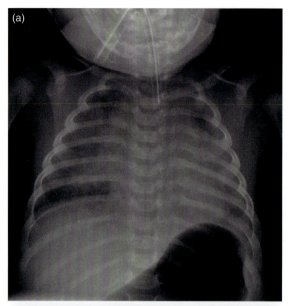

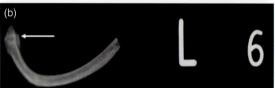

Figure 14.1 11-week-old female, unexplained death. AP chest radiograph
(a) shows posterior fractures of the left 4th, 5th, 7th, 8th, and 11th ribs and a possible fracture of the neck of the left 6th rib, which was confirmed (arrow) on high dose (faxitron) specimen radiography.
(b) The infant's skeleton must be evaluated for general bone modelling, overall proportions, outline of individual bones, and secondary ossification centres.

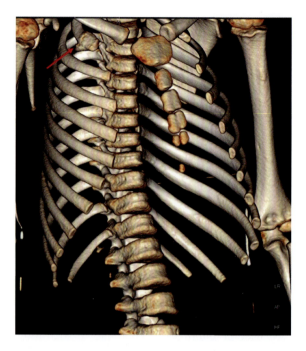

Figure 14.2 3D reconstructed PMCT in a coroner's case, confirming a fracture of the right first rib. Note the multiple sternal ossification centres – a normal finding

many of them are seen in the skeleton. Hatch et al. highlighted the importance of normal variants when using PMCT, with skeletal variants such as accessory bones, teeth, and accessory foramina being some of the more commonly seen variations.[11] Normal variants also include multiple sternal ossification centres (Figure 14.2), metaphyseal spurs and coronal cleft vertebral bodies (particularly in males). The knowledge and experience of the radiologist interpreting the images is an important factor in deciding whether these variants can be distinguished from pathological findings. Correlation with the radiographic skeletal survey is recommended, as is close collaboration with the pathologist. If identified on PMCT, consideration should be given as to whether these 'normal variants' are in fact a manifestation of an underlying skeletal dysplasia or other condition.

Intraosseous Needle Tracts

Intraosseous needle tracts and associated air and other foreign objects such as catheters are a common finding on PMCT. Needle tracts tend to be horizontally oriented and traverse the bony cortex for a relatively short distance, while vascular channels are more oblique and traverse the cortex for a longer distance (Figure 14.4). Gas may be identified within the surrounding soft tissues and/or within the needle tract. Gas embolism can be missed at autopsy and therefore the ability of PMCT to identify gas makes it a useful addition to conventional autopsy. However, care must be taken to ensure that intraosseous needle tracts and associated gas are not misdiagnosed as pathologically significant gas emboli.

It is worth noting that a bony fragment may be seen in relation to a withdrawn intraosseous needle (Figure 14.5). These fragments are not visible on the corresponding radiographs and are not necessarily directly adjacent to the exit point of the needle; therefore, the radiologist needs to be aware of this potential finding, particularly if it appears as a cortical break.

In summary, evidence suggests that PMCT may be more sensitive then radiography in the identification of skeletal abnormalities. However, PMCT has a relatively

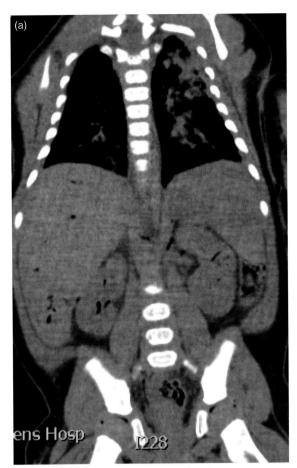

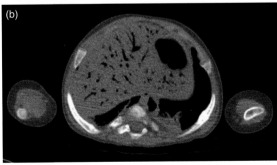

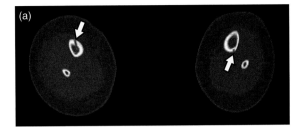

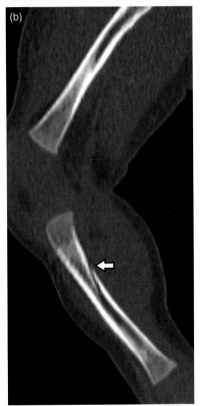

Figure 14.4 10-week-old male, SIDS
a. Axial PMCT of both tibiae.
b. Sagittal PMCT of left tibia Images show nutrient foramina – the main blood supply to bone. Note the oblique and relatively long intracortical course on the sagittal projection.

Figure 14.3 PMCT of chest and abdomen (10-week-old male, SIDS)
a. Coronal, shows post-mortem air (curvilinear low density) in the liver, kidneys, and hip joints. Note normal post-mortem patchy consolidation within the lungs.
b. Axial through the upper abdomen showing post-mortem air (curvilinear low density) in the liver.

low diagnostic accuracy for non-skeletal pathology. Care should be taken so that non-pathological findings seen on PMCT are not misinterpreted. It is important to be aware of these to prevent an incorrect diagnosis. Larger prospective comparative studies are required to fully investigate the diagnostic accuracy of PMCT in the context of SUDI.

Post-mortem Magnetic Resonance Imaging (PMMRI)

MRI scanners are now widely available throughout the UK but have a high work load and long waiting

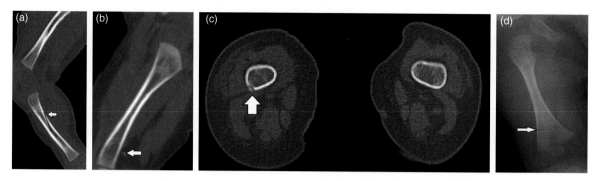

Figure 14.5 a. Sagittal PMCT of the right tibia (12-day-old female, unascertained cause of death) shows a fragment of bone (arrowhead) and soft tissue air at a distance from the interosseous needle tract (note also the nutrient foramen in the upper third of the tibia).
b. and c. Sagittal and axial PMCT (male aged 19 months who had a (probable) mitochondrial cardiomyopathy. Notice the fragment of bone (b) and cortical break.
c. Removal of an intraosseous needle which may be mistaken for a fracture.
d. Radiograph of patient in b and c; the interosseous needle tract is clearly visible, but there is no apparent cortical fragment.

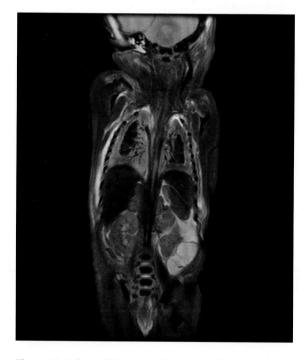

Figure 14.6 Coronal T2 weighted image of a stillborn term baby where there had been an attempt at resuscitation. Note that the central area of both lungs is darker (air filled) than the peripheral (fluid filled)

times for patients. This means that obtaining post-mortem MRI scans can be difficult and it helps if staff can be 'creative' in their work load. For example, one institution has a cold storage facility in their scanner control room that has been approved by the Human Tissue Authority, allowing them to scan cases when there are gaps or delays with other patients and not have to wait for the case to be brought to the department. Other centres scan out of normal working hours. A close collaboration between radiology and pathology staff will create the working pattern preferred for each individual department.

MRI scans provide a good quality image of the whole body with good tissue definition so the individual organs are clearly seen and assessed.

If an area of abnormality is detected at the time of the imaging, consideration should be given to performing a biopsy as would normally pertain in the clinical setting with a patient that was alive. This will give histological information that could be important to determining the cause of death.

Interpretation of the MRI scan needs to be performed with care and with understanding of the post-mortem changes that occur naturally so as not to over interpret or misdiagnose post-mortem changes with pathology prior to demise. Normal post-mortem changes include small pleural and pericardial effusions (Figure 14.6), loss of the extra axial CSF space between the brain and the skull, and changes in the pattern and lamination seen in blood clots. As with all imaging reports the clinical details should be available and relevant when reporting each case. This should include the details of the demise and any treated or resuscitation attempts made at the time. This is important as interosseous needle tracts may mimic fractures, and resuscitation of a stillbirth will cause there to be air in the lungs, which is often assumed to be a sign that the baby has breathed at some point.

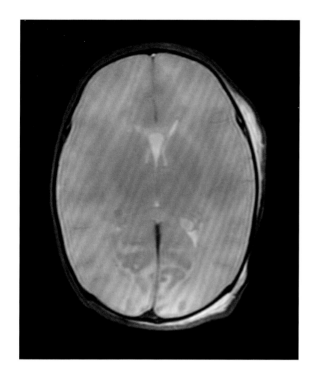

Figure 14.7 Axial section, T2 weighted image through the neonatal brain. There is loss of the normal grey white matter definition indicating hypoxia

In a large single-centre study of SUDI/SUID cases 63% remained unexplained after formal post-mortem investigations. Of those where a cause of death was found, it was dependent on the macroscopic examination in 30%, histology in 46%, microbiological investigations in 19% and clinical history in 5%.[12]

The changes that occur in the brain with hypoxia are still debated. By definition, all deaths result in hypoxia but not all have changes on imaging that are typical of hypoxia. We believe that the hypoxia that presents in a sudden death does not result in imaging changes. However, in cases where there has been an element of hypoxia sustained prior to or around the time of demise, that is prolonged enough to cause cellular changes, then there may be imaging changes too.

However, in a study imaging both neonates who died with hypoxic injury and neonates that did not (and had no hypoxic changes at autopsy) using both quantitative and qualitative approaches, all MRI images showed loss of cortical grey/white matter differentiation (Figure 14.7), loss of the normal high signal intensity (SI) in the posterior limb of the

internal capsule on T1-weighted images, and high white matter SI on T2-weighted images, thus making accurate distinction impossible.[13]

MRI will demonstrate the bones, but better information is obtained from a skeletal survey and/or CT.

MRI may not provide the cause of death but may provide essential information that allows the cause of death to be identified. This has been highlighted in a case report from Australia where the post-mortem imaging demonstrated hepatomegaly and steatosis,[14] which promoted analysis of the neonatal blood sample taken for the Guthrie test and a diagnosis of type 2 carnitine palmitoyltransferase deficiency was possible.

MRI however will exclude any major structural abnormality and in many reported studies is as good as or better, when part of a minimally invasive autopsy process, than formal autopsy for gross structural abnormalities.

It also helps exclude accidental and inflicted injury and can be used to identify areas for targeted biopsy. However, imaging cannot detect disseminated sepsis, but if this is screened for using swabs of body fluids from body cavities, blood samples, and tissue biopsy, this should be detected if present.

References

1. Olsen OE, Espeland A, Maartmann-Moe H, Lachman RS, Rosendahl K. Diagnostic value of radiography in cases of perinatal death: a population-based study. *Arch Dis Child Fetal Neonatal Ed*, 2003; **88**:F521–4.

2. Arthurs OJ, Calder AD, Kiho L, Taylor AM, Sebire NJ. Routine perinatal and paediatric post-mortem radiography: detection rates and implications for practice.*Pediatr Radiol*, 2014; **44**:252–7.

3. Yen K, Lovblad KO, Scheurer E et al. Post-mortem forensic neuroimaging: correlation of MSCT and MRI findings with autopsy results. *Forensic Sci Int*, 2007; **173**:21–35.

4. Hong TS, Reyes JA, Moineddin R et al. Value of postmortem thoracic CT over radiography in imaging of pediatric rib fractures. *Pediatr Radiol*, 2011; **41**:736–48.

5. Wootton-Gorges SL, Wexler-Stein R, Walton JW et al. Comparison of computed tomography and chest radiography in the detection of rib fractures in abused infants. *Child Abuse Negl*, 2008; **32**:659–63.

6. Le Blanc-Louvry I, Thureau S, Duval C et al. Post-mortem computed tomography compared to forensic autopsy findings: a French experience. *Eur Radiol*, 2013; **23**:1829–35.

7. Proisy M, Marchand AJ, Loget P et al. Whole-body post-mortem computed tomography compared with autopsy in the investigation of unexpected death in infants and children. *Eur Radiol*, 2013; **23**:1711–19.

8. Inoue H, Hyodoh H, Watanabe S, Okazaki S, Mizuo K. Acute enlargement of subdural hygroma due to subdural hemorrhage in a victim of child abuse. *Leg Med*, 2015; **17**:116–19.

9. Oyake Y, Aoki T, Shiotani S, Kohno M, Ohashi N, Akutsu H, Yamazaki K. Postmortem computed tomography for detecting causes of sudden death in infants and children: retrospective review of cases. *Radiat Med*, 2006; **24**:493–502.

10. Christe A, Flach P, Ross S, Spendlove D, Bolliger S, Vock P, Thali MJ. Clinical radiology and postmortem imaging (virtopsy) are not the same: specific and unspecific postmortem signs. *Leg Med*, 2010; **12**:215–22.

11. Hatch GM, Dedouit F, Christensen AM, Thali MJ, Ruder TD. RADid: A pictorial review of radiologic identification using postmortem CT. *J Forensic Radiol Imaging*, 2014; **2**:52–9.

12. Weber MA, Ashworth MT, Risdon MA, Hartley JC, Malone M, Sebire NJ. The role of post-mortem investigations in determining the cause of sudden unexpected death in infancy. *Arch Dis Child*, 2008; **93**:1048–53.

13. Montaldo P, Chaban B, Lally PJ, Sebire NJ, Taylor AM, Thayyil S. Quantification of ante-mortem hypoxicischemic brain injury by post-mortem cerebral magnetic resonance imaging in neonatal encephalopathy.*Eur J Paediatr Neurol*, 2015; **19**:665–71.

14. Bouchireb K, Teychene AM, Rigal O, et al. Post-mortem MRI reveals CPT2 deficiency after sudden infant death. *Eur J Pediatr*, 2010; **169**:1561–3.

Chapter 15

Neuropathology of SIDS

Waney Squier

Introduction

The cause of death in infants dying suddenly and unexpectedly remains a diagnostic challenge. Sudden Infant Death Syndrome (SIDS) is a diagnosis of exclusion, and as such places an even greater than usual onus on the pathologist and the neuropathologist to be increasingly stringent in the pursuit of even the most subtle pathology which may be contributory to the death. Only by performing extensive and detailed examinations in babies dying of SIDS will the causes of death eventually be unravelled.

Most of the evidence today points to a final common pathway for SIDS in the neuronal networks of the brainstem which have a critical role in cardiorespiratory control, autonomic function, sleep, and arousal and in regulation of upper airway protective reflexes. Widespread deficiencies in the caudal 5-HT system have been described, including altered neurotransmitter content of cells, neuronal immaturity, and altered neuronal numbers; detailed assessment of these changes is beyond the routine diagnostic autopsy examination and requires research methods and prospective study. As the brainstem networks undergo significant maturational changes interpretation of pathology is even more complicated in the diagnostic setting.

Neuropathological examination of SIDS babies should look beyond the brainstem. There are two main reasons: first, there are upstream influences on the brainstem which need to be considered, and second, there may be additional changes which may be either pre-existing and indicate a developmental process, or acquired, and suggest chronic or repetitive hypoxia prior to final collapse.

Autopsy Examination and Removal of the Brain

This chapter will not go into details of autopsy techniques but a few important points relating to brain

examination are worthy of mention. The parental wishes and their authority to examine the brain are paramount prior to starting a neuropathological examination. This is a sensitive topic and making the best possible diagnosis, with the opportunity for teaching and research, requires parental permission for the brain to be retained and archived.

The clinical history is the cornerstone of diagnosis and the clinical records must be carefully studied so that a full differential diagnosis can be borne in mind. A history of prematurity, seizures, apnoea (which may be a manifestation of seizure activity in the very young), and gastro-oesophageal reflux are particularly relevant. The history of the pregnancy and delivery are important; 100% of very premature babies have gliosis in the brainstem.[1] Loss or impaired function of the cells here provides a likely cause of the increased risk of sudden death in premature babies and may explain the high incidence of 'asphyxial' deaths in this group.

The infant brain has a high water content and is very soft. Removal of the brain from the skull needs very gentle handling and may be facilitated by delivery into saline to prevent mechanical disruption. It is important to preserve the caudal brainstem as this is a focus of pathology in these cases. It is extremely important to examine all the dura for evidence of dural bleeding.

The brain must be fully fixed in formalin before slicing. If the pia of the unfixed brain is damaged the soft brain will collapse. After the brain is fixed it is carefully examined externally before slicing coronally. Detailed documentation of observations with a full photographic record of findings is important. Multiple blocks are sampled for histology from standard locations as well as sampling areas of special interest. These include the brainstem – particularly the medulla, where 2–3 levels should be sampled; the hippocampus, which should be sampled at a minimum of two levels on each side; and the dura,

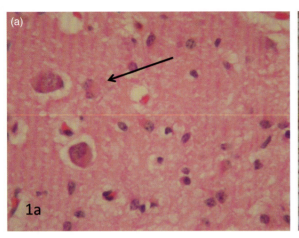
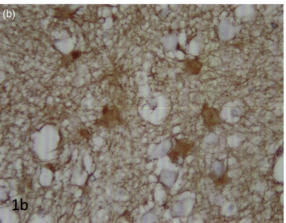

Figure 15.1 Olivary gliosis a: H&E and b: GFAP stained sections show plump reactive astrocytes, some binucleated (arrow).

where multiple blocks to include the superior sagittal sinus and parasagittal dura, the confluence of sinuses, and the parietal dura should be retained.

Skeletal muscle should be sampled and frozen for potential metabolic abnormality.

Brainstem

The Caudal Serotonin (5-HT) System

The most compelling hypothesis for sudden unexpected death in infancy is of a final common pathway in the brainstem. The caudal 5-HT system has significantly decreased levels of 5-HT and associated enzymes, alterations in 5-HT receptor, and transporter binding, altered neuronal density and neuronal maturation in in 50–75% of SIDS cases[2,3] – see Chapter 31. These observations have been made in the research setting and cannot be reproduced in routine diagnostic study. However it is important to establish that the anatomy is normal and to look for evidence of acquired damage which may compromise brainstem function.

Arcuate Nucleus

Smallness and reduced neuronal density in the arcuate nuclei have been described in babies dying unexpectedly.[4] The development of brainstem nuclei derived from the rhombic lip involves neuronal migration through the brainstem leptomeninges and excessive neurones here may indicate impairment or delay in this process.[5] Delayed maturation of the

cerebellum, manifest as increased thickness of the external granule cell layer, has been described in SIDS.[6]

Brainstem Gliosis

Brainstem gliosis has been described in some, but not all, SIDS cases.[7–9] Gliosis in the inferior olivary nucleus has been associated with risk factors for hypoxia-ischaemia during pregnancy, birth, and the perinatal period, and particularly with maternal smoking. Between 80 and 100% of very low birth-weight infants have gliosis in the pons and olive.[1] Clearly a brainstem damaged at or before birth will be less able to withstand challenges later in infancy.

Gliosis is readily demonstrated with immunocytochemistry for GFAP and is often quite prominent around the inferior olive (Figure 15.1).

Sometimes infants dying suddenly have evidence of old axonal injury; patchy axonal swellings with associated macrophage and glial responses indicate that these injuries may be survivable but can potentially contribute to later brainstem compromise (Figure 15.2).

Upstream Influences on the Brainstem

The caudal brainstem 5-HT networks are part of wider neuronal networks involving the midbrain, pons and the forebrain.[3,10] Input from peripheral sensors in the cardiovascular system, lungs, and upper airways and the oxygen-conserving reflex system are integrated here. These upstream influences may contribute to the mechanisms of sudden death and are areas where careful study may be rewarded.

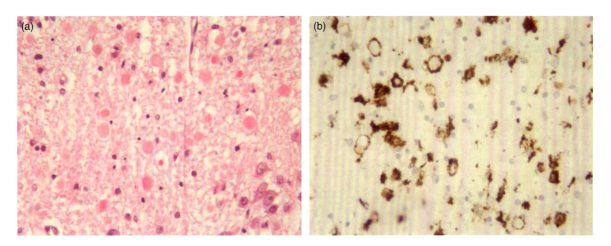

Figure 15.2 Focal brainstem axonal swelling. 2a: H&E demonstration of numerous axonal swellings. 2b: CD68 stain indicates microglial and macrophage reaction to the swellings indicating that they are at least several days old. The baby died 25 days after a traumatic ventouse delivery.

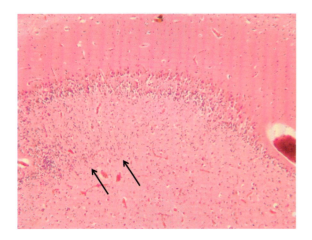

Figure 15.3 Dentate fascia showing extensive bilaminar structure and clusters of rod-shaped cells beneath it (arrows).

Hippocampus

The hippocampus generates and propagates seizures and its projections onto brainstem nuclei may be involved in sudden death due to temporary dysfunction of serotonin or 5-hydroxytryptamine (5-HT) neurones or failure of the 5-HT system to respond to stressors in the post-ictal state.[10] Hippocampal structural abnormalities have been associated with sudden death in toddlers and infants.[11,12]

A preliminary retrospective study described subtle developmental abnormalities of the hippocampus which were more frequent in, but not exclusive to, babies dying of SIDS.[12] The dentate fascia was seen to be focally bilaminar in 41% of sudden infant death babies compared with 7.7% of controls. Other associated changes included clusters of immature cells in the subgranular layer and ectopic cells in the supragranular layer of the dentate fascia (Figure 15.3). The changes described are very subtle and readers are advised to read the cited references to see their precise definition. The authors hypothesised that these changes might increase the risk of sudden death by instability of modulation of brainstem nuclei or by inducing subclinical seizure.

Clusters of rod-shaped cells, thought to be microglia, seen beneath the hippocampal dentate fascia have for many years been recognised in babies dying at less than 9 months of age and were considered to be an indication of chronic hypoxia.[13] More recent immunocytochemical studies indicate that these cells are neuronal precursors and an increase in their numbers may reflect a developmental or a reactive phenomenon.[14] Reduction in hippocampal MAP-2 positive neurones has been described in SIDS victims and babies with hypoxic-ischaemic injury but not in normal controls.[15]

Oxygen-Conserving Reflexes (OCR)

These reflexes are most pronounced in the immature infant and protect the brain against oxygen deprivation during the transition to air breathing in the first months of life. They include the laryngeal chemoreflex, the trigeminocardiac reflex, and the dive reflex. OCR are modulated and facilitated by the caudal 5-HT network and evoke dramatic bradycardia, hypotension, apnoea, and gastric hypermotility. The concept that the protective reflexes may be fatal is paradoxical but abnormal 5-HT function has been proposed as a cause of exaggerated endogenous facilitation of the OCR in SIDS victims.[16] Routine neuropathological examination is unlikely to reveal pathology in this system. However it is important also to consider pathology which may trigger hyperactivity of OCR.

The OCR are activated by stimulation of any sensory branch of trigeminal nerve; examples include airflow stimulation of the face, cold or water on the face and in the nasal passages, craniofacial surgery and dural inflammation.[17] Krous described five babies with 'SIDS while awake', in four of which nasal or laryngeal stimulation was implicated in triggering a response.[18] The dive reflex was considered to have triggered sudden death in an infant who also had brainstem gliosis.[8]

The laryngeal chemoreflex has been suggested to cause SIDS, possibly potentiated by upper respiratory infection.[18] Reflux and pooling of gastric contents around the larynx may trigger the laryngeal chemoreflex and 14% of SIDS cases have evidence of aspiration.[19]

The Dura

The responses of the trigeminal sensory afferents may be modified and enhanced if they are exposed to inflammatory mediators and become sensitised. Bleeding in the human dura produces an inflammatory response, potentially sensitises the trigeminal system and has been implicated in inducing the trigeminocardiac reflex.[17] Increased substance P immunoreactivity in the spinal trigeminal nucleus has been described in SIDS.[20]

It is important to examine the dura for evidence of bleeding; almost a third of babies who collapse with SIDS have evidence of old dural bleeding and this has been described at routine autopsy of SIDS victims.[21] The demographic features of babies with SIDS show striking overlap with babies who present with unexplained retinal and subdural bleeding.

Two studies have described dural bleeding in SIDS babies. In five cases who died of 'SIDS while awake' the dura was described in only one baby and this baby had intradural haemorrhage. In 'delayed SIDS', 12% had intradural bleeding and 4% subdural bleeding.[22,23] These may be under-representations as both were retrospective reviews of autopsy reports.

Cerebral White Matter

Abnormalities in the cerebral white matter have been described in a small proportion of babies dying unexpectedly; these include patchy rarefaction of the subcortical white matter and patchy focal necrosis of the deep white matter.[24] Although generally considered to be due to hypoxic-ischaemic injury, this pathology is probably multifactorial and includes infection and inflammation as well as prematurity.

References

1. Volpe JJ. Brain injury in premature infants: a complex amalgam of destructive and developmental disturbances. *Lancet Neurol*, 2009; **8**(1):110–24.

2. Kinney HC, Broadbelt KG, Haynes RL, Rognum IJ, Paterson DS. The serotonergic anatomy of the developing human medulla oblongata: implications for pediatric disorders of homeostasis. *J Chem Neuroanat*, 2011; **41**(4):182–99.

3. Machaalani R, Waters KA. Neurochemical abnormalities in the brainstem of the Sudden Infant Death Syndrome (SIDS). *Paediatr Respir Rev*, 2014; **15**(4):293–300.

4. Filiano JJ, Kinney HC. Arcuate nucleus hypoplasia in the Sudden Infant Death Syndrome. *J Neuropathol Exp Neurol*, 1992; **51**(4):394–403.

5. Rickert CH, Gros O, Nolte KW, Vennemann M, Bajanowski T, Brinkmann B. Leptomeningeal neurons are a common finding in infants and are increased in Sudden Infant Death Syndrome. *Acta Neuropathol*, 2009; **117**(3):275–82.

6. Cruz-Sanchez FF, Lucena J, Ascaso C, Tolosa E, Quinto L, Rossi ML. Cerebellar cortex delayed maturation in Sudden Infant Death Syndrome. *J Neuropathol Exp Neurol*, 1997; **56**(4):340–6.

7. Kinney HC, Filiano JJ, Harper RM. The neuropathology of the Sudden Infant Death Syndrome. A review. *J Neuropathol Exp Neurol*, 1992; **51**(2):115–26.

8. Matturri L, Ottaviani G, Lavezzi AM. Sudden infant death triggered by dive reflex. *J Clin Pathol*, 2005; **58**(1):77–80.

9. O'Connor TP, van der Kooy D. Cell death organizes the postnatal development of the trigeminal innervation of the cerebral vasculature. *Brain Res*, 1986; **392**(1–2):223–33.

10. Richerson GB, Buchanan GF. The serotonin axis: shared mechanisms in seizures, depression, and SUDEP. *Epilepsia*, 2011; **52** Suppl 1:28–38.

11. Kinney HC, Chadwick AE, Crandall LA, Grafe M, Armstrong DL, Kupsky WJ, et al. Sudden death, febrile seizures, and hippocampal and temporal lobe

maldevelopment in toddlers: a new entity. *Pediatr Dev Pathol*, 2009; **12**(6):455–63.

12. Kinney HC, Cryan JB, Haynes RL, Paterson DS, Haas EA, Mena OJ, et al. Dentate gyrus abnormalities in sudden unexplained death in infants: morphological marker of underlying brain vulnerability. *Acta Neuropathol*, 2015; **129**(1):65–80.

13. Del Bigio MR, Becker LE. Microglial aggregation in the dentate gyrus: a marker of mild hypoxic-ischaemic brain insult in human infants. *Neuropathol Appl Neurobiol*, 1994; **20**(2):144–51.

14. Paine SM, Willsher AR, Nicholson SL, Sebire NJ, Jacques TS. Characterization of a population of neural progenitor cells in the infant hippocampus. *Neuropathol Appl Neurobiol*, 2014; **40**(5):544–50.

15. Oehmichen M, Woetzel F, Meissner C. Hypoxic-ischemic changes in SIDS brains as demonstrated by a reduction in MAP2-reactive neurons. *Acta Neuropathol*, 2009; **117**(3):267–74.

16. Gorini C, Philbin K, Bateman R, Mendelowitz D. Endogenous inhibition of the trigeminally evoked neurotransmission to cardiac vagal neurons by muscarinic acetylcholine receptors. *J Neurophysiol*, 2010; **104**(4):1841–8.

17. Spiriev T, Tzekov C, Kondoff S, Laleva L, Sandu N, Arasho B, et al. Trigemino-cardiac reflex during chronic subdural haematoma removal: report of chemical initiation of dural sensitization. *JRSM Short Rep*, 2011; **2**(4):27.

18. Krous HF, Masoumi H, Haas EA, Chadwick AE, Stanley C, Thach BT. Aspiration of gastric contents in Sudden Infant Death Syndrome without cardiopulmonary resuscitation. *J Pediatr*, 2007; **150**(3):241–6.

19. Thach BT. Potential central nervous system involvement in Sudden Unexpected Infant Deaths and the Sudden Infant Death Syndrome. *Compr Physiol*, 2015; **5**(3):1061–8.

20. Obonai T, Takashima S, Becker LE, Asanuma M, Mizuta R, Horie H, et al. Relationship of substance P and gliosis in medulla oblongata in neonatal Sudden Infant Death Syndrome. *Pediatr Neurol*, 1996; **15**(3):189–92.

21. Rogers CB, Itabashi HH, Tomiyasu U, Heuser ET. Subdural neomembranes and Sudden Infant Death Syndrome. *J Forensic Sci*, 1998; **43**(2):375–6.

22. Krous HF, Chadwick AE, Haas E, Masoumi H, Stanley C. Sudden infant death while awake. *Forensic Sci Med Pathol*, 2008; **4**(1):40–6.

23. Krous HF, Haas EA, Chadwick AE, Masoumi H, Mhoyan A, Stanley C. Delayed death in Sudden Infant Death Syndrome: a San Diego SIDS/SUDC Research Project 15-year population-based report. *Forensic Sci Int*, 2008; **176**(2–3):209–16.

24. Takashima S, Armstrong DL, Becker LE. Subcortical leukomalacia. Relationship to development of the cerebral sulcus and its vascular supply. *Arch Neurol*, 1978; **35**:470–2.

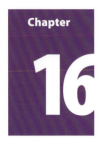
Post-mortem Microbiology: Sampling and Interpretation

Amparo Fernández-Rodríguez and Juan Alberola Enguídanos

Introduction

Post-mortem microbiology (PMM) has an important role in forensic pathology, particularly in the investigation of sudden and unexpected death in infancy (SUDI).[1–3] SUDI/SUID can be due to many causes, including infection (see Section 8). Sometimes, the rapid onset of a fulminating infection leading to death is not accompanied by significant histological inflammation. In such cases, to achieve a proper diagnose of the cause of death, the autopsy is complemented by ancillary investigations, including PMM.

In all cases of SUDI/SUID it is recommended to collect a set of samples for PMM, even when there is no clinical evidence of infection.[4–6] The minimal PMM sampling recommended is described in Table 16.1. The adequate transport media and containers, as well as the type of tests requested to rule out infection are also included. If no infection is suspected, the samples should include direct bacterial culture with antibiotic resistance studies, as well as some molecular analyses for respiratory, neurotropic, and most frequent gastrointestinal viruses.

If an infection is suspected, collection of additional specimens selected according to the clinical symptoms and gross autopsy findings should be taken. Depending on the clinical suspicion, specific analyses aimed to detect the most frequent pathogens should be done. Table 16.2 lists the specimens and investigations recommended for the different etiologies. Among them, general bacteriological cultures and polymerase chain reaction (PCR) assays for specific microorganisms are the most popular investigations.[3]

This chapter summarises guidelines developed by the ESCMID Study Group for Forensic and Postmortem Microbiology (ESGFOR) in conjunction with the European Society of Pathology (ESP).

Interpretation of Post-mortem Microbiology

The significance of isolation of a microorganism in a post-mortem sample may be very different: (i) true infection, caused by the isolated pathogen; (ii) post-mortem bacterial translocation (PMBT), which indicates the passive migration of microorganisms through mucosal surface even after circulation has stopped; and (iii) contamination, mainly due to issues during collection of samples at autopsy.[8]

For this reason, post-mortem microbiology is difficult to interpret;[9] therefore, it is very important to sample extensively and a global interpretation of the analyses performed in all the samples in the context of the clinical history and histology is required.[3] The main aim of interpretation is to identify and differentiate real pathogens from contaminants or PMBT. There are many studies including interpretation criteria based on evidence, most of them focusing on bacteriology. Many authors agree on the same criteria, the most important of which are summarised here.[2,5,10–13]

In general, the criteria to interpret post-mortem cultures should be similar to those of ante-mortem ones. Additional recommendations are needed:

- Positive results detecting the same microorganism obtained from paired blood culture samples suggest bacteraemia.[13]

- Isolation from spleen samples are believed to have the same clinical significance as blood. Consequently, the spleen can corroborate the results of a blood culture. A positive finding in both samples is usually considered as significant as a positive haemoculture in a living patient.

- A positive culture from a sample of liver or kidney may also suggest bacteraemia, especially if the

Table 16.1 Minimal sampling protocol for PMM in sudden death in infancy and childhood[1,7,14]

Laboratory	Sample	Quantity	Transport container or medium	Type of tests
Bacteriology	1. Blood	3–5 ml	Bottles for blood culture (aerobic and anaerobic)[a]	Direct bacterial culture
			Sodium citrate/SPS tube	Direct bacterial culture
			EDTA tube	Molecular analyses
	2. Serum	3–5 ml	Clot activator tube (centrifugation)	Serology
	3. Cerebrospinal fluid	3–5 ml	Sterile tube	Direct bacterial culture & Molecular analyses
	4. Nasopharyngeal swab	2	Flocked swabs (Amies medium)	Direct bacterial culture, Antigenic analyses, Direct bacterial culture & Molecular analyses
	5. Swabs from any identifiable lesion	2	Flocked swabs (Amies medium)	Direct bacterial culture & Molecular analyses
	6. Lung	>1–2 cm³	Sterile tube/container	Direct bacterial culture & Molecular analyses
	7. Spleen	>1–2 cm³	Sterile tube/container	Direct bacterial culture & Molecular analyses
	8. Intestinal content	2–3 ml	Sterile tube/container	Direct bacterial culture & Molecular analyses
Virology	1. Nasopharyngeal swab	2	Flocked swabs (Amies medium). UTM for viral cultures	1 & 2: Molecular analyses for respiratory viruses. If necessary, viral cultures
	2. Lung tissue	>1–2 cm³	Sterile tube/containar	
	3. Intestinal content	2–3 ml	Sterile tube	3. Molecular analyses for gastrointestinal viruses & Antigenic analyses
	4. Cerebrospinal fluid	3–5 ml	Sterile tube	4. Molecular analyses for Enteroviruses & group Herpes viruses. If necessary, viral cultures
Samples frozen at-80 °C for further molecular analyses	0.5 cm³ of heart, muscle, liver, brainstem, and kidney. Other tissues if relevant			5. Further molecular analyses as guided by histology

Notes: [a] Direct bacterial culture should include antibiotic resistance studies

same bacteria are isolated in other organs such as heart or spleen.

- There is a clear need for performing cultures in many different specimens, including blood, and at least five different tissues. The favourite tissues sampled are spleen, liver, heart, and both lungs. Many authors agree that a pure culture (or a predominant one) of the same pathogen found in these samples is consistent with bacteraemia and may have clinical significance.
- On the contrary, trying to interpret results in only one sample, such as blood culture, may be difficult, or at least doubtful, especially if there is a mixed culture.

- A negative post-mortem blood culture has a low negative predictive value and does not rule out the possibility of infection.
- The isolation of different bacterial species in the different tissues analysed, without correlation between them, indicates possible contamination
- A useful tip is that the pure isolation of a pathogen suggests infection, whereas a culture mixture of non-pathogenic bacteria is most likely due to post-mortem artefacts. However, this concept cannot be considered as an absolute indicator, and in some cases other confirmatory tests are required.
- Contaminated post-mortem cultures, similarly to what occurs in clinical microbiology, can be easily

Table 16.2 Additional sampling in particular situations. . (Reproduced by permission from Spring Nature: Fernández-Rodrigues et al. © Springer-Verlag Berlin Heidelberg 2015.)[6]

Clinical entity	Sample	Quantity	Transport container or medium	Type of tests
Septicaemia without an overt focus	Samples as indicated in Table 16.1 for bacteriology: mainly, blood plus 5 sterile tissues.	See Table 16.1	See Table 16.1	Tests focused on bacterial detection: direct bacterial culture, molecular analyses.
	Spleen, both lung, liver, heart	>1–2 cm³	Sterile tube/container	Mycology if immunosuppression or a fungal invasive disease is suspected
	Adrenal glands (if haemorrhagic)	>1–2 cm³	Sterile tube/container	Idem
	Skin biopsy (if petechiae)	>1–2 cm³	Sterile tube/container	Idem
	Serum	3–5 ml		Antigenic bacterial detection for *Neisseria meningitidis*, *S. pneumoniae*, *Haemophilus influenzae* serotype b, *Streptococcus agalactiae*, and *S. pyogenes*
	Pharyngeal swab (if inflammation)	2 swabs	Flocked swab (Amies medium)	Direct bacterial culture. Antigenic detection for *S. pyogenes*
	Urine, kidney if suspicion of renal urinary origin	3–5 ml/>1–2 cm³		Direct bacterial culture
Pneumonia or clear respiratory infection	Portion of the zone affected of the lung: if not clear affectation, a portion of each lobule should be taken separately	>1–2 cm³	Sterile tube/container	Direct bacterial culture and molecular analyses including respiratory viruses as well as *B. pertussis*
	Urine (children older >6 years)	3–5 ml	Sterile tube	Antigenic analyses (*S. pneumoniae*)
	Pleural liquid if empyema	3–5 ml	Sterile tube	Direct bacterial culture and molecular analyses (16S sequencing if negative culture)
	Swabbing the affected mucosae: pharyngeal, larynx, bronchial	2 (each)	Flocked swab (Amies medium)	Direct bacterial culture and molecular analyses (including *B. pertussis* in the nasopharyngeal swab)
	If flu: in the nasopharyngeal swab	2	Flocked swab (Amies medium)	Antigenic analyses (Influenza) and molecular analyses (respiratory viruses)
Bacterial peritonitis	Peritoneal fluid	3–5 ml	Sterile container (preferably anaerobic)	Direct bacterial culture aerobic and anaerobic Molecular analyses if negative culture
Soft-tissue infection	Aspiration with syringe of affected area and swabbing of lesions	3–5 ml 2 swabs	Sterile tube Flocked swab Amies medium	All samples: Direct bacterial culture aerobic and anaerobic Molecular analyses (16S sequencing) if negative culture
	Tissue sample of affected muscle	1–2 cm³	Sterile tube/container	All samples: Direct bacterial culture aerobic and anaerobic Molecular analyses (16S sequencing) if negative culture
Meningoencephalitis and myelitis	CSF, brain	3–5 ml, 1–2 cm³	Sterile tube	Direct bacterial culture and molecular analyses (bacterial and viruses). Antigenic analysis in CSF if bacterial meningitis suspicion
	Middle ears swab (after opening the petrous bones	2	Flocked swab Amies medium	Direct bacterial culture
	Pharyngeal exudates and faeces (if viral encephalitis is suspected)	2 swabs,/3–5 ml	Flocked swab Amies medium/ Sterile tube container	Molecular analyses (to detect excretion of neurotropic viruses)

Condition	Sample	Volume	Container	Analyses
Endocarditis	Sample obtained of the friable vegetations	1–2 cm³	Sterile tube/container	Direct bacterial culture, molecular analyses
Fulminant Hepatitis	Liver	1–2 cm³	Sterile tube/container	Molecular analyses (hepatitis viruses, CMV, EBV)
Abscesses	Purulent exudate (aspiration or swabbing)	1–3 ml	Sterile tube/Flocked swab (Amies medium)	Direct bacterial culture and molecular analyses
Chorioamnionitis	Samples of membranes, ovular membranes, fetal lung, amniotic fluid	1–2 cm³		Direct bacterial culture Molecular analyses
Congenital/perinatal infections: Toxoplasmosis, congenital CMV, congenital syphilis	CSF	1–3 ml		All samples: Direct bacterial culture. Molecular analyses including TORCH pathogens (Toxoplasma, Rubella, CMV, Herpes simplex, syphilis, Coxsackie, Zika etc.)
	Brain	1–2 cm³		
	If suspicion of congenital CMV, also urine and amniotic fluid (prenatal)	1–3 ml each		
	Serum	1–3 ml each		Serology (TORCH pathogens). If congenital syphilis: non-treponemal and treponemal assays in CSF/serum
	If meningitis or septic shock in neonates (<3 months)			PCR for S. agalactiae, Listeria monocytogenes
Tuberculosis	Tuberculoma (from lung or other tissue)	1–2 cm³	Sterile container	Mycobacterial culture and specific PCR
Malaria & other systemic parasitosis	Brain, liver, lung, myocardium,	1–2 cm³	Sterile container	In all samples: Specific parasite PCR
	Blood	1–3 ml	EDTA tube	In EDTA blood: Immunochromatography / ELISA / haemaglutination for Plasmodium spp. and other systemic parasites
Botulism	Faeces, exudates, tissues	1–3 ml/1–2 cm³	Sterile tube	Toxin detection, C. botulinum toxins PCR
Myocarditis confirmed by histopathology	Five pieces of myocardium tissue (2 in each ventricule, 1 in the septal wall near the apex)	5 pieces 1–2 cm³ each cryopreserved after autopsy	Sterile tube (plus RNA stabiliser)	Cardiotropic viruses molecular detection

CSF: cerebrospinal fluid; CMV: cytomegalovirus; PCR: polymerase chain reaction recognised in the laboratory because they present as polymicrobial growth.

- The isolation of pathogenic microorganisms such as *Neisseria meningitidis, Streptococcus pneumoniae*, Beta-haemolytic *Streptococcus* of Groups A or B, among others, in samples coming from sterile sites should always be reported. Semi-quantitative reports of these pathogenic bacteria are also useful for interpretation.

- The detection of some bacteria such as *Salmonella* spp. or *Mycobacterium tuberculosis*, that are not part of the normal human microbiota nor contaminants, is extremely significant.

- The presence of *Staphylococcus aureus* should always be reported, although on occasions it can be accompanied by coliforms, group *viridans* streptococci, and other microorganisms considered part of the post-mortem flora. The interpretation of the isolation of *S. aureus* is complex and should be evaluated in each case. *S. aureus* can be part of the flora, not only of the upper respiratory tract but also of skin, and therefore its finding could represent contamination during sampling.

- When a mixed culture is obtained, identifying all morphotypes that may correspond to pathogenic microorganisms is recommended.

- For each sterile fluid or tissue a semi-quantitative assessment of the amount of each of the different significant morphotypes isolated is suggested.

- Those microorganisms considered contaminants in sterile samples in clinical microbiology – a mixture of coliforms, negative coagulase *Staphylococci, viridans* group *streptococci, Enterococcus* spp., *Propionibacterium acnes* and *Bacillus* spp. different from *B. anthracis* – are also considered as such in post-mortem cultures; particularly, when in one given sample there are microorganisms from more than one of these groups.

- The isolation of gram-negative bacilli, especially when they are not in pure culture, should be evaluated in each case, as sometimes they will be contaminants (as they are part of the intestinal flora) but in others they will be responsible for acute infections. When they are isolated in pure culture or when they are the most abundant microorganism isolated from a mixture in a sterile tissue, they should be identified at species level and reported. Under such conditions, detection of the same strain in blood and other sterile specimens is

also considered of value. However, on such occasions, the final significance should be established according to the clinical background as well as the histopathological findings.

- On the contrary, the isolation in blood, or sterile tissues of most Enterobacteriaceae and other gram-negative bacilli, except *Salmonella spp., Shigella spp.* and other pathogens), as a part of a mixed flora (rather than as predominant organism), suggest a pattern of contamination, although their final interpretation requires external data. In such cases the isolation of one of these species should be reported as 'presence of coliforms', and the presence of more than one of these species as 'a mixture of coliforms'.

- It should be assumed that the lung post-mortem flora may include commensals from the upper respiratory tract. A semi-quantitative estimation of the presence of potential respiratory pathogens should be included in the report. The isolation of the same pathogen in more than one lobe and its relative amount should be taken into account for interpretation purposes, even when isolated together with commensal flora.

- Sometimes, some sterile specimens, not only of respiratory origin, can yield commensal flora from upper respiratory pathways. This should be reflected in the report, and can represent post-mortem dissemination, which may have been favoured by cardiopulmonary resuscitation.

Interpretation Criteria for Molecular Analyses

Molecular techniques offer the advantage over culture methods of their high sensitivity to detect pathogens. However, careful interpretation of molecular analyses in post-mortem specimens is required. When these techniques are used to detect viruses, precaution is essential, particularly when dealing with viruses prone to latency or persistence, although in such cases their negativity may exclude an active infection. The possibility of sample degradation affecting the detection of nucleic acids and therefore compromising the molecular detection of pathogens should also be considered. As far as respiratory viruses are concerned, their prolonged detection of some of them should be kept in mind, as sometimes their detection can be consistent with past infection, more than an active one.[5]

Another fact to evaluate when interpreting the post-mortem analyses is the possible degradation of forensic samples, which may also alter nucleic acids structure. Inadequate sample conservation or shipment to the laboratory can compromise further analyses. This can affect PCR results, yielding higher threshold cycles than expected, or even negative results. Detection of RNA viruses is also a challenge due to the easy degradation of this nucleic acid. However, degradation issues can be minimised by adding some stabiliser buffers (such as RNA-later) to the specimens at the moment of the sampling.

Paraffin sections of formalin-embedded tissues should only be considered for PMM when they are the only available specimen. Particular care should be taken when interpreting the molecular results obtained from them, as formalin can cause partial or total inhibition of PCR analyses, even yielding false negative results. However, the use of buffered formalin can improve the results, reducing these phenomena.[5]

References

1. Prtak L, Al-Adnani M, Fenton P, Kudesia G, Cohen MC. Contribution of bacteriology and virology in sudden unexpected death in infancy. *Arch Dis Child*, 2010; **95**:371–6.

2. Weber M., Klein N., Hartley J., Lock P., Malone M., Sebire N. Infection and sudden unexpected death in infancy: a systematic retrospective case review. *Lancet*, 2008 **371** (.9627):1848–53.

3. Saegeman V, Cohen MC, Alberola J, Ziyade N, Farina C, How is post-mortem microbiology appraised by pathologists? Results from a practice survey conducted by ESGFOR. *Eur J Clin Microbiol Infect Dis*, 2017; **36**:1381–5.

4. *Sudden Unexpected Death in Infancy and Childhood: Multi-agency Guidelines for Care and Investigation*, 2nd edn. London: The Royal College of Pathologists, 2016,

5. Alberola J, Cohen MC, Fernández-Rodríguez A. Procedimientos en Microbiología Clínica: análisis microbiológico post-mortem. SEIMC, 2012: **43**: https://www.seimc.org/contenidos/documentoscientificos/procedimientosmicrobiologia/seimc-procedimientomicrobiologia43.pdf (accessed 30 October 2018).

6. Fernández-Rodríguez A, Cohen MC, Lucena J, Van de Voorde W, Angelini A, Ziyade N, Saegeman V. How to optimise the yield of forensic and clinical post-mortem microbiology with an adequate sampling: a proposal for standardisation. *Eur J Clin Microbiol Infect Dis*, 2015; **34**:1045–57.

7. Cohen M. Fetal, perinatal, and infant autopsies. In: Burton J and Rutty G, eds. *The Hospital Autopsy: A Manual of Fundamental Autopsy Practice*. London: Hodder Arnold, 2010: 184–202.

8. Morris JA, Harrison LM, Partridge SM. Practical and theoretical aspects of postmortem bacteriology. *Curr Diagn Pathol*, 2007; **13**:65–74.

9. Pryce JW, Weber WA, Hartley JC, Ashworth MT, Malone, Sebire NJ. Difficulties in interpretation of post-mortem microbiology results in unexpected infant death: evidence from a multidisciplinary survey, *J Clin Pathol*, 2011; **64**:706–10.

10. Roberts FJ. A review of postmortem bacteriological cultures. *Can Med Assoc J*, 1969; **100**:70.

11. Lobmaier IVK, Vege Å, Gaustad P, Rognum TO. Bacteriological investigation-significance of time lapse after death. *Eur J of Clin Microbiol and Inf Dis*, 2009; **28**:1191–8.

12. Weber MA, Sebire NJ. Postmortem investigation of sudden unexpected death in infancy: current issues and autopsy protocol. *Diagn Histopathol*. 2009; **15**:510–23.

13. Sunagawa K, Sugitani M. Post-mortem detection of bacteremia using pairs of blood culture samples. *Leg Med (Tokyo)*, 2017; **24**:92–7.

14. Post-mortem microbiology in sudden death: sampling protocols proposed in different clinical settings. Fernández-Rodríguez A, Burton JL, Andreoletti L, Alberola J, Fornes P, Merino I, Martínez MJ, Castillo P, Sampaio-Maia B, Caldas IM, Saegeman V, Cohen MC; ESGFOR and the ESP. *Clin Microbiol Infect*. 2018; 51198–743X (18)30583–4. doi:10.1016/j.cmi.2018.08.009. [Epub ahead of print] Review.

The Investigation of Poisoning in Infants and Young Children

Robert J. Flanagan

Introduction

Although the vast majority of sudden unexpected deaths in infancy (SUDI/SUID, also known as Sudden Infant Death Syndrome – SIDS) in the Western world are not due to poisoning, exclusion of poisoning as the cause of death is nevertheless a vital part of investigating every such death.[1,2] This being said, toxicological and indeed some biochemical investigations in neonates, infants, and young children pose special problems. Although even in adults it is impossible to look for all poisons in all samples, in the case of infants and young children sample availability and sample size are almost inevitably limited, which may restrict the range of analyses that can be performed. Moreover, many drugs and other poisons, for example carbon monoxide, ethanol, and methadone[3–7] are very toxic in infants, in part because of their small size. Hence good communication with the laboratory as to any case-specific information to help guide the analysis is especially vital (Box 17.1).

It is usually advisable to contact the laboratory by telephone in advance to discuss urgent or complicated cases, if indeed complexities are apparent initially. Second, because when investigating the possibility of poisoning in children any significant findings are likely to have medicolegal implications,[9] chain-of-custody (sample security) procedures should be instituted from the outset (Box 17.2). This is again especially important since sample size restrictions usually mean that an analysis once performed cannot be repeated, and in non-fatal cases the analysis is likely to be performed by a hospital as opposed to a forensic laboratory. Finally, such samples should be protected during transport by the use of tamper-evident seals and should, ideally, be submitted in person to the laboratory by the coroner's officer or other investigating personnel.

An important aspect of all clinical work in infants and children is the ability to keep an open mind as regards the aetiology of unexpected or unusual presentations[10,11] (see Table 17.1). While in SUDI/SUID sending samples for toxicology/post-mortem biochemistry may be automatic (see Table 17.2), failure to notify the laboratory of a suspected agent, for example, may lead to that agent not being looked for if not part of the laboratory's routine 'screening' repertoire, a repertoire that is inevitably targeted towards substances commonly and sometimes not-so-commonly encountered after self-poisoning or substance abuse in adults. Carbon monoxide (as carboxyhaemoglobin), lithium, and warfarin are examples of poisons that are not looked for routinely and thus poisoning with these compounds may be missed even if toxicology screening is performed.[4,12]

A further complication is that the effects of chronic unauthorised drug administration or overdosage in children may be hard to detect. With paracetamol, for example, acute overdosage is normally without serious sequelae in children, but fatal liver damage may occur after chronic over-administration and plasma paracetamol may be 'therapeutic' or not detectable on presentation.[14] Even detection of an unusual or unexpected substance in a biological sample does not prove poisoning unless there is a clear mechanism of toxicity and quantitative information as to the duration and intensity of exposure can be provided.[15] In the case of neonates there may be concerns as to the role of drugs transferred from mother either *in utero*, or via breastmilk; in older children environmental considerations may be important, such as whether illicit drugs are used in a household, and in still older children there may be issues such as volatile substance abuse (VSA) or even deliberate self-poisoning. Iatrogenic poisoning is an especial risk in children, because first, young children are especially susceptible to the toxicity of certain compounds as noted above, and second, doses may have to be calculated on a body weight or body surface area basis giving great potential for error.

- Name, address, and telephone number of clinician/pathologist and/or coroner's officer (or equivalent), and address to which the report and invoice are to be sent. A post-mortem or registration number may also be appropriate.
- Circumstances of incident (including copy of sudden death report if available).
- Past medical history, including current or recent prescription medication, details of drugs available in the home, and relevant medical history of any parent/carer.
- Information on the likely cause, and estimated time, of ingestion/death and the nature and quantity of any substance(s) implicated.
- If the patient has been treated in hospital, a summary of the relevant hospital notes should be supplied to include details of emergency treatment and drugs given, including drugs given incidentally during investigative procedures.[8]
- Note of occupation of parents, hobbies, etc.
- A copy of any preliminary pathology report, if available.

- Name of the individual collecting the specimen
- Name of each person or entity subsequently having custody of it, and details of how it has been stored
- Date(s) the specimen was collected or transferred
- Specimen or post-mortem number
- Name of the subject or deceased
- Brief description of the specimen
- Record of the condition of tamper-evident seals

Finally, the possibility of either accidental, or deliberate overdosage of drugs given with therapeutic or indeed malicious intent may have to be considered.[16–22] Such instances may be rare but may consume vast resources, are usually very difficult to diagnose, may be associated with profound morbidity in the victims that can extend over years,[12,23] and may encompass not only pets,[24] but also adults in the family.[25]

Sample Collection, Transport, and Storage

Sampling for post-mortem biochemistry and toxicology is not always straightforward, yet is of vital importance if all subsequent analytical work is not to be invalidated. Some general guidelines as regards sample collection based on those for adults are given in Table 17.3. The use of disposable hard plastic (polystyrene) Sterilin™ tubes is recommended. If these are not available, then containers with secure closures appropriate to the specimen volumes being collected should be used, i.e. excessive headspace in the container should be avoided if possible. Preservatives should not be used except addition of 2% (w/v) sodium fluoride to a portion of (preferably) femoral blood. Some laboratories provide specimen containers for collecting post-mortem blood, urine, and other specimens. Vitreous humour is preferred for much post-mortem biochemistry because it lies in a relatively protected part of the body and is less susceptible to post-mortem change than fluids such as blood. For liver samples, the right lobe is preferred as this is furthest from the gastrointestinal tract.

All organ and tissue samples, and any tablet bottles, or scene residues, should be placed in separate containers to minimise the risk of cross-contamination of samples such as blood or vitreous humour during transport to the laboratory. When death has occurred in hospital any residual ante-mortem specimens should be obtained as a matter of urgency from the Accident and Emergency Department or pathology laboratory (not only chemical pathology and haematology, but also immunology, transfusion medicine, and virology departments may be a source of such specimens). Note that the availability of such samples should not preclude appropriate sampling at autopsy unless hospitalisation was prolonged. Intravenous giving sets, used syringes, etc. should be seized if it is thought possible that there may have been a drug administration error or that unauthorised drugs have been given.

Collecting blood by needle aspiration from a peripheral site prior to opening the body and after ligating the blood vessel proximally may help minimise the risk

Table 17.1 Some laboratory investigations commonly requested on blood, plasma, or serum that may arouse suspicion of poisoning

Investigation	Possible cause of increase	Possible cause of decrease
Sodium	MDMA [#] (malignant hyperthermia), sodium salts	Diuretics, water intoxication (acute and chronic), MDMA (very rare)
Potassium	Digoxin, potassium salts	Diuretics, laxatives (both chronic), insulin, salbutamol, sulfonylureas, theophylline
Glucose	Salicylates, theophylline	Ethanol (especially children), insulin, salicylates, sulfonylureas, valproate
Calcium	–	Ethylene glycol, fluorides, magnesium salts
Chloride	Bromide or organobromines (actually interference in method)	–
Lactate	Ethylene glycol (artefact on some blood gas analysers)	–
Magnesium	Magnesium salts	–
International normalised ratio (INR, prothrombin time)	Anticoagulant rodenticides (warfarin, brodifacoum), paracetamol (early marker of hepatic damage)	–
Anion gap ($[Na^+] + [K^+]) - ([HCO_3^-] + [Cl^-]$)	Ethanol, ethylene glycol, iron salts, isoniazid, methanol, metformin, paraldehyde, salicylates, toluene (chronic)	–
Osmolar gap [&]	Acetone, ethanol, ethylene glycol, methanol, 2-propanol, hypertonic i.v. solutions (e.g. mannitol)	–

[#] MDMA: Methylenedioxymethamphetamine

[&] Measured osmolality (freezing point depression) – calculated osmolality. Calculated osmolality = $2([Na^+] + [K^+])$ + urea + glucose (all mmol/L)

Table 17.2 Some biological samples required when investigating SUDI/SUID (modified from RCPath 2016[13])

Sample (volume)	Handling	Test
Blood (serum) (1–2 mL)	Centrifuge, store serum at −20 °C [#]	Toxicology
Urine (20 mL if available)	Centrifuge, store supernatant at −20 °C [#]	Toxicology and specialised tests for inherited metabolic diseases
Blood from Guthrie card	Ensure circle is filled. Do not put in plastic bag	Tests for inherited metabolic diseases
Skin biopsy	After discussion with paediatrician and laboratory	Tests for inherited metabolic disease, e.g. fatty oxidation flux in fibroblast culture
Muscle biopsy	After discussion with paediatrician and laboratory	If history suggests mitochondrial disorder

[#] Tightly capped with minimal headspace, but do not overfill

of sample contamination with central blood,[27,28] but will not account for changes that may have occurred during attempted resuscitation, for example. However, such precautions are not always taken (even proper documentation of the site of blood collection may be lacking) and blood sampling from a central site such as the heart, or even collection of 'cavity blood' (blood remaining in the body cavity when the organs have been removed), is not uncommon. This latter practice carries the risk of contamination of the 'blood' specimen with fluids from other sources. Sampling through tissues containing high concentrations of analyte may also lead to sample contamination. For many poisons, the blood concentrations associated with severe

Table 17.3 Sample requirements: general post-mortem biochemistry and toxicology [i]

Sample	Notes [ii]
Heart whole blood (right ventricle)	20 mL unpreserved (qualitative toxicology only) unless no other blood sample available, plain tube
Jugular vein whole blood [*]	20 mL unpreserved (qualitative toxicology only) unless no other blood sample available, plain tube
Peripheral whole blood [*]	20 mL from femoral or other peripheral site ensuring no contamination from urine or from central or cavity blood. Collect one portion into 2% w/v sodium fluoride and another into a plain tube
Urine [*]	20–50 mL if available, plain tube, no preservative unless a portion required for ethanol measurement
Gastric contents [iii]	25–50 mL, plain bottle, no preservative; keep a note of total volume
Vitreous humour	Maximum available, plain tube, separate specimens from each eye if feasible. Avoid excessive suction to minimise risk of aspirating retinal fragments. Collect one portion into 2% w/v sodium fluoride if for ethanol measurement
Cerebrospinal fluid	5–10 mL, plain tube
Pericardial fluid	Maximum available, plain tube
Synovial fluid [iv]	Maximum available, plain tube
Bile	Maximum available, plain tube
Liver and other tissues	Liver 10 g (deep inside right lobe), other tissues 10 g as appropriate, plain bottles [v]
Scene residues [vi]	As appropriate

[*] : these may be difficult to obtain in an infant

[i] See Belsey and Flanagan[26] and Dinis-Oliveira et al.[27] for detailed discussion on samples and sampling with especial reference to post-mortem biochemistry and forensic toxicology, respectively

ii Smaller volumes may often be acceptable, for example in the case of infants and very young children

iii Includes vomit, gastric lavage (stomach washout, first sample), etc.

iv Alternative if vitreous humour not available.

v As there is little information on drug distribution within solid tissues in man, collection of approximately 10 g specimens from several sites from organs such as the brain is recommended if the whole organ is available.

vi Tablet bottles, drinks containers, aerosol canisters, etc. should be packed entirely separately from biological samples, especially if poisoning with volatiles is a possibility to minimise the risk of cross-contamination

toxicity are very low, typically in the mg/L (parts per million) or even µg/L (parts per billion) range and thus even trace contamination of a peripheral blood sample with gastric contents or urine, for example, can confound the most careful analytical work. In such instances, toxicological analysis can often do little more than provide evidence of exposure to a particular substance.

As to the analysis of hair, it has been claimed that segmental analysis of head hair can give a record of drug/poison exposure dating back months or even years (head hair in adults grows on average at the rate of 1 cm/month). However, in reality there are issues such as the possibility of surface contamination, of incidental exposure in the homes of drug users, of loss of analyte by washing hair, etc. Even widely-used laboratory solvent washing procedures, said to 'decontaminate' hair by removing analyte on the hair surface prior to segmentation, have been shown to simply move analyte from the surface into the matrix of the hair.[29] Added to this is the fact that it

is impossible to estimate dose let alone biological effect from hair analysis alone. Thus, qualitative information as to drug/poison exposure that has to be viewed in the context of all the information available in a given case is usually all that can be gleaned.[6,17]

General Discussion

Poisoning in Children: Compounds Encountered

Fatal poisoning in children aged <10 years is now very rare in England and Wales[30,31] (Figure 17.1; Tables 17.4 and 17.5). Much of the decline in such deaths is due to improved fire safety in the home and elsewhere, but improved medicines safety (child-resistant closures, safer drugs, safer prescribing, improved poisons information/treatment) as well environmental safety (e.g. removal of leaded paints) has also been important. Against this is the increase in substance abuse, as reflected in the relatively high numbers of

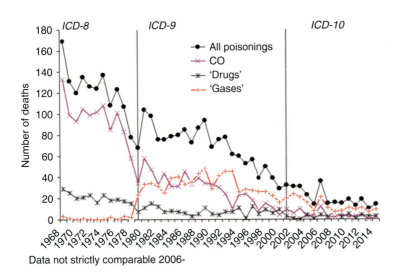

Figure 17.1 Annual numbers of deaths from poisoning aged <10 yr: England & Wales, 1968–2015

Reproduced from Handley and Flanagan[31] with permission of Taylor & Francis Ltd., www.tandfonline.com/ (N.B. 'Drugs' = poisons other than carbon monoxide and fire gases, 'Gases' = fire gases.)

Table 17.4 Drug-related poisoning deaths aged <10 yr, England & Wales, 1993–2015: age and sex

Age (years)	Male	Female
< 1	8	4
1	10	4
2	11	8
3	3	5
4	2	3
5	3	3
6	1	1
7	1	0
8	2	0
9	1	3
Totals	42	31

methadone-related deaths in England & Wales in recent years.[3] Moreover, annual numbers of non-accidental fatal poisonings in this age group were relatively constant 1968–2000 and thus in 2000 comprised a far higher proportion of fatal poisonings than in 1968.[30]

Study of fatal 'drug' poisoning data for England and Wales, 1993–2015 (poisons other than carbon monoxide and fire gases) in those aged < 10 year reveals a preponderance of deaths in males (42 vs 31) and a preponderance of deaths in those aged <3 year (45 vs 28) (Table 17.4). Of these 73 deaths,

25 were recorded as assaults, 12 as intentional self-poisoning or 'undetermined intent' (i.e. it was not clear how poisoning had occurred), and 36 as unintentional poisoning. The data include unintentional poisoning with prescribed drugs given in therapy, for example sodium nitroprusside (Table 17.5). As to the other agents involved, given that of the 10 deaths from dosulepin poisoning, 9 occurred 1993–2004, with one in 2102, the preponderance of methadone-related deaths (23 deaths, 32% of all drug poisoning deaths in this age group, 1993–2015) in such deaths in the last few years is clear (14, 1993–2004; 9, 2005–2015).[3]

Some of the problems of investigating poisoning in infants and young children have been summarised above. A further issue is that with the fragmentation of services there are no central laboratories in the UK that specialise in paediatric toxicology analogous to those that specialise in the diagnosis of inborn errors of metabolism, for example. Thus, requests for drugs or poisons screening in patients usually either go to hospital laboratories that will have variable capability in the scope and sensitivity of the analyses available, or if there is a clear need to involve the police or social services then a forensic service provider might become involved, although this does not necessarily ensure that testing is appropriate. Only in the case of a death outside hospital will an analysis go to a forensic laboratory, although this may be a hospital laboratory contracted to provide coroner toxicology services. Be

Table 17.5 Drug-related poisoning deaths aged <10 yr, England & Wales, 1993–2015: agents involved

Agent	No of deaths (no of deaths without other drugs or alcohol)
Amitriptyline	1 (1)
Amoxapine	1 (1)
Carbamazepine	1 (1)
'Chemotherapy drug'	1 (1)
Chloroform	1 (0)
Chloroquine	1 (!)
Codeine	1 (0)
Cyanide	3 (3)
Desmopressin	1 (1)
Dextropropoxyphene	1 (0)
Diamorphine/morphine	4 (2)
Dihydrocodeine	1 (1)
Dosulepin	10 (10)
'Drug'	1 (1)
Insulin	3 (2)
Iron	5 (5)
Methadone	23 (22)
Mirtazapine	1 (0)
Narcotic	1 (1)
Paracetamol	4 (2)
Phenytoin	2 (2)
Potassium	2 (0)
Quinine	1 (1)
Sodium chloride	2 (2)
Sodium nitroprusside	1 (1)
Thiopental	2 (0)
Tramadol	3 (2)
Vecuronium	1 (1)
Volatile substance abuse	1 (1)
Zopiclone	1 (0)
Total	**81 (65)**

Table 17.6 Commonly available urinary immunoassays for detection of substance abuse

Drug/Drug Group	Screening cut-off (limit of detection, μg/L)
Amphetamines (includes methamphetamine)	300
Barbiturates	200
Benzodiazepines	200
Cannabinoids	50
Cocaine metabolite (benzoylecgonine)	300
Methadone	300
Opiates (includes diamorphine/morphine)	300

Note that this latter table is only a summary and that many more compounds can be detected using these instruments, given an appropriate sample collected at an appropriate time after a pharmacologically active dose.

Malicious Poisoning

As noted above, poisoning is one way by which an illness can be fabricated or induced in a child by a carer.[35–37] The children affected are often hospitalised for long periods and may endure repetitive, painful, and expensive diagnostic attempts. Death may occur. A vast range of substances have been reported in such cases (Table 17.8), many of which (e.g. bleach, chlorpyriphos, cyanoacrylate adhesive, pepper, pine oil) will not show up on general toxicology screening of biological samples such as plasma and urine. Clinical suspicion and careful detective work, often with psychiatric input, is required in such cases. There have been tragedies such as that perpetrated by paediatric nurse Beverly Allitt.[38,39] It is beyond doubt that some cases escape detection with incalculable consequences for the victims.

Poisoning with common salt can be particularly difficult to diagnose and can even occur in a designated place of safety.[40] Common criteria used to diagnose salt poisoning focus on hypernatraemia, with high urinary concentrations of sodium and chloride. However, high urinary concentrations of sodium alone cannot distinguish salt poisoning from dehydration. The medical and legal implications of the two conditions are fundamentally different, so reliable ways to distinguish between them are

this as it may, analytical repertoires vary between laboratories.[32] This being said, with some clear exceptions as discussed above, most laboratories entrusted with this type of work will offer at the very least an immunoassay screen in urine for some groups of commonly misused drugs (Table 17.6) and a more comprehensive service nowadays usually using gas- and/or liquid chromatography linked to mass spectrometry (GC-MS and/or LC-MS)[33,34] (Table 17.7).

Table 17.7 Some drugs detectable on GC-MS and/or LC-MS screening of blood/urine within 24–48 hours of exposure (doses given in therapy)

Analgesics	Antidepressants	Anticonvulsants	Antipsychotics	Stimulants
Diclofenac	Amitriptyline	Carbamazepine	Amisulpride	Amphetamine
Ibuprofen	Citalopram	Lamotrigine	Aripirazole	Benzylpiperazine (BZP)
Lidocaine	Desipramine	Phenytoin	Chlorpromazine	Caffeine
Naproxen	Dosulepin	Topiramate	Clozapine	Cathine
Nefopam	Fluoxetine		Olanzapine	Cocaine
Paracetamol	Imipramine			Ephedrine
	Mirtazapine			Ketamine
	Nortriptyline			Methylenedioxyamphetamine (MDA)
	Paroxetine			Methylenedioxyethametamine (MDEA)
	Sertraline			Methylenedioxymethamphetamine (MDMA)
	Trazodone			
	Venlafaxine			Mephedrone
				Methamphetamine

Opiates/opioids	Other therapeutic drugs	
Codeine	Alverine	Methiopropamine
Dextropropoxyphene	Atracurium (as laudanosine)	Methylphenidate
Diamorphine/morphine	Atropine	Pseudoephedrine
Dihydrocodeine	Chlorphenamine	Trifluoromethylphenylpiperazine (TFMPP)
Methadone	Clomethiazole	
Oxycodone	Cyclizine	
Pethidine	Diltiazem	
Tramadol	Diphenhydramine	
	Promethazine	
Benzodiazepines	Propofol	
Chlordiazepoxide	Propranolol	
Diazepam	Zolpidem	
Nordazepam	Zopiclone	

needed.[41] Be this as it may, both salt poisoning and dehydration (caused by neglect) may lead to criminal or civil action. Fractional excretions (the proportions of sodium and water filtered at the glomerulus that subsequently reach the urine), calculated from the sodium and creatinine concentrations of paired plasma and associated ('spot') urine samples, can distinguish the two situations (Box 17.3). The values should be >2% in an individual who has been poisoned with salt and is volume replete and <1% when dehydrated, but with viable renal tubules. Note that the units of measurement used must be the same for plasma and urine (plasma creatinine is usually reported in μmol/L, while urine creatinine is often reported in mmol/L).

In adults, poisoning with ethylene glycol and with methanol often presents with a high anion gap metabolic acidosis, but the diagnosis is often missed.[43] Covert poisoning with ethylene glycol in children is another difficult diagnosis that may sometimes mimic an inherited metabolic disorder and may be detected by the presence of its metabolite glycolic acid in urine.[44] However, there is a report of glycolic acid detection in blood leading to a false diagnosis of

Table 17.8 Some compounds/substances reported in malicious poisoning in children

Analgesics/antipyretics (paracetamol, salicylates)	Ethylene glycol
Anticoagulants (warfarin)	Gliafenin
Anticonvulsants (carbamazepine)	Household products (oven cleaner, bleach)
Antidepressants (amitriptyline, imipramine)	Inorganic salts (potassium chloride, sodium chloride, magnesium sulfate)
Antidiabetics (insulin, phenformin, sulfonylureas)	Ipecac
Antihistamines (diphenhydramine)	Ketamine
Barbiturates (amylo/pheno/ secobarbital)	Laxatives (phenolphthalein)
Benzodiazepines (clonazepam, diazepam, midazolam, temazepam)	Lidocaine
Carbon monoxide	Methaqualone
Chloral hydrate	Opioids (codeine, methadone, propoxyphene)
Chlorpyriphos	Pancuronium
Clonidine	Paraquat
Clozapine	Pepper
Cyanide	Phenothiazines (alimemazine, chlorpromazine)
Cyanoacrylate adhesive	Phenylpropanolamine
Digoxin	Pine oil
Diuretics (furosemide, chlorthalidone)	Vitamin A
Doxylamine	Water
Ethanol	Xanthines (caffeine, theophylline)

BOX 17.3 Derivation of the fractional excretion of sodium (FE_{Na}) and water (FE_{H2O}) (adapted from Coulthard & Haycock[42] with Permission from BMJ Publishing Group Ltd.)

Fractional excretion of water, FE_{H2O}

- The FE_{H2O} is the volume of electrolyte-free water that appears as urine compared with the amount filtered
- Thus, $FE_{H2O} = V / GFR$
- Since $GFR = U_{Cr} \times V / P_{Cr}$
- $FE_{H2O} = V \times P_{Cr} / U_{Cr} \times V$
- Simplifying, $FE_{H2O} = P_{Cr} / U_{Cr}$ (then multiply by 100 to express as a percentage)

Fractional excretion of sodium, FE_{Na}

- The FE_{Na} is the amount of sodium lost in the urine compared to the amount filtered
- Thus, FE_{Na} = urinary sodium excretion/filtered sodium
- The urinary sodium excretion = $U_{Na} \times V$
- And the filtered sodium = $P_{Na} \times GFR$
- Since $GFR = U_{Cr} \times V / P_{Cr}$
- The filtered sodium = $P_{Na} \times U_{Cr} \times V / P_{Cr}$
- Therefore, $FE_{Na} = U_{Na} \times V \times P_{Cr} / P_{Na} \times U_{Cr} \times V$
- Simplifying, $FE_{Na} = U_{Na} / P_{Na} \times P_{Cr} / U_{Cr}$ (then multiply by 100 to express as a percentage)

Key: FE_{H2O}: Fractional excretion of water; V: Urine flux rate; GFR: Glomerular fractional rate; U: urinary; P: plasma; Cr: creatinine; Na: Sodium; FE_{Na}: Fractional excretion of sodium.

ethylene glycol intoxication. Only at the third admission, 2 years after the first, was the possibility of an underlying metabolic disorder considered and further investigation revealed a deficiency of complex I in the mitochondrial oxidative phosphorylation chain.[45] Misidentification of propionic acid as ethylene glycol in a patient with methylmalonic acidaemia has also been reported.[46] Clearly these misdiagnoses have serious implications not only for the health of the children concerned, but also for one, or more carers, especially if the child dies.

Finally, some carers will become obsessed with a belief that a child is being poisoned even though there is no evidence of somatic disease.[47] Such obsessions can result in mental and physical harm to the child as a result of sometimes years of unnecessary worry and investigation and must be considered a form of factitious or induced illness. Repeated comprehensive toxicological investigation can help by demonstrating the absence of specific poisons, or by showing that exposure to a specific agent such as blood lead is not unusual/worrying as compared to other apparently healthy members of the community.

Conclusions

The diagnosis of poisoning in childhood may be straightforward if the history is clear and appropriate biological samples are available for analysis. Unfortunately, reality is often different, and suspicion is all. If the diagnosis is uncertain, screening for possible poisons may be complicated because of problems of small sample size, the wide range of compounds that may be encountered, that poisoning may be chronic rather than acute, and the fact that some poisons are extremely toxic in young children. Vigilance and resources are still needed to deal with the problems caused by the increase in the prevalence of substance abuse, and with mental health issues that may become manifest as fabricated or factitious illness in a child.

References

1. Bajanowski T, Vennemann M, Bohnert M, et al; GeSID Group. Unnatural causes of sudden unexpected deaths initially thought to be Sudden Infant Death Syndrome. *Int J Legal Med*, 2005; **119**:213–16.

2. Morley SR, Becker J, Al-Adnani M, Cohen MC. Drug- and alcohol-related deaths at a pediatric institution in the United Kingdom. *Am J Forensic Med Pathol*, 2012; **330**:390–4.

3. Anderson M, Hawkins L, Eddleston M, et al. Severe and fatal pharmaceutical poisoning in young children in the UK. *Arch Dis Child*, 2016; **101**:653–6.

4. Omalu BI, Lindner JL, Janssen JK, et al. The role of environmental factors in the causation of sudden death in infants: two cases of sudden unexpected death in two unrelated infants who were cared for by the same babysitter. *J Forensic Sci*, 2007; **52**:1355–8.

5. Lamminpää A. Alcohol intoxication in childhood and adolescence. *Alcohol Alcohol*, 1995; **30**:5–12.

6. Tournel G, Pollard J, Humbert L, et al. Use of hair testing to determine methadone exposure in pediatric deaths. *J Forensic Sci*, 2014; **59**:1436–40.

7. Paul AB, Simms L, Mahesan AM. The toxicology of methadone-related death in infants under 1 year: Three case series and review of the literature. *J Forensic Sci*, 2017; **62**(5):1414–17.

8. Flanagan RJ, Saynor DA, Raper SM. Sedation for neurological investigations in children may interfere with toxicological analyses. *Lancet*, 1980; **1**(8172):830.

9. Dinis-Oliveira RJ, Magalhães T. Children intoxications: what is abuse and what is not abuse. *Trauma Violence Abuse*, 2013; **14**:113–32.

10. Flanagan RJ, Huggett A, Saynor DA, et al. Value of toxicological investigation in the diagnosis of acute drug poisoning in children. *Lancet*, 1981; **2**:682–5.

11. Hässler F, Zamorski H, Weirich S. The problem of differentiating between Sudden Infant Death Syndrome, fatal Munchausen's syndrome by proxy, and infanticide. *Z Kinder Jugendpsychiatr Psychother*, 2007; **35**:237–44; quiz 245–6.

12. Souid AK, Korins K, Keith D, Dubansky S, Sadowitz PD. Unexplained menorrhagia and hematuria: a case report of Munchausen's syndrome by proxy. *Pediatr Hematol Oncol*, 1993; **10**:245–8.

13. *Sudden Unexpected Death in Infancy and Childhood: Multi-agency Guidelines for Care and Investigation.* London: The Royal College of Pathologists, 2016,

14. Bauer M, Babel B, Giesen H, Patzelt D. Fulminant liver failure in a young child following repeated acetaminophen overdosing. *J Forensic Sci*, 1999; **44**:1299–303.

15. Lavezzi AM, Cappiello A, Termopoli V, et al. Sudden infant death with area postrema lesion likely due to wrong use of insecticide. *Pediatrics*, 2015; **136**:e1039–42.

16. White ST, Voter K, Perry J. Surreptitious warfarin ingestion. *Child Abuse Negl*, 1985; **9**:349–52.

17. Bartsch C, Risse M, Schütz H, et al. Munchausen syndrome by proxy (MSBP): an extreme form of child abuse with a special forensic challenge. *Forensic Sci Int*, 2003; **137**:147–51.

18. Holstege CP, Dobmeier SG. Criminal poisoning: Munchausen by proxy. *Clin Lab Med*, 2006; **26**:243–53.

19. Glatstein M, Garcia-Bournissen F, Scolnik D, Koren G, Finkelstein Y. Hypoglycemia in a healthy toddler. *Ther Drug Monit*, 2009; **31**:173–7.

20. Lee JC, Lin KL, Lin JJ, Hsia SH, Wu CT. Non-accidental chlorpyrifos poisoning – an unusual cause of profound unconsciousness. *Eur J Pediatr*, 2010; **169**:509–11.

21. Rajanayagam J, Bishop JR, Lewindon PJ, Evans HM. Paracetamol-associated acute liver failure in Australian and New Zealand children: high rate of medication errors. *Arch Dis Child*, 2015; **100**:77–80.

22. Gomila I, López-Corominas V, Pellegrini M, et al. Alimemazine poisoning as evidence of Munchausen syndrome by proxy: A pediatric case report. *Forensic Sci Int*, 2016; **266**:e18–22.

23. Wittkowski H, Hinze C, Häfner-Harms S, et al. Munchausen by proxy syndrome mimicking systemic autoinflammatory disease: case report and review of the literature. *Pediatr Rheumatol Online J*, 2017; **15**:19.

24. Munro HM, Thrusfield MV. 'Battered pets': Munchausen syndrome by proxy (factitious illness by proxy). *J Small Anim Pract*, 2001; **42**:385–9.

25. Vennemann B, Bajanowski T, Karger B, et al. Suffocation and poisoning – the hard-hitting side of Munchausen syndrome by proxy. *Int J Legal Med*, 2005; **119**:98–102.

26. Belsey SL, Flanagan RJ. Postmortem biochemistry: Current applications. *J Forensic Leg Med*, 2016; **41**:49–57.

27. Dinis-Oliveira RJ, Carvalho F, Duarte JA, et al. Collection of biological samples in forensic toxicology. *Toxicol Mech Methods*, 2010; **20**:363–414.

28. Lemaire E, Schmidt C, Denooz R, Charlier C, Boxho P. Postmortem concentration and redistribution of diazepam, methadone, and morphine with subclavian and femoral vein dissection/clamping. *J Forensic Sci*, 2016; **61**:1596–603

29. Cuypers E, Flinders B, Boone CM, et al. Consequences of decontamination procedures in forensic hair analysis using metal-assisted secondary ion mass spectrometry analysis. *Anal Chem*, 2016; **88**:3091–7.

30. Flanagan RJ, Rooney C, Griffiths C. Fatal poisoning in childhood, England and Wales 1968–2000. *Forensic Sci Int*, 2005; **148**:121–9.

31. Handley SA, Flanagan RJ. Drugs and other chemicals involved in fatal poisoning in England and Wales during 2000–2011. *Clin Toxicol (Phila)*, 2014; **52**:1–12.

32. Bréhin C, Cessans C, Monchaud C, et al. A pseudoencephalitis presentation of a pediatric non-intentional intoxication. *Eur J Paediatr Neurol*, 2016; **20**:418–20.

33. Flanagan RJ. Developing an analytical toxicology service: principles and guidance. *Toxicol Rev*, 2004; **23**:251–63.

34. Flanagan RJ. Postmortem biochemistry and toxicology. *Arab J Forensic Sci Forensic Med*, 2017; **1**:543–55.

35. Jones JG, Butler HL, Hamilton B, et al. Munchausen syndrome by proxy. *Child Abuse Negl*, 1986; **10**:33–40.

36. McClure RJ, Davis PM, Meadow SR, Sibert JR. Epidemiology of Munchausen syndrome by proxy, non-accidental poisoning, and non-accidental suffocation. *Arch Dis Child*, 1996; **75**:57–61.

37. Denny SJ, Grant CC, Pinnock R. Epidemiology of Munchausen syndrome by proxy in New Zealand. *J Paediatr Child Health*, 2001; **37**:240–3.

38. Repper J. Munchausen syndrome by proxy in healthcare workers. *J Adv Nurs*, 1995; **21**:299–304.

39. Marks V, Richmond C. Beverly Allitt: the nurse who killed babies. *J R Soc Med*, 2008; **101**:110–15.

40. Hospital admits errors as salt death mother jailed. *Daily Mail*, 25 February 2005; http://www.dailymail.co.uk/news/article-339204/Hospital-admits-errors-salt-death-mother-jailed.html (accessed 18 October 2018).

41. Wallace D, Lichtarowicz-Krynska E, Bockenhauer D. Non-accidental salt poisoning. *Arch Dis Child*, 2017; **102**:119–22.

42. Coulthard MG, Haycock GB, Distinguishing between salt poisoning, and hypernatraemic dehydration in children. *Br Med J*, 2003; **326**:157–60.

43. Jacobsen D, McMartin KE. Methanol and ethylene glycol poisonings. Mechanism of toxicity, clinical course, diagnosis, and treatment. *Med Toxicol*, 1986; **1**:309–34.

44. Woolf AD, Wynshaw-Boris A, Rinaldo P, Levy HL. Intentional infantile ethylene glycol poisoning presenting as an inherited metabolic disorder. *J Pediatr*, 1992; **120**:421–4.

45. Pien K, van Vlem B, van Coster R, et al. An inherited metabolic disorder presenting as ethylene glycol intoxication in a young adult. *Am J Forensic Med Pathol*, 2002; **23**:96–100.

46. Shoemaker JD, Lynch RE, Hoffmann JW, Sly WS. Misidentification of propionic acid as ethylene glycol in a patient with methylmalonic acidemia. *J Pediatr*, 1992; **120**:417–21.

47. Warner JO, Hathaway MJ. Allergic form of Meadow's syndrome (Munchausen by proxy). *Arch Dis Child*, 1984; **59**:151–6.

Chapter 18

Inherited Metabolic Disease and Sudden Unexplained Death in Infancy and Childhood: Post-mortem Samples and Investigations

Simon E. Olpin

Introduction

A coordinated plan of post-mortem investigations in cases of sudden unexpected death in infancy and childhood should include accurate clinical details and family history. Information on ethnicity, consanguinity, and previous obstetric history followed by physical examination and preliminary post-mortem findings should be assessed. This information, together with results from any pre-mortem biochemical and haematological testing may provide important clues that may help to direct the selective use of appropriate laboratory analysis. An unexplained death in an infant or child can be due to many non-metabolic causes but death due to a metabolic cause can be easily missed unless appropriate samples are taken and analysed. Any unexplained sudden death will include an infective cause as a key part of the differential diagnosis and this along with other non-metabolic causes of death must be carefully investigated and excluded wherever possible.[1,2]

Features that may suggest a metabolic cause of death include a range of dysmorphic features, some of which may suggest a specific diagnosis; e.g. microcephaly, micrognathia, anteverted nostrils, and syndactyly of second and third toes, strongly indicating the possibility of Smith-Lemli-Opitz syndrome (S-L-O).[3] Dysmorphology, particularly if it is subtle, is best assessed by a clinical geneticist. It is therefore important to carefully undertake an external examination, which must include careful evaluation and photographic documentation of any dysmorphic features.[4–7] These should be made available to the clinical geneticist when the case is discussed at a multidisciplinary meeting. Newer techniques such as PMCT or MRI may allow targeted biopsies in cases with limited consent, and in the future, some of the

subtle internal changes e.g. cerebral dysgenesis, agenesis of the corpus callosum and congenital heart anomalies may be amenable to detection by post-mortem MRI.[8–10] In cases of early neonatal death, assessment of the placenta may also yield vital information e.g. vacuolation of the syncytiotrophoblast may arise in a number of storage disorders.[11,12] Examination of tissue samples for fat deposition at an early stage of the post-mortem may give an indication for further investigations e.g. coarse vacuolation of renal tubular epithelium with fat deposition in proximal renal tubules, is highly suggestive of a fat oxidation defect.[13,14] Storage material in various organs and/or tissues may also offer other vital clues to a diagnosis.[15,16]

Samples

The collection of appropriate samples at post-mortem is of paramount importance in the investigation of metabolic disease. All too frequently, further investigations are requested in cases of unexplained death but appropriate samples are not available. It is essential to collect representative post-mortem samples and to discuss their analysis with a metabolic specialist.[14–18] Appropriate investigations on often very small samples of body fluids and tissues must be well coordinated if precious material is not to be used up unnecessarily.[14] In cases of expected death, whenever possible collect samples of blood, urine, and tissues prior to death. This applies especially to skeletal muscle biopsies and cerebrospinal fluid (CSF) for the investigation of suspected mitochondrial respiratory chain disease, as samples collected after death are highly susceptible to post-mortem deterioration.[19–22] Liver and other internal tissues undergo proteolysis quickly after death. Changes are apparent in mitochondria within two hours, and respiratory chain enzyme activity deteriorates rapidly. Consequently, for many biochemical analyses liver, heart, and skeletal muscle biopsies must be taken promptly if reliable results are to be obtained. Unless an autopsy is going to be conducted immediately, biopsies of internal organs for enzyme analysis, especially those for respiratory chain assay, should be done as soon after death as possible. Small open muscle and open liver biopsies are easily obtained.

It is most important to obtain a skin sample for fibroblast culture, as many of the enzymes known to be deficient in inborn errors of metabolism are expressed in fibroblasts, and this will frequently be the only tissue where functional confirmation of a suspected diagnosis or expression of candidate genes or protein can be investigated.[23–26] Cultured fibroblasts also provide important reference material for future prenatal diagnosis for the family concerned as these can be cryopreserved for an indefinite period in liquid nitrogen. If necessary, fibroblasts can be recovered from cryopreservation and investigated further at a later date should new information or improved techniques become available.

Urine

This should be collected by catheterisation or suprapubic puncture into a container with no preservative, as little as 100µL can be sufficient for organic acid analysis by gas chromatography mass spectrometry (GC-MS). If the sample is contaminated with blood, centrifuge the sample to remove the cells prior to freezing the urine at -20°C. Washing out the bladder with a small volume of sterile saline may also yield enough sample for organic acid analysis.

Blood

Liquid blood is frequently obtainable by cardiac puncture up to several days after death. If only small quantities of blood are available however, whole blood acylcarnitine analysis is likely to be the single most informative test that can be performed in spite of the potential problems of interpretation.[27] Spot a few drops of whole blood onto a filter paper (i.e. a Guthrie card), as this is the most convenient method of collection and, importantly, most suitable for uniformity of analytical technique. If more blood is available (in addition to the Guthrie card), collect up to 10 mL of heparinised blood as this can sometimes be successfully separated and the plasma stored at -20°C,

while the cells should be stored at $+4^0$C (*do not freeze*). If DNA analysis is likely to be required, collect a further 5 mL of whole blood (EDTA) and freeze immediately (at least -20^0C) until DNA is required. If death has occurred within the past hour or so, collect 5 mL of blood into a fluoride oxalate tube for the measurement of glucose, 3-hydroxybutyrate, and free fatty acids.

CSF

CSF may be useful in certain circumstances (e.g. organic acid analysis, acylcarnitine analysis), but is often only reliably informative (e.g. analysis of certain amino acids), if collected prior to death. Collect two 1 mL samples, one into a plain tube and one with fluoride oxalate and store these immediately at -80^0C.

Vitreous Humour

This can be collected into a fluoride bottle by needle aspiration and stored at -20^0C. It may provide valuable information regarding the electrolyte and glucose concentration.

Bile

Bile may be the only available analysable fluid in cases where the interval between death and post-mortem has been protracted. It is recommended that in all cases where there is the possibility of underlying metabolic disease a sample of bile should be obtained. Bile is most conveniently spotted onto a Guthrie card for acylcarnitine profiling. If a Guthrie card is not available bile can be collected at post-mortem into a plain tube for storage at -20^0C.

Skin or Other Samples for Culturing Fibroblasts

A skin biopsy should be a routine part of all post-mortem investigations where an infant or child has died from unknown cause. The skin biopsy should be taken with a sterile procedure. The preferred option is two punch biopsies taken from different sites and placed in separate sterile vials containing appropriate culture medium (Ham's F10, Eagle's MEM, Dulbecco's medium). It is recommended that all pathologists who undertake paediatric post-mortems should use a biopsy punch. In the absence of a punch, it should be borne in mind that small biopsies carry a lower risk of infection; two 3 mm x 3 mm full thickness biopsies are all that is required. Large pieces of skin and tissue frequently fail because of infection. It is recommended that the skin biopsy be taken at the beginning of the post-mortem to reduce the risk of contamination. Skin remains as a reliable source for culturing fibroblasts for 2 to 5 days after death, and in some cases, up to a week. However, the biopsy should be obtained as soon as practicable, as this increases the likelihood of a successful culture. The addition of Fungizone to the culture medium can help to reduce the risk of fungal infections, but it is no substitute for good aseptic technique. Alternatively, where infection is likely to be a particularly problematic or where there has been a post-mortem delay of some days and viability is likely to be low, it is worth taking small biopsies from a number of separate sites into separate containers to increase the chances of successful culture, e.g. pericardium, fascia and / or cartilage. Once the biopsies have been taken they should be sent immediately to the cell culture laboratory, but can if necessary, be stored overnight at +4⁰C *(do not freeze as this will destroy any viable cells)* prior to dispatch. In an emergency, sterile normal saline can be used instead of culture medium, but do not use agar.

Tissue Samples

The selection of organ biopsies depends on the clinical picture and is best discussed with a metabolic specialist. Liver, heart muscle, skeletal muscle and kidney are usually only suitable for biochemical analysis if taken *within 2–4 hours of death*. Open biopsies are preferable, but if not possible, two, or three needle biopsies should be taken. All such biopsies for biochemical analysis should be wrapped in aluminium foil and snap-frozen in liquid nitrogen or solid carbon dioxide. The samples should then be stored in a -80⁰ C freezer.

Tissue Samples for Histological Examination
Liver

A small piece of liver is collected into formalin for staining and light microscopy and a piece into glutaraldehyde for electron microscopy. Fat stain should be performed in a small piece of liver.

Kidney

A small piece of kidney should be obtained formalin fixed and examined with light microscopy. Fat stain should be performed in a small piece of kidney.

Muscle Biopsy

A small piece is frozen for light microscopy, fat stain, and histochemistry: thin muscle fibre, tied to a stick (to avoid contraction and preserve orientation) in 2% glutaraldehyde on ice. This is for electron microscopy.

Investigations and Analysis

The types of samples and analyses along with examples of the disorders that may be diagnosed are outlined in Table 18.1.

Blood Acylcarnitine Profiles

The introduction of acylcarnitine profiling on Guthrie card blood spots by electrospray ionisation-tandem mass spectrometry has revolutionised the investigation of metabolic disease and is the major advance in the post-mortem investigation of these disorders, facilitating the identification of a wide range of metabolic diseases in tiny samples of blood, plasma, and bile.[27] Recent advances in technology such as ultra-high-performance liquid chromatography/quadrupole time-of-flight mass spectrometry (UHPLC-Q-TOF/MS) have further improved our ability to detect and identify a wide range of potentially informative metabolites in blood and other tissue fluids.[28,29] The rapidly expanding field of metabolomics will increasingly serve to provide metabolic profiles that can be used in conjunction with molecular findings and/or other functional studies to support a putative diagnosis.[30]

Acylcarnitine profiling has the potential to detect many inherited metabolic defects including most fatty acid oxidation disorders and many organic acidaemias. Acylcarnitine profiles are likely to be more informative when expressed as ratios e.g. C8/C10 or C8/C12 ratios in the detection of medium-chain acyl-CoA dehydrogenase deficiency (MCAD) (Figure 18.1).[27] This is because post-mortem changes often lead to a non-specific rise in a number of medium- and short-chain acylcarnitines, and the expression of results as a ratio gives a more reliable indication of abnormalities resulting from specific defects in fatty acid oxidation. However, few of the profiles from post-mortem blood are in themselves reliably diagnostic and will need further investigation by molecular analysis or through functional studies, often on fibroblasts, to confirm a diagnosis (Figure 18.2). As interpretation of acylcarnitine profiles can be especially problematic in post-mortem samples it is always worth seeking out the stored newborn screening Guthrie card (if this is

Table 18.1 Samples and containers for biochemical / molecular analysis (See also [51,14,15].)

Sample	Means of preservation	Storage	Type of analysis	Examples of disorders detected
Whole blood	Guthrie card	Dry at room temperature	AC, AA	FAO, OAs AAs/UC
Bile	Guthrie card	Dry at room temperature	AC	FAO, OAs
Urine	Sterile vial	-20°C or +4°C	OA	OAs, FAO
Whole blood	Li/hep	Plasma at +4°C	AC, AA, VLCFAs, sterols	FAO, AAs Peroxisomal defects, S-L-O
Whole Blood	EDTA	-20°C	DNA	OI, MCAD, LCHAD
Skin (ellipse biopsy) or 3 mm x 3 mm	Sterile medium	Do NOT freeze +4°C or room temperature	Flux / enzyme assay, DNA, RNA	FAO, RES, OAs, PDH GSD II and IV, GA I, GA II Niemann-Pick Type C
Muscle (fresh)	Liquid nitrogen	-80°C	Enzyme assay Respiratory chain Complexes I–IV	GSD II and IV, RES
Liver (fresh)	Liquid nitrogen	-80°C	Enzyme assay Respiratory chain Complexes I–IV	OTC, CPS 1, NKH, GSD I, IV, 0 RES

Abbreviations:

AA – amino acids

AAs/UC – aminoacidopathies / urea cycle defects

AC – acylcarnitine profile

CPS I – carbamylphosphate synthase I deficiency

FAO – fatty acid oxidation defects

GA II – Glutaric aciduria type II (multiple acyl-CoA dehydrogenase deficiency)

GA I – glutaric aciduria type I (glutaryl-CoA dehydrogenase deficiency)

GSD – glycogen storage disease

LCHAD – long-chain 3-hydroxyacyl-CoA dehydrogenase deficiency

MCAD – medium-chain acyl-CoA dehydrogenase deficiency

NKH – non-ketotic hyperglycinaemia

OA – organic acid

OAs – organic acidurias

OI – osteogenesis imperfecta

OTC – ornithine transcarbamylase deficiency

PDH – pyruvate dehydrogenase deficiency

RES – mitochondrial respiratory chain disorders

S-L-O – Smith-Lemli-Opitz syndrome

available) for acylcarnitine analysis, as this is potentially more reliably informative.[31–35]

Blood-spot Amino Acid Profiles

Electrospray ionisation-tandem mass spectrometry also allows the identification of amino acid profiles in Guthrie card blood spots in a similar manner as is done with acylcarnitine analysis. This may be particularly useful in cases when larger volumes of liquid blood are not available at post-mortem. Such analysis has the potential to identify certain disorders affecting amino acid metabolism, particularly some urea cycle disorders, even on post-mortem samples e.g. argininosuccinic acid due to argininosuccinic acid lyase deficiency or citrulline in argininosuccinic acid synthase deficiency. Some other amino acid disorders

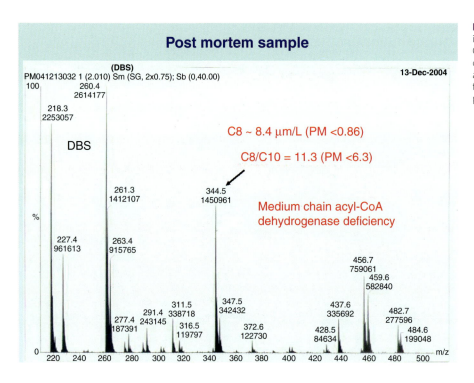

Figure 18.1 Sudden death in a neonate on day 2. Confirmed case of medium-chain acyl-CoA dehydrogenase deficiency. (Reproduced from Bove and Olpin[15] with permission.)

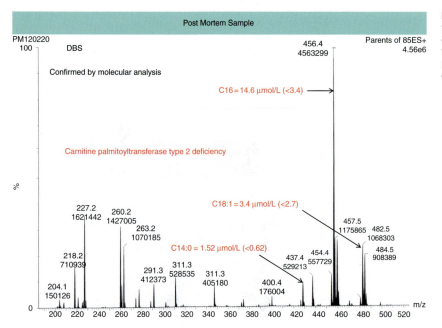

Figure 18.2 Neonatal death due to metabolic acidosis and hypoglycaemia with a molecular confirmation of carnitine palmitoyltransferase type 2 deficiency.

such as maple syrup urine disease are also potentially detectable by blood-spot amino acid profiling.[27]

Plasma Intermediary Metabolites

Blood samples collected prior to or just after death into a fluoride oxalate tube, may be useful for the measurement of intermediary metabolites, namely glucose, lactate, non-esterified fatty acids (NEFA), and 3-hydroxybutyrate (HB). Hypoglycaemic patients with fatty acid oxidation defects usually show high (>2.0) NEFA / HB ratios, while hypoglycaemic infants with hyperinsulinism show an inadequate or absent lipolytic and ketogenic response.[36]

Amino Acids in Plasma, CSF, and Urine

Aminoacidopathies and urea cycle defects will give abnormal amino acid profiles as measured by more conventional amino acid analysis in samples taken prior to death, but as with Guthrie blood spots, interpretation of post-mortem material is often problematic.[27] Abnormal elevations of certain amino acids may indicate the possibility of specific disorders, but need to be interpreted in relation to the interval between death and sampling. Suspected defects of amino acid metabolism will require enzyme / biochemical confirmation in the appropriate tissue or molecular analysis to confirm a diagnosis. It is worth noting that some of the urea cycle defects can only be enzymatically confirmed on fresh liver biopsy i.e. ornithine transcarbamylase (OTC) deficiency or in the case of carbamylphosphate synthase 1 (CPS 1) deficiency in fresh liver or colon. Mutation analysis circumvents the need for a fresh liver sample in these disorders when a specific diagnosis is strongly suspected. However, the finding of variant(s) of uncertain significance on molecular analysis requires additional biochemical/clinical/histological evidence to assess the possible significance of such findings.

Organic Acids in Urine

Organic acidurias, including many of the fatty acid oxidation defects and a significant number of other defects of intermediary metabolism will give abnormal organic acid results. Some profiles may in themselves be pathognomonic, as in the case of methylmalonic aciduria (MMA), classical isovaleric acidaemia (IVA), glutaric acidaemia type 1 (GA1) or MCAD. However, other findings may be less specific and highlight the need for further investigations.[37] The presence of

significant ketones in urine at post-mortem does *not* completely exclude a fatty acid oxidation defect.

Bile

Acylcarnitine and bile acid profiles can be measured in small quantities of post-mortem bile, but need careful interpretation and require supporting biochemical evidence for accurate diagnosis.[27] Bile acylcarnitine analysis is generally only likely to be usefully informative when interpreted in conjunction with a blood-spot acylcarnitine profile. Interpretation of post-mortem acylcarnitine profiles is best achieved by expression of acylcarnitine ratios. An example of this is in the diagnosis of MCAD (as is the case with blood) where C8/C10 or C8/C12 ratios are far more diagnostically reliable than measurement of octanoylcarnitine alone.[27]

Plasma Very-long-chain Fatty Acids and Sterols

Very-long-chain fatty acids (VLCFAs), phytanic acid and pristanic acid can be measured in plasma or serum by GC-MS in cases of suspected peroxisomal disorders. Almost all known peroxisomal defects can be detected if all 4 parameters are measured.[38] Bile salts in urine may be informative in suspected disorders of bile salt metabolism. Plasma sterol analysis can also be used to detect inherited defects of sterol metabolism e.g. 7-dehydrocholesterol for S-L-O Syndrome.[39]

Vitreous Humour

Organic acid analysis of eye fluid may be useful in the absence of urine e.g. 7-hydroxyoctanoate is elevated in cases of MCAD, as is octanoylcarnitine. Vitreous humour glucose, provided the sample was taken perimortem into a fluoride tube will reflect plasma glucose levels at that time e.g. a normal glucose result in an acute admission (provided the patient was not administered glucose prior to death) excludes hypoglycaemia as a cause of collapse.

Histochemistry and Ultrastructure

The histological or ultrastructural appearance of many tissues can be a good guide to the final diagnosis but is often non-specific.[15,40] Staining for micro and macrovesicular fat and/or glycogen deposition in muscle, heart, liver and kidney at an early stage of the post-mortem process may give an early indication of which lines of investigation to pursue. Evaluation of organ / tissue biopsy using both light and electron microscopy often provides complimentary information. Lipid inclusions suggest altered fatty acid oxidation or impaired mitochondrial function. Excess glycogen, determined by staining, or quantitative analysis, suggests altered glycogen metabolism. Increased lipids are also present in some glycogen storage diseases (GSD) e.g. GSD type I. Increased membrane-bound (i.e., lysosomal) glycogen is typical of Pompe disease. Electron microscopy may show abnormalities in mitochondriopathies such as increased size and number of mitochondria. Giant mitochondria with concentric lamellar tubular reticular or dissociated cristae are characteristic. The mitochondrial matrix may be swollen and display large spherical dense bodies, vacuoles, or crystals. Rectangular crystals may be arranged in blocks of parallel crystals with 'parking lot' configuration. However, such changes are not in isolation diagnostic of respiratory chain disease and can only be taken as indicators. Often, particularly in the case of respiratory chain disease, a final diagnosis is a 'balance of probabilities' based on cumulative clinical, histological, biochemical and molecular evidence.[14,15]

Molecular Investigations

Mutation analysis using second-generation techniques including exomic sequencing or whole-genome sequencing are rapidly becoming the first line choice for the investigation of possible inherited metabolic disease.[7,41] The rapidly expanding use of these techniques in conjunction with improved bioinformatics are facilitating the detection of a wide range of both known and newly described inherited metabolic diseases. However, with the increasing use of molecular technology there is an increasing requirement to establish the relevance of novel mutations/variants of uncertain significance.[42] Functional studies and/or additional biochemical and histological evidence are still required in such cases to establish pathogenicity.[43] DNA for molecular analysis can be most easily obtained from EDTA whole blood. Guthrie card blood spots, frozen tissue biopsies, and fibroblasts will also yield DNA. If RNA is required this can be obtained from cultured fibroblasts.

Tissue Assays

Cultured Fibroblasts

Many of the enzymes known to be deficient in inborn errors of metabolism are expressed in skin fibroblasts with the notable exception of some urea cycle and some glycogen storage enzymes. For this reason, obtaining a skin biopsy should be a routine procedure at post-mortem in cases of Sudden Infant Death Syndrome (SIDS)/Sudden Unexpected Death in Infancy (SUDI)/Sudden Unexpected Infant Death (SUID)/Sudden Unexpected Death in Childhood (SUDC). Homogenates or sonicates of cultured fibroblasts are suitable for many specific enzyme assays e.g. glutaryl-CoA dehydrogenase, or alternatively in some instances, assays using crude mitochondrial preparations or intact fibroblasts may be more appropriate e.g. the investigation of respiratory chain disorders by polarography.[44–46] Fibroblasts taken from infants with mitochondrial respiratory chain defects will often express the defect and low complex(es) II/III IV may be demonstrated; although the existing spectrophotometric methodologies are not always sensitive enough to detect reduced complexes in fibroblasts.[47,48] Newer polarographic techniques using relatively small numbers of cultured fibroblasts are significantly more sensitive and have great potential in the functional demonstration of metabolic defects particularly in the diagnosis of respiratory chain disease where current methodologies are not easily applicable to post-mortem investigation.[44,48,49]

Another particular advantage of using intact living cells is that the uptake or incorporation of various substrates into the cell or the flux of metabolites through an entire pathway can be measured.[23] Additionally cultured cells have the advantage that they are not subject to deterioration of enzyme activity or secondary loss of function, which is so frequently a problem in biopsies and particularly other post-mortem samples. An example of the use of intact cells is in the diagnosis of fatty acid oxidation disorders by tritiated release assay in cultured fibroblasts.[50] Cultured fibroblasts can also be incubated with deuterium labelled fatty acids or other suitable substrates and the resultant acylcarnitine profiles analysed by MS/MS.[24] This latter technique has proved to be particularly informative in fatty acid oxidation disorders, but also has the potential for use in a wide range of other inherited metabolic diseases.

Other Tissues

Fresh frozen muscle is often the tissue of choice for the diagnosis of mitochondrial respiratory chain disorders. Provided the muscle has been collected prior to death (or within two hours of death) complexes I, II, III, and IV of the respiratory chain can be measured. Other tissue such as heart and liver can also be used where specific involvement of these tissues is indicated e.g. mutation analysis of cardiac mitochondrial tRNAs in the case of isolated cardiomyopathy or specific enzyme assay in fresh liver for some urea cycle and glycogen storage disorders.[51]

Conclusion

The application of electrospray ionisation-tandem mass spectrometry and related technologies to clinical chemistry offers the opportunity for detailed biochemical profiling in tiny samples of post-mortem blood, plasma, and bile. This technique, coupled with recent advances in molecular genetics, now greatly improves the chances of accurate post-mortem diagnosis for a wide range of inherited metabolic diseases. This process relies on the timely collection of suitable post-mortem samples and careful review of any pre-mortem laboratory results that may be helpful in the subsequent selection of further laboratory testing.

In many cases where there is a suspicion of an underlying metabolic cause of death, it is strongly advised that, wherever possible, the neonatal screening card should be analysed for acylcarnitines and, if indicated, for amino acid analysis also. These analyses carried out on the neonatal Guthrie card blood spot generally provide a more reliable indicator of many metabolic diseases than analyses performed on post-mortem samples.

Combining all the available evidence from the clinical and laboratory investigations including the use of targeted metabolomics and where possible functional assays in fibroblasts, will provide important information to confirm or refute the pathogenic relevance of findings from next-generation sequencing.

References

1 Leach CE, Blair PS, Fleming PJ, et al. Epidemiology of SIDS and explained sudden infant deaths. CESDI SUDI Research Group. *Pediatrics*, 1999; **104**:e43.

2 *Sudden Unexpected Death in Infancy and Childhood. Multi-agency Guidelines for Care and Investigation*, 2nd edn. London: The Royal College of Pathologists, 2016.

3 Bianconi SE, Cross JL, Wassif CA, et al. Pathogenesis, epidemiology, diagnosis, and clinical aspects of Smith-Lemli-Opitz syndrome. *Expert Opin Orphan Drugs*, 2015; **3**:267–80.

4 Löwy I. How genetics came to the unborn: 1960–2000. *Stud Hist Philos Biol Biomed Sci*, 2014; **47**:154–62.

5 Dixit A, Suri M. When the face says it all: dysmorphology in identifying syndromic causes of epilepsy. *Pract Neurol*, 2016; **16**:111–21.

6 Donnai D. Dysmorphic disorders – an overview. *J Inherit Metab Dis*, 1994; **17**:442–7.

7 Yang Y, Muzny DM, Reid JG, et al. Clinical whole-exome sequencing for the diagnosis of Mendelian disorders. *N Engl J Med*, 2013; **369**:1502–11.

8 Saunders SL, Morgan B, Raj V, et al. Targeted post-mortem computed tomography cardiac angiography: proof of concept. *Int J Legal Med*, 2011; **125**:609–16.

9 Adlam D, Joseph S, Robinson C, et al. Coronary optical coherence tomography: minimally invasive virtual histology as part of targeted post-mortem computed tomography angiography. *Int J Legal Med*, 2013; **127**: 991–6.

10 Higgins S, Parsons S, Woodford N, et al. The effect of post-mortem computed tomography angiography (PMCTA) using water-soluble, iodine-based radiographic contrast on histological analysis of the liver, kidneys, and left ventricle of the heart. *Forensic Sci Med Pathol*, 2017; **13**(3):317–27.

11 Jones CJ, Lendon M, Chawner LE, et al. Ultrastructure of the human placenta in metabolic storage disease. *Placenta*, 1990; **11**(5):395–411 ; www.ncbi.nlm.nih.gov/pubmed/2127960 (accessed 31 October 2018).

12 Hulkova H, Ledvinova J, Kuchar L, et al. Glycosphingolipid profile of the apical pole of human placental capillaries: The relevancy of the observed data to Fabry disease. *Glycobiology*, 2012; **22**:725–32.

13 Howat AJ, Bennett MJ, Variend S, et al. Defects of metabolism of fatty acids in the Sudden Infant Death Syndrome. *Br Med J (Clin Res Ed)*, 1985; **290**: 1771–3.

14 Cohen MC, Yap S, Olpin SEE. Inherited metabolic disease and Sudden Unexpected Death – pathology. In: Payne-James J, Byard RW, eds. *Encyclopaedia of Forensic and Legal Medicine*, 2nd edn, vol. **2**. Oxford: Elsevier, 2016: 85–95.

15 Bove K, Olpin S. The metabolic disease autopsy. In: Cohen MC, Scheimberg I, eds. The Pediatric and Perinatal Autopsy Manual, Cambridge: Cambridge University Press: 120–38.

16 Nelson J, Kenny B, O'Hara D, et al. Foamy changes of placental cells in probable beta glucuronidase deficiency associated with hydrops fetalis. *J Clin Pathol*, 1993; **46**:370–1.

17 Rinaldo P, Yoon HR, Yu C, et al. Sudden and unexpected neonatal death: a protocol for the postmortem diagnosis of fatty acid oxidation disorders. *Semin Perinatol*, 1999; **23**:204–10.

18 Bennett MJ, Rinaldo P. The metabolic autopsy comes of age. *Clin Chem*, 2001; **47**:1145–6.

19 Valnot I, Osmond S, Gigarel N, et al. Mutations of the SCO1 gene in mitochondrial cytochrome c oxidase

deficiency with neonatal-onset hepatic failure and encephalopathy. *Am J Hum Genet*, 2000; **67**:1104–9.

20 von Kleist-Retzow J-C, Cormier-Daire V, Viot G, et al. Antenatal manifestations of mitochondrial respiratory chain deficiency. *J Pediatr*, 2003; **143**:208–12.

21 Sarzi E, Bourdon A, Chrétien D, et al. Mitochondrial DNA depletion is a prevalent cause of multiple respiratory chain deficiency in childhood. *J Pediatr*, 2007; **150**:531–4, 534.e1–6.

22 Willis JH, Capaldi RA, Huigsloot M, et al. Isolated deficiencies of OXPHOS complexes I and IV are identified accurately and quickly by simple enzyme activity immunocapture assays. *Biochim Biophys Acta – Bioenerg*, 2009; **1787**:533–8.

23 Roe CR, Roe DS. Recent developments in the investigation of inherited metabolic disorders using cultured human cells. *Mol Genet Metab*, 1999; **68**:243–57.

24 Okun JG, Kolker S, Schulze A, et al. A method for quantitative acylcarnitine profiling in human skin fibroblasts using unlabelled palmitic acid: diagnosis of fatty acid oxidation disorders and differentiation between biochemical phenotypes of MCAD deficiency. *Biochim Biophys Acta*, 2002; **1584**:91–8.

25 Robinson BH, Glerum DM, Chow W, et al. The use of skin fibroblast cultures in the detection of respiratory chain defects in patients with lacticacidemia. *Pediatr Res*, 1990; **28**:549–55.

26 Vianey-Saban C, Acquaviva C, Cheillan D, et al. Antenatal manifestations of inborn errors of metabolism: biological diagnosis. *J Inherit Metab Dis*, 2016; **39**:611–24.

27 Chace DH, DiPerna JC, Mitchell BL, et al. Electrospray tandem mass spectrometry for analysis of acylcarnitines in dried postmortem blood specimens collected at autopsy from infants with unexplained cause of death. *Clin Chem*, 2001; **47**:1166–82.

28 DiBattista A, McIntosh N, Lamoureux M, et al. Temporal signal pattern recognition in mass spectrometry: a method for rapid identification and accurate quantification of biomarkers for inborn errors of metabolism with quality assurance. *Anal Chem*, 2017; **89**(15):8112–21.

29 Wang H, Liu Z, Wang S, et al. UHPLC Q-TOF/MS based plasma metabolomics reveals the metabolic perturbations by manganese exposure in rat models. *Metallomics*, 2017; **9**:192–203.

30 Wang Y, Liu F, Li P, et al. An improved pseudotargeted metabolomics approach using multiple ion monitoring with time-staggered ion lists based on ultra-high performance liquid chromatography/quadrupole time-of-flight mass spectrometry. *Anal Chim Acta*, 2016; **927**:82–8.

31 Scaturro G, Sanfilippo C, Piccione M, et al. Newborn screening of inherited metabolic disorders by tandem mass spectrometry: past, present, and future. *Pediatr Med Chir*, 2013; **35**(3):105–9.

32 Coman D, Bhattacharya K. Extended newborn screening: An update for the general paediatrician. *J Paediatr Child Health*, 2012; **48**:E68–E72.

33 Pollak A, Kasper DC. Austrian newborn screening program: a perspective of five decades. *J Perinat Med*, 2014; **42**:151–8.

34 Garnotel R. Mass spectrometry and neonatal screening. *Ann Biol Clin (Paris)*, 2015; **73**(1):107–11.

35 Wilcken B, Wiley V. Newborn screening. *Pathology*, 2008; **40**:104–15.

36 Carragher FM, Bonham JR, Smith JM. Pitfalls in the measurement of some intermediary metabolites. *Ann Clin Biochem*, 2003; **40**:313–20.

37 Peters V, Bonham JR, Hoffmann GF, et al. Qualitative urinary organic acid analysis: 10 years of quality assurance. *J Inherit Metab Dis*, 2016; **39**:683–7.

38 Scott C, Olpin S. Peroxisomal disorders. *Paediatr Child Health*, 2015; 25(3):119–22.

39 Dempsey MA, Tan C, Herman GE. Chondrodysplasia punctata 2, X-linked. *Gene Reviews*, 2011; https://www.ncbi.nlm.nih.gov/books/NBK55062/ (accessed 30 October 2018).

40 Evason K, Bove KE, Finegold MJ, et al. Morphologic findings in progressive familial intrahepatic cholestasis 2 (PFIC2): correlation with genetic and immunohistochemical studies. *Am J Surg Pathol*, 2011; **35**:687–96.

41 Thompson K, Majd H, Dallabona CC, et al. Recurrent De Novo dominant mutations in SLC25A4 cause severe early-onset mitochondrial disease and loss of mitochondrial DNA copy number. *Am J Hum Genet*, 2016; **99**:860–76.

42 Best S, Wou K, Vora N, et al. Promises, pitfalls, and practicalities of prenatal whole exome sequencing. *Prenat Diagn*, 2018; **38**(1):10–19.

43 Olpin S, Clark S, Dalley J, et al. Fibroblast fatty acid oxidation flux assays stratify risk in newborns with presumptive-positive results on screening for very-long-chain acyl-CoA dehydrogenase deficiency. *Int J Neonatal Screen*, 2017; **3**:2.

44 Smolina N, Bruton J, Kostareva A, et al. Assaying mitochondrial respiration as an indicator of cellular metabolism and fitness. *Methods Mol Biol*, 2017; **1601**:79–87.

45 Lanza IR, Nair KS. Mitochondrial metabolic function assessed in vivo and in vitro. *Curr Opin Clin Nutr Metab Care*, 2010; **13**:511–17.

46 Jonckheere AI, Huigsloot M, Janssen AJM, et al. High-throughput assay to measure oxygen consumption in digitonin-permeabilized cells of patients with mitochondrial disorders. *Clin Chem*, 2010; **56**:424–31.

47 Theisen BE, Rumyantseva A, Cohen JS, et al. Deficiency of WARS2, encoding mitochondrial tryptophanyl tRNA synthetase, causes severe infantile onset leukoencephalopathy. *Am J Med Genet Part A*, 2017; **173**(9):2505–10.

48 Ogawa E, Shimura M, Fushimi T, et al. Clinical validity of biochemical and molecular analysis in diagnosing Leigh syndrome: a study of 106 Japanese patients. *J Inherit Metab Dis*, 2017; **40**(5):685–93.

49 Barrientos A, Fontanesi F, Díaz F. Evaluation of the mitochondrial respiratory chain and oxidative phosphorylation system using polarography and spectrophotometric enzyme assays. *Curr Protoc Hum Gen*, 2009: Unit **19**.3; https://www.ncbi.nlm.nih.gov/pmc/articles/PMC2771113/ (accessed 30 October 2018).

50 Olpin SE, Manning NJ, Pollitt RJ, et al. Improved detection of long-chain fatty acid oxidation defects in intact cells using [9,10-3 H]oleic acid. *J Inherit Metab Dis*, 1997; **20**:415–19.

51 Degoul F, Brule H, Cepanec C, et al. Isoleucylation properties of native human mitochondrial tRNAIle and tRNAIle transcripts. Implications for cardiomyopathy-related point mutations (4269, 4317) in the tRNAIle gene. *Hum Mol Genet*, 1998; 7: 347–54.

Chapter

19

Biological Factors

Fern R. Hauck

Certain biological and non-modifiable factors place infants at higher risk of SIDS. Infants are at greatest risk of SIDS between the ages of 1 and 4 months, with 90% of deaths occurring by 6 months.[1] Male infants have a 30–50% higher incidence of SIDS than female infants.[2]

An increased risk of SIDS is associated with several obstetric factors, suggesting that the in-utero environment of SIDS infants was suboptimal. SIDS infants are more commonly of higher birth order, independent of maternal age, and were born of gestations after shorter interpregnancy intervals.[2] Mothers of SIDS infants generally received inadequate prenatal care, including fewer visits and initiating care later in pregnancy.[2] Additionally, low birthweight, preterm birth, and slower intrauterine and postnatal growth rates are risk factors.[2] Infants of twin or multiple gestations are at higher risk of SIDS, explained by their generally lower birthweight.[3]

In the US, there were 3,700 sudden unexpected infant deaths in 2015; 43% were attributed to SIDS (39.4/100,000 live births), 32% to unknown cause (30.1/100,000 live births), and 25% to accidental suffocation and strangulation in bed (23.1/100,000 live births).[4] There are significant racial and ethnic disparities in SIDS and SUDI/SUID mortality rates (Figure 19.1).[4] Despite the decline in SIDS and SUDI/SUID in all races and ethnicities (Figure 19.2),[4] the rate of SUDI/SUID among non-Hispanic black (170.2 per 100,000 live births) and American Indian/Alaska Native (194.1 per 100,000 live births) infants was more than double that of non-Hispanic white infants (83.8 per 100,000 live births) in 2011–2014 [4]. Respective rates for SIDS in 2014 are 67, 91, and 39/100,000 live births).[5] SUDI/SUID and SIDS rates for Asians/Pacific Islanders and Hispanics were much lower than the rate for non-Hispanic whites. Significant disparities in SUDI/SUID and SIDS between indigenous and white

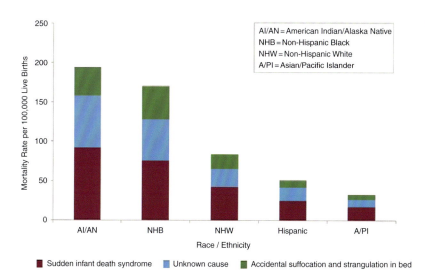

AI/AN = American Indian/Alaska Native
NHB = Non-Hispanic Black
NHW = Non-Hispanic White
A/PI = Asian/Pacific Islander

■ Sudden infant death syndrome   ■ Unknown cause   ■ Accidental suffocation and strangulation in bed

Figure 19.1 Sudden unexpected infant death by race/ethnicity, 2011–2014

Source: CDC/NCHS, National Vital Statistics System, Period Linked Birth/Infant Death Data.

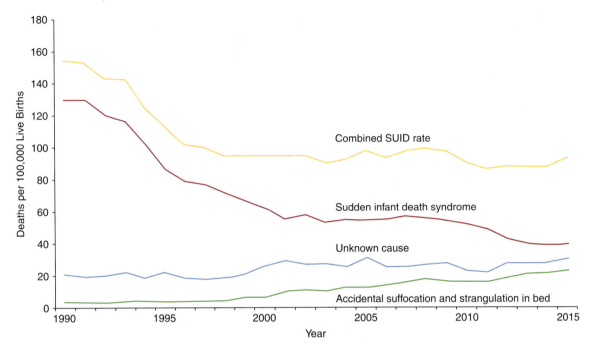

Figure 19.2 Trends in sudden unexpected infant death by cause, 1990–2015
Source: CDC/NCHS, National Vital Statistics System, Compressed Mortality File.

infants are likewise found in Canada, New Zealand, and Australia.[6] To address these persistent disparities, strategies are required that are tailored to indigenous communities and are under the leadership of, and/or are in partnership with, indigenous stakeholders.[6]

References

1. Trachtenberg FL, Haas EA, Kinney HC, Stanley C, Krous HF. Risk factor changes for Sudden Infant Death Syndrome after initiation of back-to-sleep campaign. *Pediatrics*, 2012; **129**(4):630–8.

2. Hunt CE, Hauck FR. Sudden Infant Death Syndrome. *CMAJ*, 2006; **174**(13):1861–9.

3. Malloy MH, Freeman DH. Sudden Infant Death Syndrome among twins. *JAMA Pediatrics*, 1999; **153**(7): 736–40.

4. CDC/NCHS, National Vital Statistics System, Compressed Mortality File; https://www.cdc.gov/nchs/data_access/cmf.htm (accessed 30 October 2018).

5. Data accessed from CDC Wonder Online Database, https://www.cdc.gov/sids/data.htm (accessed 16 October 2018).

6. Smylie J, Crengle S, Freemantle J, Taualii. Indigenous birth outcomes in Australia, Canada, New Zealand, and the United States – an overview. *Open Women's Health J*, 2010; **4**:7–17.

Risk of Recurrent Sudden Infant Death Syndrome in Families

Carl E. Hunt

Background

Sudden Infant Death Syndrome (SIDS) was first defined in 1969[1]. During the early years of SIDS-related research, subsequent siblings of SIDS infants were not considered to be at increased risk for SIDS, and SIDS was not considered to have genetic implications. Indeed, when recurrent sudden unexpected infant death did occur in a family, intentional suffocation (fatal child abuse, filicide) was often considered the cause.

Research results over the past several decades have expanded our understanding of both environmental and genetic risk factors contributing to risk for SIDS, including gene-environment interactions.[1,2] The increasing availability of information obtained from scene investigations has enhanced our understanding of the importance of safe-sleep environments, including the supine sleep position. Concurrently, advances in genetic technologies have led to identification of multiple polymorphisms occurring with increased frequency in SIDS compared to control infants (see Chapter 28).

Family Studies of Recurrent Infant Mortality

Multiple studies have assessed the risk for recurrent SIDS and non-SIDS in families. In aggregate, these familial recurrence studies have confirmed and quantified the risk for recurrent infant mortality in families. A recent review summarises the evidence for an increased risk of SIDS in siblings of SIDS infants and the risk for recurrence of other causes of infant mortality.[3] In a study of next siblings of first-born infants dying of SIDS, the relative risk (RR) for recurrent SIDS in the second sibling was 5.8 (p=0.002). Also of note, the RR for recurrence of the same non-SIDS cause of death in next siblings was 9.1 compared to just 1.6 for a different cause of death

(p<0.007). In another study of recurrent SIDS, the RR in the next sibling was 5.4, 95% confidence interval (CI) 2.0–14.8, a risk 4.6 times greater than expected by parity. Again of note, the risk for recurrence of a non-SIDS cause of death in the next sibling was similar, RR 6 (p<0.001). In a population-based case-control study of all unexpected infant deaths, among SIDS infants the odds ratio (OR) for a prior SIDS death was 3.82 (95% CI 1.58–9.22). Of note, the OR for prior infant death in infants with explained sudden unexpected death was also significant, OR 5.96 (CI 1.29–27.6). Overall, the recurrence risk for SIDS in all subsequent siblings was increased to a similar and significant extent for the next sibling, and the recurrence risk for same non-SIDS cause of infant mortality was similar to the recurrence risk for SIDS. The risk for SIDS was also similar when analysed for prior siblings. The risk for recurrent SIDS in surviving twins is also increased, but the risk is not greater than for non-twin SIDS siblings.

Individually, the various studies of recurrent SIDS mortality in infants are subject to a variety of limitations. Especially in the earlier studies, autopsy rates were not consistently 100%, especially for the index case. In most studies, scene investigation information was not available, and most studies did not include an expert panel review or multidisciplinary confidential inquiry committee. Most studies did not include any information regarding epidemiological risk factors including, for example, race, sex, cigarette smoking, socio-economic status, or gestational age. Despite selected limitations in individual studies, however, each study also had specific strengths. Collectively, the results have been remarkably consistent in observing a significant risk for recurrent SIDS and for recurrent non-SIDS in families. None of these studies, however, provided any insights as to the relative importance of environmental and genetic mechanisms to explain this increased familial risk for recurrent infant mortality.

Recurrent SIDS in Families Before and After Safe-Sleep Campaigns

A recent study based on the Utah Population Database confirmed the increased risk for recurrent SIDS and non-SIDS in siblings.[4] Of particular note, this study also compared SIDS rates before and after the back-to-sleep recommendations of 1992–4 and therefore provided new insights regarding the relative importance of genetic and environmental influences on risk for recurrent SIDS and non-SIDS in families.

The Utah study included over 1,700 SIDS deaths from 1975–2013.[4] Post back-to-sleep SIDS cases were defined as occurring after 1994. During these thirty-eight years, the incidence of SIDS decreased eight-fold, with no change in the ratio of male to female deaths. The files of SIDS infants were linked to other family members, and the odds ratio for SIDS and non-SIDS was assessed in siblings, aunts, uncles, nieces, nephews, and first cousins. The investigators also included deaths coded as 'other' or 'unknown' when SIDS occurred in a relative (Table 20.1).

As summarised in Table 20.1, the OR for recurrent SIDS in siblings in all years (1968–2013) was 4.2, similar to the increased risk for siblings in previous publications.[3] Also, the OR was similar (4.8) for other or unknown causes of death in relatives of SIDS infants. The aggregate OR for recurrent SIDS for all years was less in first to third degree relatives than in siblings, but was still significantly increased. Of particular note, when the analysis for aggregate OR for recurrent SIDS was restricted to births after 1994, there was a three-fold increase compared to all years. Based on this increase after versus before implementation of back-to-sleep campaigns, the authors hypothesised that post back-to-sleep SIDS deaths, especially recurrences in families, were 'enriched' for genetic causes as the frequency of environmental risk factors related to unsafe sleep environments, including non-supine sleep position, significantly decreased after 1992–4.

Summary

Multiple studies have assessed the risk for recurrent SIDS in siblings and in families.[3,4] All studies have reported a significant increase in risk for recurrent SIDS, with a RR ranging from 3.7 to 10.0, similar to recurrence risk for non-SIDS causes of infant mortality. Although none of these studies assessed potential mechanisms for this increased risk, the causes of SIDS are likely related to interactions between environmental and genetic risk factors.[1] Of particular note in this regard, the recent Utah study results are consistent with an 'enrichment' of recurrent deaths due to genetic risk factors (see Chapter 28) following implementation of back-to-sleep campaigns and subsequent reductions in environmental risk factors related to unsafe sleeping.[4] To put this increased recurrence risk in perspective, however, it is important to note that most subsequent siblings of a prior SIDS infant will not be affected; assuming a population risk of 0.4 SIDS deaths/1,000 live births or less and a five-fold increased RR for recurrence, for example, at least 99.8% of subsequent siblings will be unaffected and hence survive.

Table 20.1 Recurrence rates in Sudden Infant Death Syndrome (SIDS) in families before and after back-to-sleep campaigns implemented in the United States in 1992–4*

Time-period for deaths	Relationship	Cases versus controls	
		Odds Ratio	95% Confidence Interval
SIDS 1968–2013	Siblings	4.2	2.50–7.05
	Aggregate**	2.95	2.18–4.0
SIDS 1995–2013	Aggregate**	9.29	2.62–32.96
1968–2013: Other/ unknown cause of death	SIDS Relatives	4.84	1.68–13.95

* Adapted from Christensen et al with permission from John Wiley and Sons.[4]

** Siblings, aunts, uncles, nieces, nephews, 1st cousins

References

1. Hunt CE, Darnall RA, McEntire BL, Hyma BA. Assigning cause for sudden unexpected infant death. *Forensic Sci Med Pathol*, 2015; **11**:283–8.

2. Opdal SH, Rognum TO. Gene variants predisposing to SIDS: current knowledge. *Forensic Sci Med Pathol*, 2011; 7:26–36.

3. Hunt CE. Sudden Infant Death Syndrome and other causes of infant mortality: diagnosis, mechanisms, and risk for recurrence in siblings. State of the art. *Am J Resp Crit Care Med*, 2001; **164**:346–57.

4. Christensen ED, Berger J, Alashari MM, Coon H, Robison C, Ho H-T, et al. Sudden Infant Death Syndrome – insights and future directions from a Utah population database analysis. *Am J Med Genet*, 2017; **173**(1):177–82 https://onlinelibrary.wiley.com/doi/pdf/10.1002/ajmg.a.37994 (accessed 30 October 2018).

Prenatal and Postpartum Nicotine Exposure

Adèle C. Engelberts

Smoking is one of the most important factors associated with SIDS. It was identified as a potential risk factor in the 1960s, about the same time that SIDS was recognised as an entity. Infant death rates from all causes are associated with deprived socio-economic circumstances and while tobacco exposure is a marker for social deprivation, the risk of tobacco exposure associated with SIDS far exceeds that.

There are pitfalls in pooling studies reporting on smoking and SIDS such as differences in autopsy rates, smoking definitions, control data, and confounding variables. However, there has been great consistency in the increased SIDS risk associated with maternal smoking. A meta-analysis published in 2013 examined 35 case-control studies encompassing more than 30,000 cases and almost 6,000,000 controls.[1] Prenatal maternal smoking carried an odds ratio (OR) of 2.25 (95% CI 2.03–2.50) and postnatal maternal smoking an OR of 1.97 (95% CI 1.77–2.19). Heavy smoking increased the risk. There is also some evidence that cessation of smoking during pregnancy reduces the risk of SIDS.[2] These considerations all support a causal relationship between SIDS and tobacco exposure before and after birth.

Biochemical validation of smoking status is the most reliable parameter for smoking status but most epidemiological studies rely on self-reporting. The actual prevalence of smoking is underreported, more so in pregnant than in non-pregnant women. In studies in the United States and Scotland, nondisclosure of smoking by pregnant women when comparing self-reporting to cotinine levels was about 25%.[3] If nondisclosure varies with outcome, as would seem likely, the bias in retrospective studies may even be greater. This bias would lead to an underestimation of the risk, however, so that the odds ratios associated with smoking are even more striking in their consistency and magnitude.

There are several epidemiological difficulties in separating the effect of prenatal and postnatal smoking on SIDS risk. Almost all women who smoke in pregnancy will continue to do so after giving birth. Therefore, it is difficult to separate the effect of prenatal smoking from postnatal exposure. To explore the effect of postnatal smoking only, it would be ideal to study a group of women who do not smoke in pregnancy but start after birth; but this is an almost non-existent group. Another way to look at the influence of postnatal smoking is to look at paternal smoking and control for maternal smoking or to look at the risk associated with paternal smoking if mother is a non-smoker. Mitchell and Milerad found a pooled relative risk of 1.49 (95%CI 1.25–1.77) for paternal smoking if mother is a non-smoker.[4] Fleming and Blair found an increase in risk associated with a higher number of smokers in the household. Furthermore, when families were asked to estimate the number of hours their baby was exposed to smoke there was also a clear dose response curve: the greater the duration of exposure, the greater the associated risk.[5] This leads to the conclusion that although maternal smoking in pregnancy carries the greatest increase in risk associated with exposure to tobacco smoke, there is a separate effect of postnatal smoking.

Studies that looked at different ethnic groups found that the odds ratios appear consistent even if smoking rates vary widely. This also seems to apply to different socio-economic groups. The New Zealand Cot Death Study found that although smoking rates vary widely between social groups, with higher rates in the lower socio-economic groups, the magnitude of the risk was similar.[4]

Smoking interacts with other risk factors for SIDS. Effect modification exists if one risk factor, such as smoking, influences the magnitude of the risk of SIDS associated with another risk factor. Several studies have found an interaction between smoking and time of day when the death occurs, with the risk associated with smoking being greater in deaths that occur at night. In part this may be due to the fact that there is a strong interaction between the risk associated with sharing a bed with an infant, usually a night-time occurrence, and smoking. Bed-sharing increases the risk only slightly if there has been no tobacco exposure, but is a major risk factor if parents smoke. An interaction with another postnatal factor, the prone sleeping position, shows contradictory results. The Nordic study found the highest OR for SIDS if infants slept prone and mother smoked[6] while the New Zealand study found a lower risk of SIDS for smoking mothers if their infant slept prone.[4]

The Westphalian Perinatal Inquiry conducted in Germany between 1990 and 1994 also found an interaction between smoking and several prenatal risk factors.[7] Few prenatal visits, low birthweight, and preterm birth only increased the risk of SIDS among smoking mothers but not in non-smokers. This suggests that for infants born of non-smoking mothers, postnatal risk factors play the greatest role.

After the back-to-sleep campaigns and the decline in prevalence of prone sleeping, the population attributable risk of smoking increased. It was estimated that 23–34% of SIDS deaths in the US in 2002 could have been avoided if prenatal smoking were eliminated.[8] This makes tobacco exposure of infants, prenatally and postnatally, the most important modifiable risk factor for SIDS. But in practice, tobacco addiction is not so readily modified. In 2007 smoking was banned in both the workplace and enclosed public places in the United Kingdom. This was associated with an immediate reduction of 7.8% in stillbirths, a reduction of 3.9% of low birthweight and a 7.6% reduction in overall neonatal mortality. Surprisingly, there was no overall reduction in SIDS or post-neonatal mortality.[9] Perhaps the fact that over 50% of adults already worked in a smoke-free environment before the ban led to an underestimation of the effect. Also there is always the possibility of misclassification since SIDS is a diagnosis of exclusion: if this were the case, however, one would still expect to see an effect on the post-neonatal mortality and this was not observed. It is interesting that another study showed that although smoking bans did not affect SIDS rates, raising the price of tobacco did: this could indicate that only an intervention that targets actually reducing smoking by pregnant women themselves is effective in reducing SIDS.[10]

There has also been some concern that banning smoking in public places may actually lead to more smoking in the home. This is particularly relevant for the incidence of SIDS, as this would lead to more second-hand exposure of pregnant women and infants. However, there is evidence that this is not the case in both higher-income and middle- to low-income countries. Thus on a more positive note, smoke-free legislation could even change social norms about smoking and lead to more smoke-free homes. There is evidence that although the exposure to environmental tobacco smoke as measured by urinary cotinine levels is still 5–7 times higher in families that are trying to protect their infant by smoking outdoors compared to non-smoking families, infants whose family members smoke indoors are subjected to 3–8 times higher exposures than infants of outdoor smokers.[11] This implies that besides encouraging parents to quit smoking, trying to lessen exposure seems effective in lowering cotinine levels; if it is also effective in lessening the incidence of SIDS is unknown. During pregnancy it is also important to lessen the exposure of (non-smoking) pregnant women to second-hand smoke. Studying the risk of smoke exposure is further complicated by the fact that being in close proximity while a cigarette is being smoked is the most obvious source of exposure, but vapour components are deposited on objects – furniture, walls, and curtains – and re-emitted into the air in the course of hours to months. There is little known about the contribution of this third-hand exposure to the risk of SIDS.

Even less is known about possible risks associated with the use of alternative tobacco products and the risk of SIDS. Although cigarette use has declined, there is an upcoming market for non-cigarette tobacco products such as water pipes/hookahs and smokeless tobacco (such as snuff and chewing tobacco). Hookah use is perceived to be less harmful, but a single water pipe session can equate to smoking up to 100 cigarettes. It is very popular among women in non-Western societies. Studies from Lebanon have shown that hookah use in pregnancy is associated with about a 2.5 increased odds of a low-birthweight baby. There are no SIDS studies that have included data on e-cigarettes; a recent US study showed these seem to be primarily used by smokers, however, with a little less than 4% exclusive e-cigarette use.[12] It is noteworthy that electronic delivery systems have not been shown to be effective in smoking cessation.

A Cochrane review of smoking cessation in pregnancy found that there was evidence that nicotine replacement therapy added to behavioural therapy increased smoking cessation rates, but if potentially biased non-placebo trials were eliminated, replacement therapy was no more effective than placebo.[13] This is in contrast with the effect of replacement therapy outside of pregnancy. There was no evidence that nicotine replacement therapy influenced birth outcome; one trial suggested a positive effect on neurological development. Adherence to the medication was generally low, and most of the women did not use a large proportion of the replacement therapy. Another explanation for the lack of success of replacement therapy in pregnancy is that nicotine metabolism is increased in pregnancy so that higher doses might be necessary. A very promising approach towards effective cessation seems to be offering financial incentives.[14]

As prenatal and postnatal smoking is now the largest potential modifiable risk factor for SIDS, research efforts should be directed at effective ways to motivate and support pregnant women to stop smoking, and to eliminate their second- and third-hand tobacco exposure if they themselves do not smoke. Extrapolating data from studies in non-pregnant women is not valid, however. It would be possible to take a big step forward in SIDS prevention if effective methods to save infants from both prenatal and postnatal tobacco exposure were developed.

References

1. Zhang K, Wang X. Maternal smoking and increased risk of Sudden Infant Death Syndrome: a meta-analysis. *Legal Medicine*, 2013; **15**:115–21.

2. Alm B, Milerad J, Wennegren G, Skjaerven R, Oyen N, Norvenius G, et al. A case-control study of smoking and Sudden Infant Death Syndrome in the Scandinavian countries, 1992–1995. *Arch Dis Child*, 1998; **78**(4): 329–34.

3. Dietz PM, Homa D, England LJ, Burley K, Tong VT, Dube SR, Bernert JT. Estimates of nondisclosure of cigarette smoking among pregnant and non-pregnant women of reproductive age in the United States. *Am J Epidemiol*, 2011; **173**:355–9.

4. Mitchell EA, Milerad J. Smoking and the Sudden Infant Death Syndrome. *Rev Environ Health*, 2006; **21**(2):81–103.

5. Fleming P, Blair PS. Sudden Infant Death Syndrome and parental smoking. *Early Hum Dev*, 2007; **83**(11):721–5.

6. Oyen N, Markestad T, Skjaerven R, Irgens LM, Helweg-Larsen K, et al. Combined effects of sleeping position and prenatal risk factors in Sudden Infant Death Syndrome: the Nordic epidemiological study. *Pediatrics*, 1997; **100**:613–21.

7. Schellscheidt J, Oyen N, Jorch G. Interactions between maternal smoking and other prenatal risk factors for Sudden Infant Death Syndrome (SIDS). *Acta Paediatr*, 1997; **86**:857–63.

8. Dietz PM, England LJ, Shapiro-Mendoza CK, Tong VT, Farr SL, Callaghan WM. Infant morbidity and mortality attributable to prenatal smoking in the US. *Am J Prev Med*, 2010; **39**(1):45–52.

9. Been JV, Mackay DF, Millett C, Pell JP, van Schayck O, Sheikh A. Impact of smoke-free legislation on perinatal and infant mortality: a national quasi-experimental study. Sci Rep, 2015; **5**:13020; https://www .ncbi.nlm.nih.gov/pmc/articles/PMC4534797/ (accessed 30 October 2018).

10. King C, Markowitz S, Ross H. Tobacco control policies and Sudden Infant Death Syndrome in developed nations. *Health Econ*, 2015; **24**(8):1042–8.

11. Matt GE, Quintana PJE, Hovell MF, Bernert JT, Song S, Novianti N, et al. Households contaminated by environmental tobacco smoke: sources of infant exposures. *Tobacco Control*, 2004; **13**:29–37.

12. Wilson FA, Wang Y. Recent findings on the prevalence of e-cigarette use among adults in the US. *Am J Prev Med*, 2017; **52**(3):385–90.

13. Coleman T, Chamberlain C, Davet MA, Cooper SE, Leonardi-Bee J. Pharmacological interventions for promoting smoking cessation during pregnancy. *Cochrane Database Sys Rev*, 2015; **12**:CD010078; https ://www.cochranelibrary.com/cdsr/doi/10.1002/146518 58.CD010078.pub2/full (accessed 30 October 2018).

14. Tappin D, Bauld L, Purves D, Boyd K, Sinclair L, MacAskill S, et al. Financial incentives for smoking cessation in pregnancy: randomized controlled trial. *BMJ*, 2015; **350**:h134.

Misuse of Drugs in Pregnancy

Marta C. Cohen and Robert Coombs

Many drugs are known to be teratogenic to the developing fetus but few are associated with SIDS, and it is often difficult to distinguish between an effect of the drug the mother has taken and the reason she may have been prescribed it.

Clearly the most important drug taken by the mother associated with SIDS is tobacco and its products (see Chapter 21). Maternal postnatal alcohol consumption is well recognised as a significant risk factor and rarely goes without preceding alcohol consumption in pregnancy.[1] The risk of SIDS is highest when a maternal alcohol diagnosis (indicating heavy prenatal alcohol exposure) is recorded during pregnancy or within 1 year post-pregnancy (1). While the teratogenic effects of smoking have been found in the brains of SIDS infants,[2,3] there are no described associations between the teratogenic effects of alcohol and SIDS, though developmental changes in the corpus callosum using imaging techniques have been described in infants exposed to heavy maternal alcohol consumption.[4]

Several case-control studies have looked for associations with other drugs and substances. In New Zealand, heavy maternal caffeine intake, defined as 400 mg/day or more (equivalent to four or more cups of coffee per day), was associated with a small increased risk of SIDS,[5] while in a Nordic case-control study where heavy caffeine intake was defined as greater than 800 mg/day there was a significant association which was, however, no longer significant after controlling for smoking, maternal age, parity, and education.[6] Caffeine is frequently used postnatally to treat apnoea of prematurity, and while SIDS is more frequent in the small preterm population, the timing of this occurrence does not seem to suggest a direct effect of treatment with caffeine. Rather, the higher incidence of SIDS in this population seems to be an effect of prematurity or its cause.

The majority of SIDS infants in the UK have multiple known risk factors often associated with poor parental compliance with advice, and social deprivation. This may be the historic reason that SIDS was also noted to be increased in the offspring of drug-using mothers. The results of the National Institute of Child Health and Human Development SIDS Cooperative Epidemiologic Study identified a two-fold increase in SIDS risk (p<0.001) with misuse of drugs during pregnancy, when birthweight and black race were controlled.[7] Studies comparing the SIDS rate in New York drug users from 1979–89 to non-drug-using mothers found that the SIDS rate was significantly increased in mothers using methadone and heroin.[8,9] There was a much lower effect for cocaine. Similar findings were reported from Australia where the SIDS rate for methadone-using mothers was 9.2/1000 live births compared to a rate of 0.4/1000 live births for the non-drug-using population.[10]

In the UK, the CESDI (Confidential Enquiry into Stillbirth and Death in Infancy) study found that 14% of parents of infants who died of SIDS had consumed narcotics in the previous 24 hours, compared with 6% of parents from the control group. However, the combination of alcohol or drug use before bed-sharing (infant sharing the same bed or sofa with an adult or child) was nine times more prevalent among the parents of SIDS infants than among those of the random control infants and six times more prevalent than among those of the high-risk control infants.[11] However, for methadone there may be other factors at play in addition to the well-known environmental risk factors. Methadone prolongs the QT interval on the electrocardiogram (ECG).[12] At birth, infants have similar plasma levels of methadone to their mothers and a recent study showed significant prolongation of the QT interval in a cohort of babies born to substance-misusing mothers.[13] This prolongation decreased back to the controls' range over the first few days of life. None of the infants had any symptoms, though the authors had previously noted an infant of a methadone-using mother with bradycardia. Methadone crosses into breastmilk, so that about 3% of a mothers' dose may be absorbed by a breastfeeding infant. In both the UK and USA, breastfeeding is encouraged in this population to improve mother–infant bonding and to help manage any narcotic withdrawal. Little is known about the infant's ability to excrete methadone.

We have recently described a population of infants dying suddenly and unexpectedly within the first 14 days of life.[14] This is an unusual age for SIDS with approximately 18% of SIDS deaths in England and Wales occurring in this age group. Within this group, over a third had a history of maternal use of methadone or of other drugs of addiction. Not surprisingly, most infants had multiple risk factors. All deaths occurred in the first two weeks of life, all mothers for whom there were data smoked, often heavily, and half of the cases had a history of withdrawal syndrome at birth. The vast majority of sudden deaths occurred in the presence of their mothers and three-quarters were sharing a sleep surface with them.

In summary, infants born to drug-using mothers are a growing population. They are at increased risk of low birthweight, prematurity, and possible long-term neurodevelopmental problems. They also seem to be at an increased risk of SIDS during the early neonatal period. In our experience, 37.5% of sudden neonatal deaths had a history of maternal prescription of methadone or were known to have misused drugs of addiction during pregnancy.[14]

References

1. O'Leary CM, Jacoby PJ, Bartu A et al. Maternal alcohol use and Sudden Infant Death Syndrome and infant mortality excluding SIDS. *Pediatrics*, 2013; **131**:e770–82.

2. Bublitz MH, Stroud LR. Maternal smoking during pregnancy and offspring brain structure and function: review and agenda for future research. *Nicotine & Tob Res*, 2012;**14**(4):388–97.

3. Cornelius MD, Day NL. Developmental consequences of prenatal tobacco exposure. *Curr Opinion Neurol*, 2009;**22**:121–5.

4. Boronat S, Sánchez-Montañez A, Gómez-Barros N, et al. Correlation between morphological MRI findings and specific diagnostic categories in fetal alcohol spectrum disorders. *Eur J Med Genet*, 2017; **60**:65–71.

5. Ford RP, Schluter PJ, Mitchell EA, et al., Heavy caffeine intake in pregnancy and Sudden Infant Death Syndrome. New Zealand cot death study group. *Arch Dis Child*, 1998 **78**:9–13.

6. Alm B, Wennergren G, Norvenius G, et al. Caffeine and alcohol as risk factors for Sudden Infant Death Syndrome. *Arch Dis Child*, 1999; **81**:107–11.

7. Hoffman HJ, Damus K, Hillman L, Krongrad E. Risk factors for SIDS. Results of the National Institute of Child Health and Human Development SIDS Cooperative Epidemiological Study. *Ann N Y Acad Sci*, 1988; **533**:13–30.

8. Kandall SR, Gaines J. Maternal substance use and subsequent Sudden Infant Death Syndrome (SIDS) in offspring. *Neurotoxicol Teratol*, 1991; **13**:235–40.

9. Kandall SR, Gaines J, Habel L et al. Relationship of maternal substance abuse to subsequent Sudden Infant Death Syndrome in offspring. *J Pediatr*, 1993; **123**:120–6.

10. Burns L, Conroy E, Mattick RP. Infant mortality among women on a methadone program during pregnancy. *Drug Alcohol Rev*, 2010; **29**:551–6.

11. Blair PS, Sidebotham P, Evason-Coombe A et al. Hazardous cosleeping environments and risk factors amenable to change: case-control study of SIDS in southwest England. *BMJ*, 2009;**339**:b3666.

12. Stringer J, Welsh C, Tommasello A. Methadone-associated Q-T interval prolongation and torsades de pointes. *Am J Health Syst Pharm*, 2009; **66**:825–33.

13. Parikh R, Hussain T, Holder G, et al. Maternal methadone therapy increases QTc interval in newborn infants. *Arch Dis Child Fetal Neonatal Ed*, 2011; **96**:F141–3.

14. Cohen MC, Morley SR, Coombs RC. Maternal use of methadone and risk of sudden neonatal death. *Acta Paediatr*, 2015;**104**:883–7.

Environmental Risk Factors for SIDS

Michael Goodstein

The triple-risk theory of SIDS focuses on three components whose point of intersection leads to the greatest risk of SIDS for any given infant.[1] With the possible exception of electrocardiograms to identify infants with cardiac channelopathies, there are currently no standardised screening methods of identifying the infant who has intrinsic risk factors making him more vulnerable to SIDS. As a result, education efforts to reduce the risk of SIDS have focused on extrinsic risk factors or environmental influences. Since it would be unethical to perform randomised, controlled trials to determine SIDS risk or protective factors, the highest quality research available are case-control studies. These studies compare the environments of infants dying of SIDS with those of a cohort of live infants matched for demographic factors such as age, race/ethnicity, and socio-economic status. Such case-control studies are limited in that they identify associations, but do not provide information on causation. As such, researchers must use other data to tie these results into our understanding of the pathophysiology of SIDS. This section will review the environmental factors that have been associated with increased and reduced risk of SIDS.

Sleep Position

Prior to 1992, infants in the US routinely were placed to sleep in the prone position, with the thought that supine positioning put the infant at risk for aspiration. However, the New Zealand Cot Study found a three-fold increased risk of death for infants sleeping prone.[2] These data, as well as data from Great Britain, led the American Academy of Pediatrics to recommend that infants be placed either supine or on the side for sleep.[3] As more babies were placed on their sides for sleep, reports found this position to be an independent risk factor for SIDS (adjusted OR 2.0, 95% CI 1.2–3.4).[4] The side position is inherently unstable; infants placed on the side who roll to prone are at much greater risk for SIDS (adjusted OR 8.7.[4] Additionally, infants who are unaccustomed to prone sleep and are placed prone have an 8–45-fold increased risk of death compared to infants who are routinely placed on the stomach for sleep.[5]

In 1994, the National Institutes of Health in conjunction with other stakeholders initiated the back-to-sleep campaign. Over a ten-year period, the US SIDS rate dropped by 52% (Figure 23.1).[6] Data from numerous other industrialised countries have demonstrated consistently dramatic falls in SIDS rates when the population follows the recommendation to place infants supine for sleep. Conversely, data from Norway demonstrated a rise in the rate of SIDS when the prone sleep position was recommended, to promote developmental milestones. The rates returned to baseline when public policy was revised to recommend supine positioning again.[7]

After the rapid decline in the incidence of SIDS in the US in the late 1990s through the mid-2000s, rates have stagnated and this corresponds with a peak in the rate of routine supine sleep at 78%. Both the National Infant Sleep Position study (NISP) and Pregnancy Risk Assessment and Monitoring System (PRAMS) show white infants placed supine for sleep at rates of 75–80%, while for black infants the rates were 53–4%.[8,9] This disparity corresponds with the much higher rate of SIDS seen in black infants compared to white infants in the US (172 vs. 84 per 100,000 live births).[5]

Multiple etiologies have been implicated in explaining the increased risk of SIDS in the prone position. The triple-risk hypothesis suggests that SIDS is the result of a sequence of progressive asphyxia secondary to a failure of arousal.[10] Infants who sleep prone have longer periods of deep sleep, experience less movement, have higher arousal thresholds, and can experience sudden decreases in blood pressure and heart-rate control. These alterations in autonomic cardiovascular control can lead to reduced cerebral oxygenation, especially around two

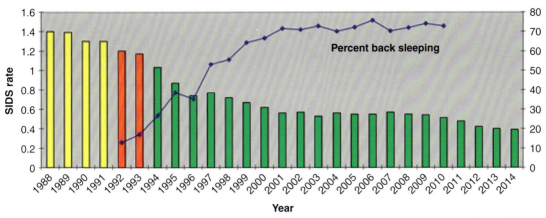

Figure 23.1 SIDS rate* (1998–2014) and Infant Sleep Position (1988–2010)

*Rate = number of SIDS deaths per 1,000 live births

Sources: Xu JQ, Kochanek KD, Murphy SL, Tejada-Vera B. Deaths: Final data for 2007. National vital statistics reports; vol 58 no 19. Hyattsville, MD: National Center for Health Statistics. 2010.
National Infant Sleep Position Study. https://www.nichd.nih.gov/research/supported/Pages/nisp.aspx

to three months of age. Thus, the increased risk of SIDS with prone positioning can be explained by impaired cerebral oxygenation resulting in the increased likelihood of a failure to arouse to a threat in the environment.

Alternatively, prone positioning is known to increase body temperature by decreasing the rate of heat loss as compared to supine positioning.[11] Overheating has been associated with an increased risk of SIDS and could represent the trigger in the vulnerable infant placed in the prone position.[12,13] In addition to promoting hyperthermia, prone positioning increases the chance of upper airway obstruction or rebreathing expired gases, resulting in hypoxia and hypercapnia.[14–16] Finally, the lack of developmental motor skills (i.e., the inability to lift and turn the head in response to an environmental threat) may predispose the vulnerable infant in the prone sleep position.

Sleep Devices/Sleep Surfaces

Infants should always sleep in their own safety-approved sleep 'device' to minimise the risk of SIDS. Cribs or cots, bassinets, and play yards have firm surfaces which are designed to avoid the potential hazards of other sleep surfaces such as the adult bed, couches, bean bag chairs, and recliners. Firmness is defined as a lack of deformability of the surface such

that it will not conform to the infant's head when placed on the surface. Firmness should not be confused with the tautness of the sheet over the sleep surface.

Unfortunately, there is no universally accepted definition of a firm sleep surface or way to test the firmness of a sleep surface. Manufacturers comply with voluntary safety standards, such as those established by the American Society and Testing and Materials. However, these standards are proprietary and not easily accessible to the public. Ron Somers, a researcher in Australia, has devised a tool that replicates one of the standard measurement devices using common household items to measure the depression made into the surface of a mattress, but it has not undergone formal testing.[17]

Soft surfaces can increase the risk of death five-fold.[18] Additionally, when placed prone on a soft surface, the risk of SIDS increases 21-fold.[13] Soft surfaces can allow the infant's head to sink into the surface. If the infant is placed or turns to the prone position, a soft surface can create a pocket of air which when rebreathed will lead to hypoxia and hypercarbia. Sofas, couches, cushioned arm chairs are some of the most dangerous places for an infant to sleep, with odds ratios for SIDS ranging from 5.1 to 66.9.[5]

In addition to the issue of firmness, child, and adult beds are dangerous for multiple other reasons.

Infants can become entrapped between the mattress and head or foot boards, as well as between the mattress and walls. Other injuries may occur if the child should roll out of the bed. Portable bed rails are not recommended due to risk of entrapment and suffocation. An extensive discussion about bed-sharing can be found elsewhere in this volume (Chapter 26).

Crib slats should be no wider than $2\frac{3}{8}$ inches to prevent entrapment of the head. Drop rail cribs are not recommended due to numerous device failures resulting in asphyxia from entrapment. The crib mattress should fit snugly in the crib. Gaps can lead to entrapment of the infant and asphyxia. Special mattresses are marketed promoting increased air permeability as a potential benefit to infants found in the prone position during sleep. However, there is no epidemiologic evidence that these mattresses reduce the risk of SIDS. The use of a 'breathable' mattress can be an acceptable alternative if it meets all other safety manufacturing requirements. There is no evidence to support the hypothesis that SIDS is related to release of toxic gases (such as antimony or arsenic) from mattresses.

Other devices have been developed for infant sleep, including co-sleepers, and baby boxes. Co-sleepers can be divided into bedside and in-bed sleepers. Bedside sleepers or side cars attach to the parental bed. Although the US Consumer Product Safety Commission (CPSC) recently developed safety standards for bedside sleepers, they have not been established in many other countries. Additionally, CPSC standards do not exist for in-bed sleepers, also called sleep enablers. In August 2017, Health Canada released an advisory against the use of baby nests (also known as baby pods) for infant sleep, due to suffocation risk from the padded sides. A baby nest is a small, portable bed that has been promoted by manufacturers for multiple uses, including bed sharing. Health Canada recommends that babies should never be left unattended in a nest, nor should the nests be placed inside another product, such as a crib or bassinet.[19] Recent data from New Zealand suggest that SIDS rates have declined in areas that have implemented programmes that include the use of one of two devices developed by the indigenous Māori community, the wahakura and Pēpi-Pod[TM][20] Because these programmes provide extensive education and community outreach, it is difficult to determine which element is responsible for the improvement.

Baby boxes have become extremely popular in the US and other countries, attempting to replicate the low infant mortality rate of Finland, where the concept originated. However, there are no studies evaluating the use or safety of the device. Other industrialised countries have shown similar dramatic falls in infant mortality over the twentieth century without the use of the baby box. The reasons are numerous, including improved nutrition, sanitation, immunisations, antibiotics, perinatology, and intensive care nurseries. Currently, there is not enough evidence to comment on the potential benefit or dangers of using these devices.

Car seats and other reclining devices do not provide a safe-sleep surface. Babies should sleep on a flat surface, as inclined surfaces can allow infants to roll into an unsafe sleep position. Sitting devices can worsen gastro-oesophageal reflux by pushing up on abdominal contents. Additionally, young infants with poor motor control of head and neck muscles can develop airway compromise if the head should fall forward while asleep.

Infants often fall asleep during travel; however, they should be moved to a safe-sleep environment as soon as it is feasible. It is unsafe to leave the infant in the car seat for sleep. It is especially dangerous to leave the infant in an unbuckled seat. In one study of deaths related to sitting and carrying devices in children under the age of two, 46 of 47 deaths were due to positional asphyxia or strangulation and 52% of deaths associated with car seats were attributed to strangulation from straps.[21]

Bedding (Soft or Loose Objects)

Bedding is a risk factor for SIDS, independent of sleep position. Unsafe materials in the sleep area include: pillows, quilts, comforters, plush toys, sheepskin, crib bumpers, and loose bedding such as blankets and non-fitted sheets. Use of a pillow has been shown to increase the risk three-fold, jumping to twelve-fold when combined with prone positioning.[18] Soft bedding can be a hazard either under the infant or loose in the sleep area. Death from SIDS or suffocation can occur with obstruction of the airway. Infants dying of SIDS in the supine position are often found with the head or face covered. Although the prevalence of soft bedding use has decreased in the US, it is still commonplace, having dropped from 86% to 55% between 1993 and 2010.[22] Rates are particularly high in teen mothers (83.5%), as well as those of non-white race (75.3%) and those with less than high school qualifications (81.9%).

Reasons why parents choose to use soft bedding include an extrapolation of their own feelings of comfort and warmth and a misunderstanding that soft and taut is not the same as firm.[23] Additionally, some parents mistakenly use blankets, pillows and rolls as a safety strategy to prevent falls from beds and other unsafe surfaces for infant sleep. However, soft bedding is the most important risk factor for infants 4 to 12 months old.[24] It is possible that some infants roll into the bedding and then cannot extract themselves.

Bumper pads were once used to help prevent infants from slipping between crib slats with head entrapment and asphyxia. However, with manufacturer regulations limiting the distance between slats to $2\frac{3}{8}$ inches, the risk of entrapment was eliminated. Bumper pads continued to be used to prevent other injuries, such as limb entrapment, or bumps and bruises. But a review of CPSC data discovered several infants dying from three mechanisms involving bumper pads: 1) suffocation involving soft, 'pillow-like' bumper pads; 2) asphyxia from entrapment between the bumper and the crib mattress; and 3) strangulation from long bumper ties. Some agencies have disagreed with the interpretation of the data, suggesting that other environmental factors were responsible for the deaths, rather than the bumper pads. An update on the original report increased the total number of deaths to 77, noting an increased frequency of cases being reported.[25] It is unclear if the increased number of deaths represents better reporting, diagnostic shift, or a true increase in deaths. Newer devices have been developed, such as 'breathable' bumpers and individual wraps for each slat, but no data are available regarding their safety. Since crib bumpers have been associated with SIDS and have not been shown to prevent significant injury in young infants, their use is not recommended.[5]

Overheating

It has been suggested that overheating of the infant is a risk factor for SIDS. This is based on data showing that SIDS risk is elevated when infants are heavily bundled with clothes or blankets.[26,27] There is also the previously described risk with prone positioning which leads to heat retention. The notion of overheating is difficult to sort out, though, from the risk related to loose bedding and head covering. It is unclear whether the risk is due to the temperature elevation, airway obstruction, or rebreathing. Studies have shown head covering to result in more frequent episodes of hypoxemia and rebreathing of carbon dioxide. Other studies have shown derangement of autonomic control of respiratory and cardiovascular systems with head covering. Additionally, studies have demonstrated impaired arousal from sleep when the face is covered.

Limited data suggest that room ventilation may be important, with one study showing an increased risk of SIDS with bedroom heating and another showing a decreased risk with good ventilation.[28,29] A third study suggested the use of a fan may be protective, but when other risk factors were controlled for, the benefit was lost.[30]

It is recommended to keep the room temperature comfortable for a normally dressed adult. Some countries give specific recommendations for actual room temperature. Babies can be dressed in layers, but should not be over-bundled. Due to concerns of potential face covering, blankets can be replaced with wearable blankets or infant sleeping sacks. It is important that sacks fit appropriately so that the infant's head cannot slip into the sack. If a blanket is necessary, it should be lightweight, and firmly tucked in and no higher than the axilla. Additionally, some countries recommend that the infant be placed with feet at the foot of the crib to prevent blankets from riding up over the face. Head coverings are not recommended for sleep.

Swaddling

Swaddling of infants is a practice that has existed for thousands of years across many cultures. Benefits of swaddling include providing warmth, decreasing fussiness, and promoting supine sleep positioning. However improper swaddling can result in numerous hazards for the newborn. An excessively tight swaddle can result in an increased respiratory rate. Restriction of leg movement can exacerbate developmental dysplasia of the hips. A swaddle that comes loose can become a suffocation hazard or increase the risk of SIDS. Recently, two articles were released questioning whether swaddling increases the risk of SIDS. The first, a review of reports to the Consumer Product Safety Commission involving blankets and swaddling devices (wearable blankets), found that of the 10 deaths involving wearable blankets, 80% of the deaths were due to positional asphyxia from prone sleeping and in 70% of the cases there were additional risk factors.[31] In the 12 deaths with regular blankets,

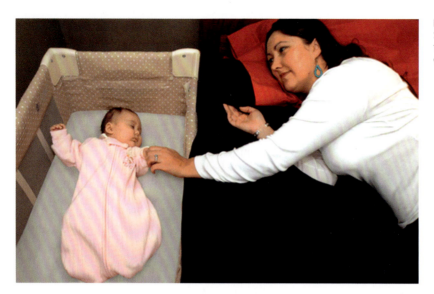

Figure 23.2 Examples. of Safe Infant Sleep Environments. Image courtesy of the Safe to Sleep® campaign, for educational purpose only.

58% were diagnosed as positional asphyxia from prone sleeping and 92% had additional risk factors. It is unclear as to what role swaddling played in these deaths. The study was further limited by a lack of a denominator to determine how common these events are in relation to the overall use of swaddling devices.

The second, a meta-analysis on swaddling, and SIDS risk found a slightly increased risk, with a pooled odds ratio of 1.38 (1.05–1.80).[32] However, there were dramatic differences in risk based on infant sleep position. The odds ratio in the prone position was 12.99 and in the side position it was 3.16. The risk was least in the supine position, 1.93. Age also played a role, with a 2-fold increased risk of death with swaddling beyond the age of 6 months. The study had significant limitations, including heterogeneity of studies in the meta-analysis, a lack of consistent definition of swaddling, and the possibility of other unidentified, confounding risk factors. Based on the current evidence, it is recommended that if infants are swaddled, they should be maintained in the supine sleep position and that swaddling should be discontinued once infants start to roll over.

Conclusion

In conclusion, many environmental factors have been identified that increase the risk of SIDS, and modifying the sleep environment accordingly has resulted in the prevention of thousands of deaths throughout industrialised countries. Examples of safe infant sleep environments, as recommended by the American Academy

of Pediatrics and multiple other international organisations, are shown in Figure 23.2.[5] However, 3,700 infants in the US continue to die each year from SIDS and other sleep-related causes.[33] There has been little reduction in these numbers since 2001 and this stagnation indicates there is still much work to be done.

References

1. Filiano JJ, Kinney HC. A perspective on neuropathologic findings in victims of the Sudden Infant Death Syndrome: the triple-risk model. *Biol Neonate*, 1994;**65**(3–4):194–7.

2. Mitchell EA, Stewart AW, Becroft DM, Taylor BJ, Ford RP, et. al. Results from the first year of the New Zealand cot death study. *N Z Med J*, 1991; **104**(906):71–6.

3. American Academy of Pediatrics Task Force on Infant Positioning and SIDS. Positioning and SIDS. *Pediatrics*, 1992; **89**(6):1120–6; http://pediatrics.aappu blications.org/content/pediatrics/89/6/1120.full.pdf (accessed 31 October 2018).

4. Li DK, Petitti DB, Willinger M, et al. Infant sleeping position and the risk of Sudden Infant Death Syndrome in California, 1997–2000. *Am J Epidemiol*, 2003; **157**(5):446–55.

5. Moon RY. Task force on Sudden Infant Death Syndrome, SIDS and other sleep-related infant deaths: evidence base for 2016 updated recommendations for a safe infant sleeping environment. *Pediatrics*, 2016; **138**(5):e20162940.

6. Moon, R. Y. SIDS and other sleep-related infant deaths: expansion of recommendations for a safe infant sleeping. *Pediatrics*, 2011; **128**(5):1030–9.

7. Irgens LM, Markestad T, Baste V, Schreuder P, Skjaerven R, Oyen N. Sleeping position and Sudden Infant Death Syndrome in Norway 1967–91. *Arch Dis Child*, 1995; **72**:478–82.

8. Colson ER, Rybin D, Smith LA, Colton T, Lister G, Corwin MJ. Trends and factors associated with infant sleeping position: the National Infant Sleep Position Study, 1993–2007. *Arch Pediatr Adolesc Med*, 2009; **163**(12):1122–8.

9. Centers for Disease Control. Pregnancy Risk Assessment and Monitoring System (PRAMS); https://www.cdc.gov/prams/index.htm (accessed 31 October 2018).

10. Kinney HC, Thach BT. The Sudden Infant Death Syndrome. *N Engl J Med*, 2009; **361**:795–805.

11. Ammari A, Schulze KF, Ohira-Kist K, et al. Effects of body position on thermal, cardiorespiratory, and metabolic activity in low birthweight infants. *Early Hum Dev*, 2009; **85**(8):497–501.

12. Tuffnell CS, Petersen SA, Wailoo MP. Prone sleeping infants have a reduced ability to lose heat. *Early Hum Dev*, 1995; **43**(2):109–16.

13. Fleming PJ, Gilbert R, Azaz Y, et al. Interaction between bedding and sleeping position in the Sudden Infant Death Syndrome: a population-based case-control study. *BMJ*, 1990; **301**(6743):85–9.

14. Kanetake J, Aoki Y, Funayama M. Evaluation of rebreathing potential on bedding for infant use. *Pediatr Int*, 2003; **45**(3):284–9.

15. Kemp JS, Thach BT. Quantifying the potential of infant bedding to limit CO2 dispersal and factors affecting rebreathing in bedding. *J Appl Physiol (1985)*, 1995; **78**(2):740–5.

16. Patel AL, Harris K, Thach BT. Inspired CO(2) and O(2) in sleeping infants rebreathing from bedding: relevance for Sudden Infant Death Syndrome. *J Appl Physiol (1985)*, 2001; **91**(6):2537–45.

17. Consumers' Federation of Australia. At-home consumer test makes it possible to identify dangerously soft baby mattresses (22 April 2015); http://consumersfederation.org.au/at-home-consumer-test-makes-it-possible-to-identify-dangerously-soft-baby-mattresses/ (accessed 31 October 2018).

18. Hauck, FR, Herman SM, Donovan M, Iyasu S, Merrick Moore C, et. al. Sleep environment and the risk of Sudden Infant Death Syndrome in an urban population: the Chicago Infant Mortality Study. *Pediatrics*, 2003; **111**(5):1207–14.

19. Health Canada. Consumer product update: Health Canada warns Canadians of health and safety risks of baby nests (Children's Products Advisory RA-64318). 27 August 2017; http://healthycanadians.gc.ca/recall-alert-rappel-avis/hc-sc/2017/64318a-eng.php (accessed 31 October 2018).

20. Mitchell EA, Cowan S, Tipene-Leach D. The recent fall in postperinatal mortality in New Zealand and the Safe Sleep programme. *Acta Paediatrica*, 2016; **105**:1312–20.

21. Batra EK, Midgett JD, Moon RY. Hazards associated with sitting and carrying devices for children two years and younger. *J Pediatr*, 2015; **167**(1):183–7.

22. Shapiro-Mendoza CK, Colson ER, Willinger M, Rybin DV, Camperlengo L, Corwin MJ. Trends in infant bedding use: national infant sleep position study, 1993–2010. *Pediatrics*, 2015; **135**(1):10–17.

23. Ajao TI, Oden RP, Joyner BL, Moon RY. Decisions of black parents about infant bedding and sleep surfaces: a qualitative study. *Pediatrics*, 2011; **128**(3):494–502.

24. Colvin JD, Collie-Akers V, Schunn C, Moon RY. Sleep environment risks for younger and older infants. *Pediatrics*, 2014; **134**(2); www.pediatrics.org/cgi/content/full/134/2/e406 (accessed 4 October 2018).

25. Scheers NJ, Woodard DW, Thach BT. Crib bumpers continue to cause infant deaths: a need for a new preventive approach. *J Pediatr*, 2015; **169**(2):93–7.

26. Ponsonby A-L, Dwyer T, Gibbons LE, Cochrane JA, Jones ME, McCall MJ. Thermal environment and Sudden Infant Death Syndrome: case-control study. *BMJ*, 1992; **304**(6822):277–82.

27. Fleming PJ, Gilbert R, Azaz Y, et al. Interaction between bedding and sleeping position in the Sudden Infant Death Syndrome: a population-based case-control study. *BMJ*, 1990; **301**(6743):85–9.

28. Ponsonby AL, Dwyer T, Kasl SV, Cochrane JA. The Tasmanian SIDS case-control study: univariable and multivariable risk factor analysis. *Paediatr Perinat Epidemiol*, 1995; **9**(3):256–72.

29. McGlashan ND. Sudden infant deaths in Tasmania, 1980–1986: a seven-year prospective study. *Soc Sci Med*, 1989; **29**(8):1015–26.

30. Coleman-Phox K, Odouli R, Li DK. Use of a fan during sleep and the risk of Sudden Infant Death Syndrome. *Arch Pediatr Adolesc Med*, 2008; **162**(10):963–8.

31. McDonnell E, Moon RY. Infant deaths and injuries associated with wearable blankets, swaddle wraps, and swaddling. *J Pediatr*, 2014; **164**(5):1152–6.

32. Pease AS, Fleming PJ, Hauck FR, et al. Swaddling and the risk of Sudden Infant Death Syndrome: a meta-analysis. *Pediatrics*, 2016; **137**(6):e20153275.

33. Centers for Disease Control and Prevention. *Sudden Unexpected Infant Death and Sudden Infant Death Syndrome*. www.cdc.gov/sids/data.htm (accessed 31 October 2017).

The Relationship Between Breastfeeding and SIDS

John M. D. Thompson

Introduction

Breastfeeding has always been the essence of feeding of mammalian offspring, and continues to be so among all species for whom survival without it would essentially be impossible, with the exception of humans. Maternal feeding of the infant creates natural bonds with the mother, protection from danger, and transfer of evolutionarily developed nutrients essential for the survival of the species.

As a consequence of technolgcial advances and modern medicine, along with cultural beliefs that have shifted, breastfeeding rates in developed as well as developing countries have declined.[1-3] The World Health Organisation (WHO) and the United Nations Children's Fund (UNICEF) implemented a global campaign named Baby Friendly Hospital Initiative (BFHI). This initiative has been implemented in most Western countries and the continued promotion has been shown to increase breastfeeding rates. Currently breastfeeding rates around the world still vary significantly with the highest rates seen in Scandinavian countries[4,5] and New Zealand,[6,7] while the United Kingdom[8] and United States[9] have lower rates. The reasons for this large variability in rates across countries is unknown.

Association of Breastfeeding and Risk of SIDS

Breastfeeding is unique in relation to SIDS as it is one of the few factors that not only meets the criteria for likely being causally related, but imparts a protective effect. Hence messages about brestfeeding are not around risk avoidance or risk minimisation but encouraging mothers to partake in a natural practice to increase the chance of survival of their offspring.

As early as 1965 Carpenter and Shaddick found that SIDS cases had a history of early bottle feeding.[10] The late 1980s and the 1990s saw a plethora of case-control studies around the world including New Zealand,[7,11] Australia,[12] the United Kingdom,[13] Scandinavia,[14-16] United States,[17-19] and numerous European countries.[20] The majority of these studies found that in univariable analyses breastfeeding was protective against SIDS. In the early 2000s two meta-analyses were carried out showing reduced risks, but both had methodological issues that led to somewhat inconclusive evidence.

In 2011 Hauck and colleagues carried out a meta-analysis[21] using data from all published case-control studies of SIDS where data were available. This analysis showed that for all studies, except for a small number with limited power, the univariable odds ratio for any breastfeeding was protective and the aggregated effect size was 0.40 (95%CI=0.35, 0.44). Fewer studies had multivariable analyses available but the combined effect of the multivariable odds ratios (given the issue that they had controlled for different factors) was 0.55 (95%CI=0.44, 0.69). Fewer studies investigated exclusive breastfeeding, though all showed statistically significant univariable odds ratios with a combined protective effect of 0.27 (95% CI=0.24, 0.31). A multivariable combined effect was not able to be carried out due to lack of availability of multivariable results. The major limitation of this work was the lack of ability to assess the effect of duration of breastfeeding due to the differing definitions across studies.

A very recent analysis was conducted by the same group. They gathered individual patient level data that were available from case-control studies across the world to enable assessment of the association of duration of breastfeeding and SIDS.[22] This analysis has shown that any breastfeeding was protective against SIDS, with the risk decreasing further as the length of breastfeeding increased: the combined odds ratio was 0.61 (95%CI=0.54, 0.69) for less than two months and decreased to 0.13 (95%CI=0.10, 0.18) for greater than 6 months. After controlling for potential confounders these odds ratios all moved towards unity with breastfeeding less than 2 months not showing a significantly protective effect, but the pattern of a decreased risk with longer duration continuing for those breastfeeding for 2–4 months (OR 0.60, 95% CI-0.44–0.82) to 0.36 (95% CI-0.22–0.61) for those breastfeeding longer than 6 months, in a model that controlled for a maximum number of potential confounders. Similarly, in relation to exclusive breastfeeding the magnitude of the protective effect increased with longer duration. Again, the effects were reduced in multivariable analyses and breastfeeding duration under 2 months was found to not be associated with a significantly reduced risk. Of particular note and interest also was the fact that the effect of exclusive breastfeeding was no more protective than any breastfeeding.

In conclusion, the evidence clearly suggests a protective effect of breastfeeding in relation to SIDS. The most current evidence would suggest that breastfeeding needs to have a duration of at least 2 months to convey a protective effect, and that exclusive breastfeeding is not necessary to convey this effect.

Mechanisms

The main question that remains around breastfeeding is that of the mechanism of protection against SIDS. An initial proposal which still remains today was made in 1975 by Tonkin,[23] who suggested that the vulnerability of the infant was at the oropharyngeal level between the soft palate and the base of the skull. One of the potential reasons proposed for this vulnerability was that a large tongue with a strong suckling action as the result of artificial feeding could cause occlusion of the airway.

There has also been a wide range of other suggested mechanisms, many of which relate to the gastrointestinal tract, from suggestions of toxigenic intestinal infections such as infant botulism through formula ingestion[24] to more contemporary hypotheses around gut microbiome differences.[25] Similarly these toxigenic bacteria have also been said to be more common in the nasal flora of SIDS infants, though not in relation to bottle feeding.[26] Studies have shown that breastfeeding appears to enhance the infants' immunological status at a time when they are transitioning from maternal levels to their own production.

Similarly, there have been numerous studies relating to the arousability of infants as a possible

mechanism, suggesting that particularly in active sleep, breastfed infants are more easily aroused than formula-fed infants.[27,28] It has also been shown that docosohexanoic acid in the brain cortex is higher in breastfed infants,[29] which may also relate to increased arousability.

Controversies in Relation to Breastfeeding

There are two main factors related to both breastfeeding and SIDS that raise debate, namely the use of pacifiers/dummies (another factor shown to have a protective effects against SIDS) and bed-sharing (one of the most significant risk factors, particularly in combination with smoking, for SIDS).

Pacifiers/Dummies

It has been suggested that one consequence of pacifier use may be to reduce breastmilk production and shorten duration of breastfeeding, though there are limited data around this. A recent Cochrane review found that pacifier use had no effect of the proportion of infants exclusively or partially breastfed at 3 or 4 months of age.[30] (See Chapter 25 for futher discussion.)

Bed-sharing

Proponents of bed-sharing suggest that in routine bed-sharing situations. the number of breastfeeding events and duration of breastfeeding are increased. However from an opposing point of view, falling asleep with the infant (particularly while breastfeeding) increases the risk of rolling onto the infant and producing a dangerous environment. (See Chapter 26 for further discussion.)

The Future

There is a need to carry on the promotion of BFHI around the world with an emphasis not just on initiation of breastfeeding but the continuation of breastfeeding well into infancy. The WHO recommends exclusive breastfeeding until 6 months; however, this target will need significant work in the Western world. Fortunately, the statistically reduced risk of SIDS appears to be in place after only two months of breastfeeding. Future research may advance our understanding of the mechanisms leading to the large protective effect that breastfeeding—whether exclusive or partial—confers against SIDS.

References

1. Baumgartel KL, Sneeringer L, Cohen SM. From royal wet nurses to Facebook: the evolution of breastmilk sharing. *Breastfeed Rev*, 2016; **24**:25–32.

2. Daglas M, Antoniou E. Cultural views and practices related to breastfeeding. *Health Sci J*, 2012; **6**:353–61.

3. Stevens EE, Patrick TE, Pickler R. A history of infant feeding. *J Perinat Educ*, 2009; **18**:32–9.

4. Alm B, Wennergren G, Norvenius SG, et al. Breast feeding and the Sudden Infant Death Syndrome in Scandinavia, 1992–95. *Arch Dis Child*, 2002; **86**:400–2.

5. Lindgren C, Thompson JM, Haggblom L, et al. Sleeping position, breastfeeding, bedsharing, and passive smoking in 3-month-old Swedish infants. *Acta Paediatr*, 1998; **87**:1028–32.

6. Ford RP, Mitchell EA, Scragg R, et al. Factors adversely associated with breastfeeding in New Zealand. *J Paediatr Child Health*, 1994; **30**:483–9.

7. Mitchell EA, Tuohy PG, Brunt JM, et al. Risk factors for Sudden Infant Death Syndrome following the prevention campaign in New Zealand: a prospective study. *Pediatrics*, 1997; **100**:835–40.

8. Gilbert RE, Wigfield RE, Fleming PJ, et al. Bottle feeding and the Sudden Infant Death Syndrome. *BMJ*, 1995; **310**:88–90.

9. Centers for Disease Control and Prevention (CDC). Breastfeeding trends and updated national health objectives for exclusive breastfeeding – United States, birth years 2000–2004. *MMWR Morb Mortal Wkly Rep*, 2007; **56**:760–3.

10. Carpenter RG, Shaddick CW. Role of infection, suffocation, and bottle-feeding in cot death; an analysis of some factors in the histories of 110 cases and their controls. *Br J Prev Soc Med*, 1965; **19**:1–7.

11. Mitchell EA, Taylor BJ, Ford RP, et al. Four modifiable and other major risk factors for cot death: the New Zealand study. *J Paediatr Child Health*, 1992; **28**:S3-8.

12. Ponsonby AL, Dwyer T, Kasl SV, et al. The Tasmanian SIDS case-control study: univariable and multivariable risk factor analysis. *Paediatr Perinat Epidemiol*, 1995; **9**:256–72.

13. Fleming PJ, Blair PS, Bacon C, et al. Environment of infants during sleep and risk of the Sudden Infant Death Syndrome: results of 1993–5 case-control study for confidential inquiry into stillbirths and deaths in infancy. Confidential enquiry into stillbirths and deaths regional coordinators and researchers. *BMJ*, 1996; **313**:191–5.

14. Alm B, Norvenius SG, Wennergren G, et al. Changes in the epidemiology of Sudden Infant Death Syndrome in Sweden 1973–1996. *Arch Dis Child*, 2001; **84**:24–30.

15. Daltveit AK, Oyen N, Skjaerven R, et al. The epidemic of SIDS in Norway 1967–93: changing effects of risk factors. *Arch Dis Child*, 1997; **77**:23–7.

16. Irgens LM, Markestad T, Baste V, et al. Sleeping position and Sudden Infant Death Syndrome in Norway 1967–91. *Arch Dis Child*, 1995; **72**:478–82.

17. Hauck FR, Herman SM, Donovan M, et al. Sleep environment and the risk of Sudden Infant Death Syndrome in an urban population: the Chicago Infant Mortality Study. *Pediatrics*, 2003; **111**:1207–14.

18. Hoffman HJ, Hillman LS. Epidemiology of the Sudden Infant Death Syndrome: maternal, neonatal, and postneonatal risk factors. [Review]. *Clin Perinatol*, 1992; **19**:717–37.

19. Klonoff-Cohen HS, Edelstein SL. A case-control study of routine and death scene sleep position and Sudden Infant Death Syndrome in Southern California. *JAMA*, 1995; **273**:790–4.

20. Carpenter RG, Irgens LM, Blair PS, et al. Sudden unexplained infant death in 20 regions in Europe: case-control study. *Lancet*, 2004; **363**:185–91.

21. Hauck FR, Thompson JMD, Tanabe KO, et al. Breastfeeding and reduced risk of Sudden Infant Death Syndrome: a meta-analysis. *Pediatrics*, 2011; **128**:103–10.

22. Thompson JMD, Tanabe K, Moon RY, et al. Duration of breastfeeding and risk of SIDS: an individual participant data (IPD) meta-analysis. *Pediatrics published online*, 30 October 2017.

23. Tonkins S. Sudden Infant Death Syndrome: hypothesis of causation. *Pediatrics*, 1975; **55**:650–61.

24. Arnon SS. Breast feeding and toxigenic intestinal infections: missing links in crib death? *Rev Infect Dis*, 1984; **6**(Suppl 1):S193-201.

25. Highet AR, Berry AM, Bettelheim KA, et al. Gut microbiome in Sudden Infant Death Syndrome (SIDS) differs from that in healthy comparison babies and offers an explanation for the risk factor of prone position. *Int J Med Microbiol*, 2014; **304**:735–41.

26. Blackwell CC, MacKenzie DA, James VS, et al. Toxigenic bacteria and Sudden Infant Death Syndrome (SIDS): nasopharyngeal flora during the first year of life. *FEMS Immunol Med Microbiol*, 1999; **25**:51–8.

27. Horne RS, Parslow PM, Ferens D, et al. Comparison of evoked arousability in breast- and formula-fed infants. *Arch Dis Child*, 2004; **89**:22–5.

28. Horne RS, Parslow PM, Harding R. Respiratory control and arousal in sleeping infants. *Paediatr Respir Rev*, 2004; **5**:190–8.

29. Byard RW, Makrides M, Need M, et al. Sudden Infant Death Syndrome: effect of breast and formula feeding

on frontal cortex and brainstem lipid composition. *J Paediatr Child Health*, 1995; **31**:14–16.

30. Jaafar SH, Ho JJ, Jahanfar S, et al. Effect of restricted pacifier use in breastfeeding term infants for increasing duration of breastfeeding. *Cochrane Database Syst Rev*, 2016; **8**:CD007202. https://www.cochranelibrary.com/cdsr/doi/10.1002/14651858.CD007202.pub4/full (accessed 31 October 2018).

Pacifier Use and SIDS

Alejandro Gustavo Jenik

Pacifier (also known as dummy) use has always been a controversial topic. The aim of this chapter is to provide a comprehensive summary of current relevant evidence about pacifier use in relation to breastfeeding and SIDS.

Pacifiers: Protecting Against SIDS

In 1993, a landmark study showing the connection between SIDS and pacifiers was published. The use of a pacifier in the last sleep of SIDS cases was significantly less than in matched living controls.[1] Subsequently, eleven case-control studies have confirmed the work by Mitchell et al., showing a risk reduction of about 50% if the infant used a pacifier. Two meta-analyses reported approximately the same summary odds ratio of about 0.5.[2,3] Hauck et al. found that in studies where a variety of factors were controlled, 'usual' pacifier use was associated with an approximately 30% reduction in the risk of SIDS.[2] An approximately 50% reduction in risk was associated with 'pacifier use at last sleep' among studies using univariate analysis, and a 60% reduction was found using multivariate analysis. In a second meta-analysis that included many of the same studies, Mitchell et al. found a 17% reduction in risk associated with 'routine' pacifier use and a 50% risk reduction associated with use at the last sleep.

Using a pacfier at the onset of sleep is protective, even when the pacifier falls out of the mouth after the infant falls asleep. The reduced risk of SIDS associated with its use appears to be greater with adverse sleep conditions (such as sleeping prone or on the side, and sleeping with a mother who smokes).[4] In relation to this, Blair et al. showed that the protective effect of the pacifier was mainly confined to those who bed-share (OR – 0.3) although it was barely significant for those who did not (OR – 0.8).[5] The way in which a pacifier can reduce the risk of SIDS is still unclear. Box 25.1 lists possible proposed mechanisms for pacifier protection.

In conclusion, advocating the use of pacifiers for infants in high-risk populations may have the potential to further reduce the incidence of SIDS. The use of the pacifier is recommended only when the infant is placed to sleep (all naps and night-time sleep) and to comfort the infant. The recommendation is to phase out the use of the pacifier after one year.[6]

The Pacifier Debate: Are Pacifiers Associated with Early Weaning from Breastfeeding?

Historical Background

There is ample evidence that breastfeeding and pacifier use reduce the risk of SIDS. The BFHI is a global campaign launched by WHO and UNICEF which recognises that implementing best practice in health services is crucial to the success of breastfeeding programmes. Best practice is represented by The Ten Steps to Successful Breastfeeding ('The Ten Steps'), which were first published in *Protecting, Promoting and Supporting Breastfeeding: The Special Role of Maternity Services* – a joint WHO/UNICEF Statement in 1989.[7] Step 9 of the statement recommends total avoidance of artificial teats or pacifiers for breastfeeding infants.

There was no epidemiological evidence of an association between pacifier use and breastfeeding at the time The Ten Steps were published in 1989. We must take into consideration that Victora et al. published the first observational study which concluded that pacifiers are causally associated with weaning in the *Lancet* in 1993.[8] The investigation regarding pacifiers and breastfeeding continued. The same negative correlation between the use of pacifiers and successful breastfeeding was found in most, but not all, large observational studies carried out with. the use of pacifiers associated with shortening of the breastfeeding

BOX 25.1 Mechanisms of possible pacifier protection

1. Improves autonomic control
2. Prevents the infant from rolling into the prone position
3. Alters the infant's sleeping environment favourably (by the pacifier's external handle)
4. Helps maintain upper airway patency
5. Increases sleeping blood pressure
6. Increases arousability (controversial)
7. Induces a forward movement of the mandible

period. Nevertheless the cause and effect relationship is not clear. Observational studies cannot determine if pacifier use causes breastfeeding cessation; these studies therefore can be used only to describe associations between the behaviours.[9]

Ten steps to Successful Breastfeeding have been revised in April 2018 and updated in line with the evidence-based guidelines. Steps 9 of the Statement have been changed to "Counsel Mothers on the use and risks of feeding bottles, teats and pacifiers". As a conclusion, nowadays WHO guidelines do not call for absolute avoidance of feeding bottles, teats and pacifiers.

The Reconciliation

Does pacifier use have an adverse effect on breastfeeding? Or is it simply a marker of breastfeeding difficulties or of an attempt to wean the baby? Evidence of causation is bettter supplied by randomised controlled trials. Results from four randomised controlled trials (RCT) revealed no difference in breastfeeding outcomes with different types of pacifier interventions: in preterm infants,[10] pacifiers introduced at fifteen days of age,[11] and educational programmes for mothers emphasising avoidance of pacifiers[12] and a BFHI environment.[13] Only one RCT found an increased risk of early weaning. In a multivariate analysis, Howard et al. found that pacifier use in the first five days versus pacifier use after 4 weeks postpartum was associated with shorter breastfeeding duration.[14]

Lactation consultants, who are likely to be familiar with observational studies, may disagree with the RCT's conclusion that did not find reduction of the duration of breastfeeding with the use of a pacifier.

In 2011, Jaafar conducted a meta-analysis to determine the effect of restricting or not using pacifiers on the duration of breastfeeding (Cochrane Review).[15] This review included in their final analysis two RCTs studies carried out by Jenik[11] and Kramer.[12] Jenik et al. published a large RCT (n=1021) of pacifier use in breastfed infants; they showed that offering a pacifier at fifteen days of age does not reduce the prevalence or duration of breastfeeding. This RCT from Argentina was a multicentre trial from five hospitals and the inclusión criteria were mothers with well-established lactation at 2 weeks and highly motivated to breastfeed for three months.

Kramer et al. performed a randomised controlled trial involving 281 healthy, breastfeeding mothers that were either counselled to avoid a pacifier or given no specific counselling on pacifer use. When analysed with 'intention to treat' (i.e. according to randomisation), there were no differences in weaning by three months between the groups.[12] However, in another study when randomisation was ignored for analysis, a strong association was found between exposure to daily pacifier use and weaning by three months. The authors argue that breastfeeding and pacifier use are complex behaviours that are influenced by many factors that are difficult to measure and therefore to control for in observational studies and that causality can only be assessed through well-designed randomised trials. Victora et al. found that mothers used pacifiers to lengthen the interval between feedings and to assist with weaning, suggesting that pacifier use is a marker, but not a cause, of breastfeeding difficulties or reduced breastfeeding.[8] Jafaar concluded that the use of pacifiers in healthy term breastfeeding infants, started from birth, or after lactation is established, did not affect the prevalence or duration of exclusive and partial breastfeeding up to four months of age.[15]

Clinical Commentary

The RCT published by Jenik et al. clearly shows that the use of a pacifier introduced at fifteen days of infant age in motivated mothers does not support the claim that pacifiers lead to a decreased breastfeeding duration.[11] O'Connor et al. in a systematic literature review concluded that the 'strongest current evidence on pacifiers and breastfeeding indicates that pacifier use is not detrimental to breastfeeding outcomes'.[9]

Final recommendations, which are consistent with recommendations from the American Academy of Pediatrics,[6] are as follows:

- Use of a pacifier/dummy is associated with lower SIDS rates and parents may consider offering a pacifier/dummy when settling the baby to sleep
- If the mother chooses to breastfeed, breastfeeding should be established before the pacifier/dummy is introduced
- A pacifier/dummy can be introduced in formula-fed infants as soon as desired

References

1. Mitchell EA, Taylor BJ, Ford RP, Stewart AW, Becroft DM, Thompson JM, et al. Dummies and the Sudden Infant Death Syndrome. *Arch Dis Child*, 1993; **68**(4):501–4.

2. Hauck FR, Omojokun OO, Siadaty MS. Do pacifiers reduce the risk of Sudden Infant Death Syndrome? A meta-analysis. *Pediatrics*, 2005; **116**(5):e716–23.

3. Mitchell EA, Blair PS, L'Hoir MP. Should pacifiers be recommended to prevent Sudden Infant Death Syndrome? *Pediatrics*, 2006; **117**(5):1755–8.

4. Li DK, Willinger M, Petitti DB, Odouli R, Liu L, Hoffman HJ. Use of a dummy (pacifier) during sleep and risk of Sudden Infant Death Syndrome (SIDS): population-based case-control study. *BMJ*, 2006; **332**(7532):18–22.

5. Blair PS, Sidebotham P, Pease A, Fleming PJ. Bed-sharing in the absence of hazardous circumstances: is there a risk of Sudden Infant Death Syndrome? An analysis from two case-control studies conducted in the UK. *PLoS One*, 2014; **9**(9).

6. AAP Task Force on Sudden Infant Death Syndrome. SIDS and other sleep-related infant deaths: updated 2016 recommendations for a safe infant sleeping environment. *Pediatrics*, 2016; **138**(5):e2016293.

7. World Health Organization and UNICEF. *Protecting, Promoting and Supporting Breastfeeding: The Special Role of Maternity Services. A Joint WHO/UNICEF Statement*. Geneva: WHO, 1989; http://apps.who.int/iris/bitstream/handle/10665/39679/9241561300.pdf?sequence=1 (accessed 31 October 2018).

8. Victora CG, Tomasi E, Olinto MT, Barros FC. Use of pacifiers and breastfeeding duration. *Lancet*, 1993; **341**(8842):404–6.

9. O'Connor NR, Tanabe KO, Siadaty MS, Hauck FR Pacifiers and breastfeeding: a systematic review. *Arch Pediatr Adolesc Med*, 2009; **163**(4):378–82.

10. Collins CT, Ryan P, Crowther CA, McPhee A, Paterson S, Hiller J. Effect of bottles, cups, and dummies on breast feeding in preterm infants: a randomised controlled trial. *BMJ*, 2004; **329**(7459): 193–8.

11. Jenik AG, Vain NE, Gorestein AN, Jacobi NE. Does the recommendation to use a pacifier influence the prevalence of breastfeeding? *J Pediatr*, 2009; **155**(3): 350–4.

12. Kramer MS, Barr RG, Dagenais S, Yang H, Jones P, Ciofani L, et al. Pacifier use, early weaning, and cry/fuss behavior: a randomized controlled trial. *JAMA*, 2001; **286**(3):322–6.

13. Schubiger G, Schwarz U, Tonz O. UNICEF/WHO baby-friendly hospital initiative: does the use of bottles and pacifiers in the neonatal nursery prevent successful breastfeeding? Neonatal Study Group. *Eur J Pediatr*, 1997; **156**(11):874–7.

14. Howard CR, Howard FM, Lanphear B, Eberly S, deBlieck EA, Oakes D, et al. Randomized clinical trial of pacifier use and bottle-feeding or cupfeeding and their effect on breastfeeding. *Pediatrics*, 2003; **111**(3):511–18.

15. Jaafar SH, Ho JJ, Jahanfar S, Angolkar M. Effect of restricted pacifier use in breastfeeding term infants for increasing duration of breastfeeding. *Cochrane Database Syst Rev*, 2016 (**8**):CD007202 https://www.cochranelibrary.com/cdsr/doi/10.1002/14651858.CD007202.pub4/full (accessed 31 October 2018).

Chapter

26

Bed-sharing: What is the Evidence?

Peter S. Blair, David Tipene-Leach, and Eve R. Colson

Bed-sharing and SIDS

Prolonged physical contact between parents and infants during sleep is a normal infant care behaviour in many different cultures and is commonly practised in Western society. In England, almost half of all neonates bed-share at some time with their parents, and a fifth of infants are brought into the parental bed on a regular basis over the first year of life.[1] In the United States, about 21% of all mothers and more than 25% of Hispanic mothers report bed-sharing for some or all of the night.[2] Postulated physiological benefits of close contact between infants and caregivers include improved cardiorespiratory stability and oxygenation, fewer crying episodes, better thermoregulation, increased prevalence and duration of breastfeeding, and enhanced milk production.[3] Even in modern Western societies infant mortality is significantly lower among breastfed infants.[4] Although commonly known as 'cot death' or 'crib death', SIDS can occur in any infant sleeping environment and has increasingly been discovered to occur in shared sleeping spaces more often than expected. Recent observational case-control studies suggest as much as half of the SIDS deaths take place when infants sleep alongside an adult.[5] This rather alarming proportional rise in SIDS deaths outside the cot, along with consistent data from case-control studies, has led some countries to recommend against bed-sharing including the American Academy of Pediatrics (AAP) since 2005.[6] A meta-analysis of 11 SIDS case-control studies published in 2012 showed a pooled risk associated with bed-sharing of 2.89 [95% CI 1.99–4.18], with increased risk if the infant was exposed to maternal tobacco smoke or was younger than 12 weeks but did not reach significance in older infants or those not exposed to tobacco smoke.[5] The recommendations of the AAP is that the safest sleep location to prevent SIDS is to room-share without bed-sharing,[7] while other countries such as the UK recommend against bed-sharing in certain hazardous environments.

The Fall in SIDS Rates

Longitudinal data from Avon in England of 300 consecutive SIDS deaths over a 20-year period show that the proportional rise in bed-sharing SIDS deaths does not equate to an increase in the prevalence of these deaths.[8] The national 'back-to-sleep' campaign in 1991 was first initiated in Avon by Fleming and colleagues in 1989 and showed a striking reduction (sevenfold) in deaths occurring in the cot (crib) (Figure 26.1).[8] SIDS deaths in the parental bed also fell by half over this time-period but not as dramatically, while the rare event of a sofa-sharing death became slightly more common. This is particularly important to observe because any carer who wants to avoid the potential risk of bringing the baby into bed to breastfeed and inadvertently falling asleep may put the infant at greater risk by getting out of bed and sitting in a chair or on a sofa. Ironically the proportional rise in bed-sharing SIDS deaths and concerns raised by this practice is largely due to the tremendous success we have had in reducing solitary deaths occurring in a cot or crib. Why the 'back-to-sleep' campaign was less effective among bed-sharing deaths is not clear although data from the Avon cohort[8] and subsequent studies[9] suggest placing infants prone to sleep was far more common among those sleeping alone than those sleeping with someone. This may partly explain the inherent protection of breastfeeding against SIDS in that to initiate or enable such a process infants are more likely to be placed supine and that the exposure of risk while bed-sharing may thus lay elsewhere.

Significant Interactions Providing Hazardous Exposure to the Infant

The interaction between maternal smoking and bed-sharing as a risk for SIDS was first identified by Mitchell et al's large New Zealand study in 1993.[10] The risk among infants bed-sharing next to mothers who smoked was more than four-fold (OR 4.55 [95%

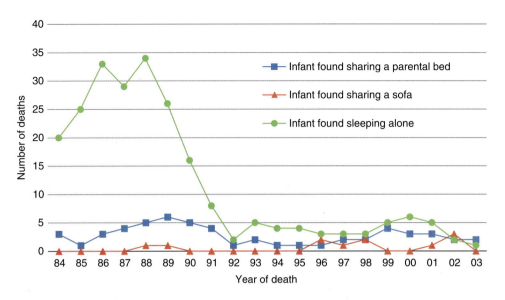

Figure 26.1 SIDS deaths by sleeping environment (300 consecutive SIDS deaths in Avon, UK between 1984, and 2003)

CI 2.63–7.88]) compared to no risk among infants sleeping next to non-smoking mothers (OR 0.98 [95% CI 0.44–2.18]). Similar findings were observed in subsequent studies. It is not clear why this exposure would put the infant at risk; innate vulnerability due to fetal exposure of tobacco smoke during pregnancy, postnatal prolonged passive exposure or a proxy marker for some other unmeasured risk-taking parental behaviour have all been postulated but little further evidence has been provided. Significant interactions have also been observed between bed-sharing and parental use of alcohol or drugs prior to the last sleep and using a sofa to sleep with the infant.[11] A combined analysis from two English studies[9] suggest an 18-fold increase in SIDS deaths if an infant sleeps next to an adult who drinks more than two units of alcohol or if an infant sleeps with an adult on a sofa (Table 26.1). Both hazardous circumstances are suggestive that overlaying is a potential causal explanation for these SIDS deaths although it is difficult to verify such a causal classification using current post-mortem techniques. Noticeably, the exposure of these two hazardous circumstances was very rare among the controls (<1%) suggesting such practices are potentially lethal. An observational study of nearly 8,000 sleep-related infant deaths in 45 US states from 2004 to 2012 showed that 11% occurred while the infants slept with an adult on a sofa.[12] The diagnoses of these deaths were fairly evenly split between SIDS (R95), ill-defined (R99) and accidental suffocation and strangulation in bed (ASSB, W75) suggesting the prevalence of sofa-sharing deaths is far higher than first reported in SIDS studies. Bed-sharing SIDS victims are younger than those infants found in cots/cribs and other potential characteristics that may lead to increased risk include the use of pillows near the infant, parental exhaustion, vulnerable low birthweight or premature infants and lack of provision for a cot/crib although further evidence is needed for these factors.

The Risk of Bed-sharing in Non-hazardous Circumstances

The combined analysis from England suggests there is no risk of bed-sharing in the absence of the hazards described (Table 26.1). A subgroup analysis limited to younger infants (under 3 months) increases the observed risk (OR 1.62 [95% 0.96–2.73]) but this did not quite become significant.[9] In contrast, a similar combined analysis of 5 studies with 1,472 SIDS cases and 4,679 control infants showed a five-fold increased risk associated with younger infants (under three months) bed-sharing in non-hazardous circumstances although the idealised reference group used (breastfed infants placed on their back to sleep in a separate room by non-smoking parents in the absence of any other risk factors) would inflate any observed SIDS risk factor.[13] This combined analysis

Table 26.1 The risk associated with bed/sofa-sharing overall and by different sleeping environments

	SIDS		Controls		Multivariable Risk[†]	
Overall	N	(%)	N	(%)	OR [95% CI]	P-value
Slept alone	255	(63.8%)	1173	(84.6%)	1.00 [Ref Group]	
Bed/sofa shared for the last sleep	145	(36.3%)	213	(15.4%)	3.91 [2.72–5.62]	<0.0001
By sleeping environment						
Slept alone	255	(63.8%)	1173	(84.6%)	1.00 [Ref Group]	
Slept with adult on a sofa or chair[*]	33	(8.3%)	7	(0.5%)	18.34 [7.10–47.35]	<0.0001
Bed-shared next to adult (>2 units of alcohol)	29	(7.3%)	12	(0.9%)	18.29 [7.68–43.54]	<0.0001
Bed-shared next to adult who smoked	59	(14.8%)	63	(4.5%)	4.04 [2.41–6.75]	<0.0001
Bed-shared in the absence of these hazards	24	(6.0%)	131	(9.5%)	1.08 [0.58–2.01]	0.82

[*] All but one was a sofa

[†] Adjusted for infant age and whether a day or night sleep as well as infant characteristics: birthweight <2500 g, preterm, male gender, and currently breastfeeding, maternal characteristics: larger families (≥3 children), younger mothers (≤ 21 years) and poor maternal education (< General Certificate of Secondary Education or no qualification) factors at the time of the last sleep: infant unwell (scoring 8 or more on the Babycheck), infant placed prone or side, infant swaddled, use of a duvet, use of a dummy, and infant found with head covered
The logistic regression model used 1700/1786 (95.4%) individuals from the cohort

did not report the risk using the standard reference group of non-bed-sharing infants and relied heavily on imputation as many of the studies involved did not have data on parental alcohol consumption. Both analyses, despite combining data from different studies, were limited by small sample size for subanalyses. The AAP, in their review of the evidence to support their 2016 guidelines, concluded that the data from these two different analyses do not support a definitive conclusion that bed-sharing among the youngest infants is safe, even under less hazardous circumstances.[7] In contrast a 2014 review of these two analyses by the independent body NICE (National Institute for Health and Care Excellence) in the UK concluded that bed-sharing in itself is not causal and that parents need to be informed of the specific hazards associated with this practice.[14] It is not clear whether infants sleeping next to an adult in a parental bed who has not consumed alcohol or drugs and does not smoke are at risk. If so, this risk is small when compared to the risk for infants in some hazardous circumstances which are a magnitude higher than other reported SIDS risk factors.

Risk-reduction Strategies

Different strategies have been adopted to advise parents on bed-sharing over the last decade. One is to advise against bed-sharing, which has been adopted in countries such as the US since 2005. This has the advantage of being a clear direct message to the public and perceived to be an easier one to get across. However, the US (AAP and National Institutes of Health Safe to Sleep Campaign) in its most recent set of guidelines (2016) has been more nuanced; although they do not recommend bed-sharing they do recommend room-sharing for at least the first six months, to facilitate breastfeeding and comforting.[15] In addition, the AAP acknowledges that mothers often fall asleep while breastfeeding their babies in bed, and advise that the parental bed should be prepared to avoid hazardous bedding should this occur. The latest guidelines also advise that it is safer to breastfeed in bed at night-time, compared with on sofas or armchairs, and strongly advise against the latter.

Despite campaigns to decrease bed-sharing in some states, bed-sharing has increased in the US in recent years, especially among black and Hispanic communities.[16] This practice may be responsible in part for recent trends in SIDS and SUDI. Taking into account the potential diagnostic shift currently happening in the US from SIDS (R95) to ASSB (W75), the combined SUDI/SUID rate appears to have stopped decreasing over the last five years (Figure 26.2).

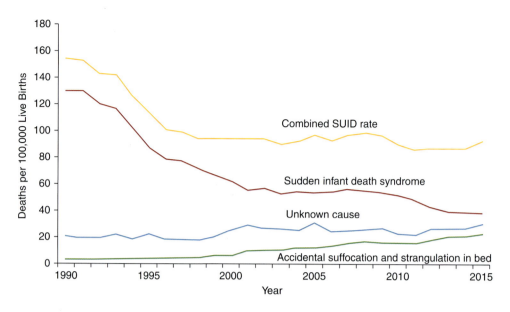

Figure 26.2 US Trends in SIDS and SUDI/SUID (1990–2015)

Source: CDC/NCHS, National Vital Statistics System, Compressed Mortality File. Available at: https://www.cdc.gov/sids/data.htm

There is now recognition that current AAP recommendations on bed-sharing are not being followed as widely as hoped due to the complexity of the practice and reasons for choosing it; bed-sharing is a culturally ingrained infant care practice and in some low-income communities, used to keep infants safe,[17] while others choose to bed-share to facilitate breastfeeding. In one trial using enhanced messaging with high-risk families to avoid bed-sharing, the prevalence of bed-sharing increased rather than decreased during the trial.[18] In a more recent randomised trial at 16 hospitals across the US, researchers found that delivering advice to parents to room-share but not bed-share via short videos through text messages or email significantly increased this behaviour (82.8%) compared with the control group (70.4%). This study suggests that using targeted communication methods can positively influence parental behaviour change.[19]

Another strategy, adopted in some countries such as the UK, is to acknowledge that bed-sharing occurs either intentionally or unintentionally and discuss the circumstances when it would be risky to bed-share. Although this lacks the same simplicity as the US approach, acknowledging that bed-sharing happens means it can be discussed without judgement and specific hazardous situations or environments can be highlighted. Since many of the risks to be avoided should already be known to the parents, the discussion should include reminding them how to create a safer environment if choosing to sleep with their infant by following the other safe-sleeping guidelines.[20] In the UK both the SIDS rate and combined SUDI/SUID rate have fallen over the last 10 years (Figure 26.3), although this may be due to many different factors.

In New Zealand, the interaction between bed-sharing and maternal smoking was demonstrated in 1993[21] and, in discussion of an appropriate policy, the authors later concluded that there 'could be a marginal cost (against its acceptance) by including infants of non-smoking mothers in the recommendation not to bed-share'.[22] After the plateau in SUDI/SUID rates became apparent in the 2000s and the five-fold disparity in Māori SUDI/SUID rates had proven persistent,[23] Māori SUDI/SUID researchers developed an intervention based on the premise that the provision of a separate sleep surface deployed in a shared sleep environment would reduce the risk of bed-sharing where the mother smoked in pregnancy. The wahakura, a woven flax bassinet-like structure and the Pēpi-Pod[TM], a plastic box of similar proportions, were introduced into SIDS/SUDI/SUID prevention efforts in 2006 and 2011, respectively.[24] The intervention involves the distribution of these devices in high SUDI/SUID risk situations like

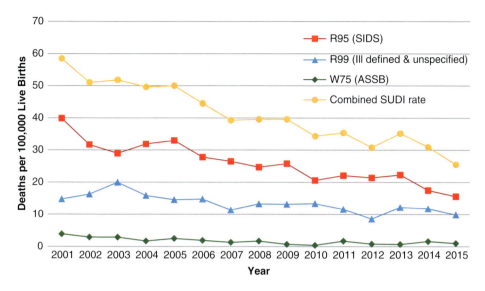

Figure 26.3 England and Wales trends in SIDS and SUDI/SUID (2000–2015)
Source: Office of National Statistics for England & Wales

smoking in pregnancy, and the provision of one-on-one advice that heightens awareness of risk and promotes 'Safe Sleep'. Importantly, the acceptability of this change to a culturally valued practice has been enhanced by the appeal of 'reclaiming' a - traditional Māori infant care practice[25] and the fact that this device, placed in the shared bed, maintains the highly valued proximity of mother and infant. The high SIDS and SUDI/SUID rates in New Zealand have fallen dramatically since 2009, especially among Māori infants and in the areas with the most intensive Safe Sleep programmes.[26] Based on these results, the New Zealand Ministry of Health has recently adopted the Safe Sleep programme as national policy.

On the face of it, it seems that the provision of a walled, flat surfaced, culturally acceptable sleeping space in a bed-sharing environment offers improved safety for an infant whose respiratory system has been impacted upon by cigarette smoking in pregnancy. The recent publication in New Zealand of an adjusted odds ratio of 32.8 (95%CI 11.2–95.8) for exposure to both risk factors confirms this thinking,[27] and although disentangling whether the sleeping device actually decreases risk is not simple, it is safe to say that such devices do not increase risk.[28,29] Jurisdictions in other countries are following this

lead in developing similarly targeted interventions with safe-sleeping devices and safe-sleep education.

The Way Forward

Different risk-reduction strategies have been used in different populations although there are signs that a mixed-strategy approach targeting certain populations may be more beneficial in the future. What is clear is that we need to emphasise the magnitude of risk surrounding unsafe sleeping practices involving alcohol, drugs, and sofas and have a more coordinated approach with other public health strategists on how to best care for the infants as well as keep them safe.

References

1. Blair PS, Ball HL. The prevalence and characteristics associated with parent-infant bed-sharing in England. *Arch Dis Child*, 2004; **89**(12):1106–10.

2. Smith LA, Geller NL, Kellams AL, Colson ER, Rybin DV, Heeren T, Corwin MJ. Infant sleep location and breastfeeding practices in the United State: 2011–2014. *Acad Pediatr*, 2016; **16**:540–9.

3. Anderson GC. Current knowledge about skin-to-skin (kangaroo) care for preterm infants. *J Perinatol*, 1991; **11**:216–26.

4. Chen A, Rogan WJ, Breastfeeding, and the risk of post-neonatal death in the United States. *Pediatrics*, 2004; **113**:e435–9.

5. Vennemann MM, Hense HW, Bajanowski T, Blair PS, Complojer C, Moon RY, Kiechl-Kohlendorfer U. Bed sharing and the risk of Sudden Infant Death Syndrome: can we resolve the debate? *J Pediatr*, 2012; **160**(1):44–8.

6. American Academy of Pediatrics. The changing concept of Sudden Infant Death Syndrome: diagnostic coding shifts, controversies regarding the sleeping environment, and new variables to consider in reducing risk. *Pediatrics*, 2005; **116**:1245–55.

7. Moon RY. Task Force on Sudden Infant Death Syndrome. SIDS and other sleep-related infant deaths: evidence base for the 2016 updated recommendations for a safe infant sleeping environment. *Pediatrics*, 2016; **138**:e20162940.

8. Blair PS, Sidebotham P, Berry PJ, Evans M, Fleming PJ, Major epidemiological changes in Sudden Infant Death Syndrome: a 20-year population-based study in the UK. *Lancet*, 2006; **367**:314–19.

9. Blair PS, Sidebotham P, Pease A, Fleming PJ. Bed-Sharing in the absence of hazardous circumstances: is there a risk of Sudden Infant Death Syndrome? An analysis from two case-control studies conducted in the UK. *PLoS One*, 2014; **9**(9):e107799.

10. Scragg R, Mitchell EA, Taylor BJ, Stewart AW, Ford RP, Thompson JM, Allen EM, Becroft DM. Bed sharing, smoking, and alcohol in the Sudden Infant Death Syndrome. New Zealand Cot Death Study Group. *BMJ*, 1993; **307**(6915):1312–18.

11. Blair PS, Sidebotham P, Evason-Coombe C, Edmonds M, Heckstall-Smith EM, Fleming P. Hazardous cosleeping environments and risk factors amenable to change: case-control study of SIDS in south-west England. *BMJ*, 2009; **339**:b3666.

12. Rechtman LR, Colvin JD, Blair PS, Moon RY. Sofas and infant mortality. *Pediatrics*, 2014; **134**(5):e1293–300.

13. Carpenter R, McGarvey C, Mitchell EA, Tappin DM, Vennemann MM, Smuk M, Carpenter JR. Bed sharing when parents do not smoke: is there a risk of SIDS? An individual level analysis of five major case-control studies. *BMJ Open*, 2013; **3**:e002299.

14. NICE. Postnatal care up to 8 weeks after birth. 2014; https://www.nice.org.uk/Guidance/CG37/Evidence (accessed 31 October 2018).

15. American Academy of Pediatrics Task Force on SIDS. SIDS and other sleep-related infant death: updated 2016 recommendations for a safe infant sleeping environment. *Pediatrics*, 2016; **138**(5):e20162938.

16. Colson ER, Willinger M, Rybin D, Heeren T, Smith LA, Lister G, Corwin MJ. Trends and factors associated with infant bed sharing, 1993–2010: the National Infant Sleep Position Study. *JAMA Pediatr*, 2013; **167**(11):1032–7.

17. Joyner BL, Oden RP, Ajao TI, Moon RY. Where should my baby sleep: a qualitative study of African American infant sleep location decisions. *J Natl Med Assoc*, 2010; **102**(10):881–9.

18. Moon RY, Mathews A, Joyner BL, Oden RP, He J, McCarter R. Health messaging and African-American infant sleep location: A randomized controlled trial. *J Community Health*, 2017; **42**(1):1–9.

19. Moon RY, Hauck FR, Colson ER, Kellams AL, Geller NL, Heeren T, Kerr SM, Drake EE, Tanabe K, McClain M, Corwin MJ. The effect of nursing quality improvement and mobile health interventions on infant sleep practices: a randomized clinical trial. *JAMA*, 2017; **318**:351–9.

20. UNICEF UK, *Baby Friendly initiative. Leaflet and Guidelines for Caring for Your Baby at Night*, 2016. www.unicef.org.uk/babyfriendly/baby-friendly-resources/leaflets-and-posters/caring-for-your-baby-at-night / (accessed 4 October 2018).

21. Scragg R, Mitchell EA, Taylor BJ, Stewart AW, Ford RP, Thompson JM, et al. Bedsharing, smoking, and alcohol in the Sudden Infant Death Syndrome. New Zealand Cot Death Study Group. *BMJ*, 1993; **307**:1312.

22. Scragg R, Stewart AW, Mitchell EA, Ford RP, Thompson JM. Public health policy on bed sharing and smoking in the Sudden Infant Death Syndrome. *NZ Med J*, 1995; **108**(1001):218–22.

23. *Te Rōpū Arotake Auau Mate o te Hunga Tamariki, Taiohi. Third Report to the Minister of Health: Reporting Mortality 2002–2004*. Wellington: Child and Youth Mortality Review Committee, 2006; https://www.hqsc.govt.nz/assets/CYMRC/Publications/Third-CYMRC-Report-2002-2004.pdf (accessed 31 October 2018).

24. Abel S. Tipene-Leach D. SUDI prevention: a review of Māori safe-sleep innovations for infants. *NZ Med J*, 2013; **1379**:126.

25. Abel S, Stockdale-Frost A, Rolls R, Tipene-Leach D. The wahakura: a qualitative study of the flax bassinet as a sleep location for New Zealand Māori infants. *NZ Med J*, 2015; **128** (1413):12–19.

26. Mitchell EA, Cowan S, Tipene-Leach D. The recent fall in postperinatal mortality in New Zealand and the Safe Sleep programme. *Acta Paediatr*, 2016; **105**(11): 1312–20.

27. Mitchell E, Thompson J, Zuccollo J, MacFarlane M, Taylor B, Elder D, et al. The combination of bedsharing and maternal smoking leads to a greatly increased risk of sudden unexpected death in infancy: the

New Zealand SUDI Nationwide Case Control study. *NZ Med J*, 2017; **130**(1456):52–64.

28. Baddock SA, Tipene-Leach D, Williams SM, Tangiora A, Jones R, Iosua E, et al. Wahakura versus bassinet for safe infant sleep: a randomized trial. *Pediatrics*, 2017;**139**:e20160162; http://pediatrics .aappublications.org/content/139/2/e20160162.long (accessed 31 October 2018).

29. Baddock SA, Tipene-Leach D, Williams SM, Tangiora A, Jones R, Mącznik AK, Taylor BJ. Physiological stability in an indigenous sleep device: a randomised controlled trial. *Arch Dis Child*, 2018; **103**(4):377–82.

Child-care Environment

27

Chapter 27

Rachel Moon

Data on sudden and unexpected infant death occurring in child-care settings are currently available from the United States and the Netherlands. This phenomenon has not been reported in other countries, most likely because in countries with longer durations of paid parental leave, young infants typically are not cared for by child-care providers during the period of highest risk for SIDS and other sleep-related infant deaths.

The first reports of SIDS in child-care settings were published in 1997. In this US cohort, approximately 20% of SIDS deaths occurred while infants were in child care.[1] The majority of these deaths occurred in child-care centres or family child-care homes (in which non-relative providers care for children in their homes, usually for pay). In this study, infants who died in child-care settings were more likely to be older and non-African-American, with more educated mothers. Further analysis revealed that many of the SIDS deaths occurred during the first week of child care (and often on the first or second day of child care), and that infants who died of SIDS in a child-care setting were more likely to have been in the unaccustomed prone position.[1] Mitchell and Thach et al. have reported that infants who are unaccustomed to the prone position are at extremely high risk for SIDS if they are either placed in or roll to the prone position.[2] Because surveys revealed that many child-care providers were unaware of the association between SIDS and prone sleeping position and that many of the infants in child care were being placed prone,[3] there was a concerted effort by the American Academy of Pediatrics, the back-to-sleep campaign, and other organisations to educate child-care providers about the importance of sleep position.[4] Additionally, many US states have implemented child-care regulations that stipulate supine positioning and a safe-sleep environment.

A subsequent study found that, although 16% of infants who died of SIDS did so in child-care settings,

infants in child care were no more likely to be placed or found prone and no more likely to be on an unsafe sleep surface.[5] Similarly, a Netherlands cohort found that 10.5% of SIDS deaths occurred in child-care settings; however, there was no association with sleep position.[6] Indeed, in that study, infants who died of SIDS in a child-care setting were more likely to be found in safe-sleep environments than those who died at home. It has been hypothesised that changes in routine care and the accompanying stress may contribute to the risk.[6]

Most recently, a cross-sectional analysis of 11,717 sleep-related infant deaths reported to the US National Child Fatality Review and Prevention database found that 20% of these deaths occurred out of the infant's home; 60% occurred at relatives' homes, and 22.3% occurred in child-care settings. Infants who died in out-of-home settings were more likely to be in a stroller or car seat (adjusted odds ratio 2.6; 95% confidence interval 2.1–3.4, p <0.001) and other locations (aOR 1.9, 95% CI 1.02–1.27, p=0.02), and less likely to be in a bed-sharing arrangement (aOR 0.7; 95% CI 0.6–0.7, p<0.001).[7]

Anyone who provides care for infants, including child-care providers, family members, friends, and babysitters should receive information about safe-sleep environments. Further studies to investigate other factors that may increase the risk for infants attending child care are needed.

References

1. Moon RY, Patel KM, Shaefer SJ. Sudden Infant Death Syndrome in child care settings. *Pediatrics*, 2000; **106**(2 Pt 1):295–300.

2. Mitchell EA, Thach BT, Thompson JMD, Williams S. Changing infants' sleep position increases risk of Sudden Infant Death Syndrome. *Arch Pediatr Adolesc Med*, 1999; **153**:1136–41.

3. Gershon NB, Moon RY. Infant sleep position in licensed child care centers. *Pediatrics*, 1997; **100**(1):75–8.

4. Moon RY, Kotch L, Aird L. State child care regulations regarding infant sleep environment since the Healthy Child Care America–Back to Sleep campaign. *Pediatrics*, 2006; **118**(1):73–83.

5. Moon RY, Sprague BM, Patel KM. Stable prevalence but changing risk factors for Sudden Infant Death Syndrome in child care settings in 2001. *Pediatrics*, 2005; **116**(4):972–7.

6. de Jonge GA, Lanting CI, Brand R, Ruys JH, Semmekrot BA, van Wouwe JP. Sudden Infant Death Syndrome in child care settings in the Netherlands. *Arch Dis Child*, 2004; **89**(5):427–30.

7. Kassa H, Moon RY, Colvin JD. Risk factors for sleep-related infant deaths in in-home and out-of-home settings. *Pediatrics*, 2016; **138**(5): e20161124.

Chapter

28

The Genetics of Sudden Infant Death Syndrome

James Steer and Srinivas Annavarapu

Introduction

Sudden Infant Death Syndrome (SIDS) has been defined as the sudden and unexplained death of an infant less than 1 year of age which remains unexplained after a thorough case investigation, including performance of a complete autopsy, examination of the death scene, and review of clinical history.[1,2] Thus, it is a diagnosis of exclusion.

Despite the success of the 'back-to-sleep' campaign, which has reduced the incidence of SIDS deaths by over 50–80% in the Western world,[3–5] SIDS still remains the leading cause of post-neonatal mortality.[6–10] About 2,000 babies born in the United States die each year from SIDS. The incidence of SIDS halved in the US from 1.2 deaths per 1000 live births in 1992 to 0.57 deaths per 1000 live births in 2006 [9; 10]. In England and Wales, there were 214 reported cases of unexplained infant deaths in 2015 (0.28 deaths/1,000 live births) of which around 60% were recorded as SIDS.[5] The major difficulty in collating statistics on SIDS is the lack of consistency in the way pathologists apply the diagnosis of SIDS, which can be appreciated by looking at the disparity in the incidence of SIDS across various regions in a small country like the UK.[5] This difficulty is further compounded by the fact that it is very challenging to separate true SIDS deaths from those of asphyxia associated with accidental suffocation and/or overlaying, especially when there is evidence of co-sleeping with a parent who has consumed alcohol and/or illicit drugs.[7]

The most widely accepted theory for the causation of SIDS is the so-called 'triple-risk hypothesis' which proposes that SIDS occurs when there is convergence of three overlapping risk factors – a vulnerable infant, a critical development period, and an exogenous environmental stressor.[11] Thus, if a vulnerable infant in his critical developmental period (1–6 months) encounters environmental stressors such as smoking, bed-sharing (especially on sofas), alcohol or drugs/medication, it may have a significant risk of dying from SIDS.[12–17] Overlap of the three critical risk factors is thought to be crucial in the causation of SIDS.[7,8,18]

According to this model, SIDS deaths occur in infants with intrinsic vulnerability that normal infants do not have and thus these susceptible infants may die upon encountering an environmental stressor that unmasks their underlying disease process.[19–21] SIDS is more common in male infants and is more common in winter months. There are racial differences in the incidence of SIDS. In the US, it is much more common in African-American and Native-American infants than in Caucasian, Hispanic, and Asian infants;[18] in the UK, the incidence appears to be higher in Caucasian infants as compared to Asian infants.[5]

Current data suggests that even after a thorough post-mortem examination, in almost 60–80% cases of sudden unexpected infant deaths, the cause of death remains elusive.[5,7,22] Although a number of studies have attempted to identify SIDS-associated genes, which have resulted in a vast network of genes and their encoded proteins, there is still a big gap in our understanding of the mechanisms underpinning SIDS.

Genetic Basis of SIDS

Recent advances in molecular and genetic studies indicate that around one-third of SIDS cases may have a genetic/hereditary basis. However, currently there are no specific genetic markers that can accurately detect or predict SIDS. It is interesting to note that most of the genetic defects (mutations or polymorphisms) associated with SIDS, are clustered around cardiac defects, defects in the serotonin pathway, immune dysfunction, inborn errors of metabolism and nicotine response receptors.[7,18,22,23] It appears that there is a complex interplay of aberrant physiological responses to environmental stressors compounded by impairment of arousal reflex leading to fatal asphyxia.[24]

This chapter will introduce the genetic basis of SIDS. Other chapters in this section will analyse in-depth current knowledge of particular genetics aspects.

Cardiac Defects

Over the last decade, there has been a significant advancement in our understanding of the sudden infant deaths resulting from underlying cardiomyopathies and cardiac channelopathies.[25,26]

Cardiomyopathies in Infancy

Although rare, infantile cardiomyopathies can cause sudden unexpected death in infants under the age of 1 year. Morphologically these can be divided into dilated cardiomyopathy (DCM) and hypertrophic cardiomyopathies (HCM).

- DCM in infancy is related mostly to Barth Syndrome and mitochondrial defects such as Kearns-Sayre syndrome. There are no definitive diagnostic histopathological features of DCM and genetic investigations are necessary for diagnosis.[18,22,23]
- Hypertrophic cardiomyopathies (HCM) are related to genetic conditions like Noonan Syndrome or underlying metabolic diseases such as Pompe's disease (AR, acid maltase deficiency) mitochondrial defects (complex I, II, III, IV deficiency) and fatty acid oxidation disorders (MCAD is most common). In HCM, there is marked asymmetric septal/ventricular hypertrophy at autopsy. Histologically, myocyte disarray, and interstitial fibrosis can be seen. Genetic investigations are necessary to identify underlying genetic defects.[18,22,23]
- Rarely, infants may die from arrhythmogenic right ventricular cardiomyopathy (ARVC), characterised histologically by excessive fibrofatty infiltration of the right ventricle with subsequent heart failure.[23]

Channelopathies

Channelopathies are inherited syndromes caused by mutations in genes encoding for ion channels, their subunits, or associated proteins.[27] Cardiac ion channels are multimeric transmembrane proteins responsible for conduction of ions such as sodium, potassium and calcium across the cell membrane of the cardiac myocytes. The ion channels consist of

various subunits which are encoded by different genes and serve different functions. Depolarisation of the cell membrane is critical for the generation of action potential that results in cardiac impulse. If any of the subunits are defective, there may be a risk of cardiac arrhythmias or epilepsy.[28]

The common ion channelopathies that cause sudden, unexpected death in infancy (SUDI) include Long QT syndrome (LQTS), Brugada syndrome (BS) and catecholaminergic polymorphic ventricular tachycardia (CPMVT).[21,27] For a detailed account of channelopathies in SIDS please see Chapter 29.

Long QT Syndrome

LQTS is a group of disorders characterised by prolongation of the QT interval secondary to delayed cardiac repolarisation which in turn predisposes to fatal polymorphic ventricular tachycardia and cardiac arrest. It should be considered in all infants who die suddenly and unexpectedly in their sleep. The main subtypes include LQT1 ($KCNQ1$—alpha subunit of $K_v7.1$ associated with I_{Ks}), LQT2 ($KCNH2$—alpha subunit of $K_v11.1$ associated with I_{Kr}) and LQT3 ($SCN5A$—alpha subunit of $Na_v1.5$ associated with I_{Na}).[21,29]

In various studies, LQT gene defects were found in 11–20% of SIDS cases.[30–35] Other studies have reported variants within $SCN5A$ gene or within genes encoding key regulatory subunits of the sodium channel including genes for caveolin-3 ($CAV3$),[36] GPD1-L ($GPD1-L$),[37] α1-syntrophin ($SNTA1$)[38,39] and the sodium channel beta subunits encoded by $SCN1B$, $SCN2B$, $SCN3B$ and $SCN4B$.[40]

Wang et al. (2007) comprehensively characterised seven missense variants (S216L, R680H, T1304M, F1486L, V1951L, F2004L, and P2006A) and one in-frame deletion allele (delAL586-587) of $SCN5A$. All variants exhibited significant defects in the kinetics and voltage dependence of inactivation.[41] Three alleles (delAL586-587, R680H, and V1951L) exhibited increased persistent current only under conditions of internal acidosis. This provides a compelling evidence of arrhythmia susceptibility in SCN5A variants which may be causally linked with SIDS deaths.[41] Interestingly, specific polymorphisms (S1103Y) in $SCN5A$ have been shown to increase the risk for SIDS in the African-American population.[42,43]

Brugada Syndrome

Brugada syndrome is characterised by typical electrocardiogram (ECG) changes (J-point elevation, coved-type

ST segment and negative T-wave) in the right precordial leads, seen most commonly in East and Southeast Asian infants who die in their sleep and is the result of defects in the cardiac sodium channel.[21] Severely defective Nav1.5 channel, caused by the Q1832E mutation in *SCN5A* gene, is the major mechanism for fatal cardiac arrhythmias and cardiac arrest. Recently, a novel variant in *SCN5A* gene has been reported. This is a nonsense mutation that produces a premature stop codon and a C-terminal truncation (R1944Δ).[44]

Catecholaminergic Polymorphic Ventricular Tachycardia

CPMVT is disorder of ryanodine receptor gene *RyR2*, which leads to abnormal conduction and predisposes the heart to ventricular tachycardia and sudden death. RyR2 encodes for the cardiac ryanodine receptor and mutations within this gene cause CPVT.[21] Tester et al. performed targeted mutational analysis of RyR2 on the genomic DNA from 134 SIDS cases and found two novel missense mutations (R2267 H and S4565 R) localised to functional domains of the receptor.[45] They proposed that these mutations could potentially alter the response of the channels to sympathetic nervous system stimulation (such that during stress) and could potentially trigger fatal cardiac arrhythmias.[45]

Rare Channelopathies

Hof et al. screened for mutations in the *transient potential melastatin 4 gene* (*TRPM4*) in a cohort of LQTS patients (n=178) where there were no mutations in the 3 major LQTS genes (*KCNQ1, KCNH2, and SCN5A*), and found four potential disease-causing *TRPM4* variants.[46] Thus, *TRPM4* gene defects may account for a small number of LQTS. Others LQTS genes included *KCNJ2* (Andersen syndrome), *CACNA1 C* (Timothy syndrome) and connexin-43 (GJA1).[46] Lastly, *nitric oxide synthase 1 adaptor protein* (*NOS1AP*) genetic variants have been positively correlated with variations in the QT interval duration and sudden cardiac death in four studies.[47–50]

Evidence for Channelopathies in SIDS

In a meta-analysis of sixteen studies looking into the correlation between SIDS and channelopathies, Norstand et al. found a positive correlation in over 80% of the studies that found novel mutations

associated with Long QT syndrome (LQTS), Brugada syndrome and CPVT.[7] In a recent study, a Swiss group demonstrated channelopathies in 9% of their cases (n=192) by whole-exome sequencing.[23] This was similar to the previous study by Arnestad et al. who examined seven LQTS-susceptibility genes and reported an incidence of 9.5% (19 of 201) in their study which looked at three major LQTS-susceptibility genes, which harboured the vast majority of mutations (SCN5A – 50%; KCNQ1 & KCNH2 – 38%).[51] Hertz et al. investigated coding regions of 100 genes associated with inherited channelopathies and cardiomyopathies in 47 SIDS cases and found that in 34% cases there was evidence of variants with likely functional effects.[26]

Overall, the body of literature suggests that up to 10% of SIDS may result from cardiac arrhythmias undiagnosed during the first year of life, of which cardiac sodium channelopathies are the most frequent[7] and should be tested in all SUDI/SUID cases. In cases where the autopsy appears negative, it is crucial that the pathologist takes appropriate and adequate biologic samples for genetic studies to test for genetic cardiac defects.

Central Nervous System Pathways

Another area of active SIDS research is to understand the role of CNS pathways involved in cardiovascular homeostasis, respiratory control, and sleep.[52] Defective CNS pathways in the brainstem can result in defective arousal reflex in the face of asphyxia and hypercapnia (from rebreathing exhaled CO_2 that gets trapped in the bedding while sleeping in a face-down position) leading to sudden infant death.[53] For a more detailed analysis, see Chapters 30–32.

Serotonin (5-hydroxytryptamine) Pathways

Serotonin (5-hydroxytryptamine/5-HT) is an important neuromodulator and neurotransmitter that regulates the brainstem autonomic pathways, especially the ponto-medullary[54] and thalamo-cerebral circuits.[55] Most of the serotonin in the body is produced by the raphe nuclei of the medulla oblongata which in turn regulates body temperature, cardiorespiratory centres, and circadian rhythm.[18] Serotoninergic neurons are stimulated by carbon dioxide and thus are known to activate arousal response in response to hypercapnia.[55] Impairment of this response may contribute to sleep apnoea, SIDS, and sudden unexpected death in epilepsy (SUDEP).[55] Some of the main genes that regulate serotonin pathways in the CNS include TPH2, the serotonin transporter SLC6A4, and the serotonin receptor HTR1A.[18,56–59] Defects in these regulatory genes may predispose the baby to SIDS.

The *5-HTT* gene, encoding the serotonin transporter, has been reported to show copy number variations of a 20–23 base pair repeat unit within its promoter region.[7,56,59] Narita N et al. investigated *5-HTT* promoter gene polymorphisms in the 5' regulatory region from 27 SIDS cases and 115 age-matched controls. Three variations in the *5-HTT* gene promoter were observed – a shorter allele/S (14 copies), a long allele/L (16 copies) and an extra-long allele/XL (18–20 copies).[56,57] The L and XL alleles were more frequently found in SIDS cases than in age-matched control participants.[56] The longer allele L was shown to be associated with decreased 5-HT concentrations at the nerve endings in the brain.[9] Similar results were obtained by Opdal et al. in their study when they investigated 5-HTT gene polymorphisms in the promoter region of 163 cases of SIDS and 243 age-matched controls using PCR and gel electrophoresis. LL genotype was more common in the SIDS cases compared to the controls.[60] Accordingly, high serum 5-HT has been proposed as a potential biomarker in infants with SIDS with serotonergic defects.[52]

Defects in the Central Nervous System

Arcuate nucleus is an important region of the brain that regulates cardiorespiratory homeostasis, body temperature, and sleep-arousal processes. Filiano and Kinney identified severe developmental hypoplasia of the arcuate nucleus in a subset of infants who died of SIDS.[61] They hypothesised that arcuate neurons may be involved in the response to hypercarbia. They supported their finding by data from functional MRI in adults exposed to hypercarbia in which CO_2 responsivity was localised to arcuate nucleus.[61] Expectedly, babies with defects in this region may be unable to respond to a hypoxic trigger, unlike normal babies who may wake up and take evasive action. A similar mechanism may operate in hyperthermia. Under normal circumstances, if a baby is too hot, it will be aroused from sleep but if a baby has a defect in the arcuate nucleus, the brain may not perceive danger signals, increasing the risk for SIDS.[62,63]

Sleep arousal requires mature and functional neuronal respiratory networks. An important centre regulating this is the pontine Kölliker-Fuse nucleus

(KFN). It has established connections with serotonin and noradrenaline neurons in the brainstem. Orexin is a neuropeptide synthesised by lateral hypothalamic neurons and has major interconnections with brainstem raphe nuclei and locus coeruleus, both of which also play a crucial role in sleep-wake transition. Hence, breakdown of KFN pathways can lead to sleep apnoea and may predispose to SIDS.[64]

PHOX2B Gene Polymorphism

Phox2B gene is expressed in the hindbrain and controls the differentiation of neuronal progenitor cells into branchiomotor (bm) neurons (innervating muscles originating from branchial arches) and visceral motor (vm) neurons (innervating ganglia of autonomic nervous system).[65,66] Liebrechts-Akkerman et al. studied variations in *PHOX2B* gene in 195 SIDS cases and 846 age-matched healthy controls in the Dutch population. They found evidence of statistically significant length variation of the polyalanine repeat in exon 3 of the PHOX2B gene with SIDS.[67] It is possible that abnormalities in the *Phox2B* gene expression may interfere with autonomic nervous system as they confer susceptibility to SIDS.

Pituitary Adenylate-Cyclase-Activating Polypeptide (PACAP)

PACAP and its complementary receptor, PAC1, are crucial in central respiratory control.[68,69] PACAP is a protein that mediates vasopressin signalling and is expressed throughout the autonomic control centres. Reduced PACAP expression is associated with an increased incidence of spontaneous neonatal death.[18] PACAP-knockout (KO) mice exhibit a SIDS-like phenotype, with an inability to overcome noxious insults, compression of baseline ventilation, and death in the early post-neonatal period.[70] PAC1 KO demonstrates similar attributes to PACAP-null mice, but with the addition of increased pulmonary artery pressure, consequently leading to heart failure and death.[7] Frequent gene polymorphisms have been identified in SIDS infants within genes involved in thermoregulation by brown fat and neuronal signalling, most importantly in *monoamine oxidase A (MAOA)*,[71,72] *PHOX2B* [67,73] and *SLC6A4* genes.[18,60,74,75] *MAOA* gene is X-linked; hence it may offer some insights as to why male babies have a greater susceptibility to SIDS than age-matched female babies.[18,76]

Immune Dysfunction

There is mounting evidence linking the pathogenesis of SIDS deaths with altered immune responses to subclinical infections.[76–81] An exaggerated immunological response or cytokine storm related to subclinical infection has been suggested since almost 50% of the infants who die of SIDS have had some recent history of mild infection in the days preceding their death.[80,81]

Genes encoding proteins involved in modulating immune function have shown genetic polymorphism in IL-10,[82] IL-6,[83] Tumour necrosis factor alpha (TNF-α)[84] and interferon-γ.[85] The most commonly investigated *IL-10* polymorphisms in SIDS are the promoter variants at positions -1082*A, -819*T, and -592*A.[82,86] IL-10 is a very important immune regulator since it opposes the pro-inflammatory cytokines (IL-6, TNF-α) and maintains the critical balance between pro-inflammatory and humoral responses. Breakdown of this regulation can lead to a heightened pro-inflammatory state.[87,88] IL-1 and IL-6 are acute phase proteins that are pro-inflammatory and mediate pyrexia.[87,88] TNF-α is a transmembrane protein that is produced by the body in response to bacterial toxins.[88]

Positive correlation has also been proposed between SIDS and VEGF, IL-1α, IL-1 receptor antagonist genes and *TNF-α* promoter region.[18] Since most babies who die of SIDS have some prior mild infection and raised IL-6 CSF levels, a link was suggested between CNS and the laryngeal immune system.[89] This link assumes much greater significance when one notes that there is a concomitant increased IL-6 receptor expression on serotonergic cells in brainstem nuclei of SIDS victims, as compared to the control group, which is involved in regulation of respiration and protective responses to hypercapnia.[89] Studies by two European groups highlighted a possible association between partial deletions of complement genes (either C4A or C4B gene) with mild infection prior to death.[90,91]

Weber et al. identified a high rate of positive cultures from SIDS infants (n=470) as compared to controls. They found a high proportion of pathogens, particularly *Staphylococcus aureus* and *Escherichia coli*, in otherwise unexplained cases of SUDI/SUID and suggested that these bacteria could be associated with SIDS.[92] It was hypothesised that in the critical age window of 2–3 months (peak time for SIDS), babies start to lose the passive immunity provided by mother's antibodies, hence they might not be able to stave off infection and may probably succumb from it.[92]

Another mechanism of death in SIDS may be infection with viruses (such as RSV, Metapneumovirus) that not only cause severe respiratory distress in infants due to acute bronchiolitis, but also cause respiratory arrest by causing central apnoea and predispose infants to secondary bacterial infections. The brain's respiratory control centre is located in the so-called pre-Bötzinger complex. If there is inhibition of this region, the breathing during sleep becomes imbalanced and there is failure to give the correct signal to inhale, causing respiratory arrest in sleep. This may be a mechanism operative in SIDS.[93]

Inborn Errors of Metabolism

Inborn errors of metabolism (IEM) may account for approximately 1–2% of SIDS cases.[94] Medium-chain acyl-CoA dehydrogenase (MCAD) deficiency, is the most common defect and homozygous mutations in the *MCAD* gene can present with sudden infant death, most common mutation being G985A.[95,96] Other fatty acid oxidation disorders are very rare in SIDS deaths. As described previously, IEM can present with cardiomyopathies associated with mitochondrial defects, which can be of DCM phenotype as in Kearns-Sayre syndrome or the HCM phenotype as seen in Pompe's disease, mitochondrial defects (complex I, II, III, IV deficiency) and fatty acid oxidation disorders.[7] See Chapter 34.

Nicotine Response

There is an established association between the SIDS and exposure to cigarette smoke as a risk factor.[59,97] See Chapter 21, Poetsch et al.[98] investigated for the presence of genetic polymorphisms (that are known to impair nicotine metabolism) in the nicotine metabolising enzyme gene *FMO3* (coding for flavin-monooxygenase 3), in 159 SIDS cases with matched controls from Germany. They found common polymorphism 472 G >A resulting in amino acid change E158 K that was over-represented in SIDS cases where mothers were heavy smokers (≥10 cigarettes per day) during pregnancy as compared with controls. The study provides a viable argument for the interaction between genetic susceptibility (genetic variant known to impair nicotine metabolism) and an environmental hazard (cigarette exposure) in SIDS.[98] Moreover, nicotinic acetylcholine receptors are expressed in the serotoninergic medullary raphe neurons in the brain.[99] It has been observed that exposure to cigarette smoke causes inhibition of the medullary raphe serotoninergic neurons in rats.[100] Furthermore, nicotine exposure reduces immunoreactivity of the serotonin receptors 5-HT1A (HTR1A) and 5-HT2A (HTR2A) in several nuclei of the brainstem.[18,101]

Inner-Ear Defects

Researchers from Seattle Children's Hospital investigated arousal response (assessed by how well the mice could move or react when they experienced hypoxia or hypercarbia during sleep) in mice with inner-ear defects and appropriate controls. They found that mice that had a hearing suppression did not move away when faced with hypoxia or hypercarbia during sleep whereas the control mice made vigorous movements and took evasive action by moving their heads away to get fresh air. Thus, there appears to be a link between inner-ear dysfunction and SIDS.[102,103] A collaborative US–UK study called 'Oto-Acoustic Signals in SIDS' (OASIS) was launched in May 2016 to investigate a possible association between SIDS and hearing defects on the newborn hearing screen test.[104]

Previously, Rubens et al. [105] observed that each of the 31 SIDS babies included in their study showed some inner-ear defect that may have compromised the baby's ability to adjust the respiratory system when there was hypercarbia.[106] Further research is needed to confirm whether inner-ear abnormality can act as a marker for identifying babies at risk for SIDS. See also Chapter 33.

Genetic Analysis

There are a number of technologies that have been, and have become, available for genetic investigation following a case of sudden infant death. The following is a brief precis of the most common core technologies and their utility in this context.

Karyotype

Karyotyping is the process of analysing chromosomes using light microscopy at 1000x magnification. The DNA in nucleated cells is packaged into chromosomes which during the mitotic cycle become condensed. In vitro cell culture techniques are used to capture cells at the prometaphase stage of mitosis.

Fixed cells are stained and banded in situ on glass slides for microscopic analysis. Many centres may now use an automated scanning platform to scan and digitally capture appropriate metaphase chromosome preparations for analysis on screen rather than by looking down the microscope.

This is a relatively simple whole-genome screen and the sensitivity and utility is in terms of detection of chromosome aneuploidy (loss or gain of a chromosome or chromosomes) such as trisomy 18 or 21, polyploidy (multiples of haploid set) such as triploidy and chromosome rearrangements which can be apparently balanced (no loss or gain of genetic material) such as a balanced translocation; or unbalanced with an inherent loss or gain of genetic material, for example deletions, or duplications. Maximum sensitivity is approximately 5-10mb DNA. Utility is limited to those cases where there are sufficient syndromic phenotypic features to indicate genetic investigation. Karyotyping has often been used in the past as a basic exclusion test as it is relatively cheap, however the abnormality rate is likely to be low in an otherwise phenotypically normal patient group and microarray is a more viable baseline option. Viable tissue is required for cell culture, which may be a limiting factor especially if post-mortem is delayed.[107]

FISH/QF-PCR

Fluorescent In Situ Hybridisation (FISH) utilises fluorescently labelled DNA-based probes to target and label specific regions of interest in the genome either in interphase or metaphase cells. This requires very specific probes, therefore can only be used as a very targetable test. Utility is as an adjunct to karyotyping to check for deletion of specific loci, or can be used on paraffin embedded tissue (PET) slides to check for common chromosomal aneuploidies related to major syndromes. Quantitative fluorescence–polymerase chain reaction (QF-PCR) allows quantification of PCR products to detect chromosomal aneuploidy as above, but from DNA extracted from tissue, including from PET.

Chromosomal Microarray (CMA)

There are different types of array but the term chromosomal microarray or CMA covers all types of array-based genomic copy number analysis; including array comparative genomic hybridisation (aCGH) and single nucleotide polymorphism (SNP) arrays. The key principle in CMA is the competitive hybridisation between two differentially fluorescently labelled DNA sequences: the patient and a normal reference, to the target sequence on the array. The array is scanned and fluorescence intensity measured for each target sequence. Difference from expected patient:reference 1:1 ratio is plotted against sequence position to give a map of genetic imbalance.[108]

CMA performs a similar function to karyotyping but at an increased resolution for the detection of genomic imbalance in terms of Copy Number Variants (CNV). The resolution is dependent on the density and distribution of the probe sequences compared to the DNA backbone but for diagnostic arrays is in the region of 50–500kb, which is sufficient to detect all known recurrent microdeletion and microduplication syndromes mediated by segmental duplication architecture. SNP arrays also detect areas of homozygosity which may represent uniparental disomy. CMA will not detect balanced rearrangements or low-level mosaicism. Abnormality detection rates are higher than karyotyping, especially in selected referral groups (for example in patients with congenital abnormality and developmental delay, or prenatal testing with raised nuchal translucency or abnormal scan[109,110] and therefore this technique will have higher clinical utility in the SIDS referral group compared to karyotyping. Certainly, this is one of the more common technologies employed for the investigation of fetal loss samples in miscarriage. However, this technique is still limited by resolution at the molecular level and there is the additional challenge of determining the clinical significance of Variants of Uncertain Clinical Significance (VOUS). Requirement for testing is DNA which can be extracted from viable fresh, fresh frozen, or paraffin embedded tissue.

Specific Sequencing/Genotyping

Only if there is suspicion of specific genetic diagnosis is there utility for targeted sequencing or genotyping for a particular genetic disorder. The limitations are that sequencing/genotyping of this type requires a highly differential referral as the testing itself is limited to very specific loci. In general, this type of testing only has clinical utility in terms of patients presenting with specific symptoms/phenotype, prior family history, or convincing evidence from post-mortem investigation.

The abnormalities detected using these techniques are single-base pair changes and small insertions or deletions at the molecular level. It may be used as a followup confirmatory or familial test after diagnosis using one of the following technologies. Requirement for testing is DNA which can be extracted from viable fresh, fresh frozen, or paraffin-embedded tissue.[111]

Next-Generation Sequencing (NGS) Technologies

NGS utilises massively parallel sequencing technology to sequence many thousands of DNA fragments at once, usually from multiple patients, followed by a number of quality control, filtering, analytical, and interpretation stages as part of a bioinformatics 'pipeline', to deliver data on a diagnostically interpretable scale for final interpretation and reporting by a scientific team. Following DNA extraction from either fresh, fresh frozen, or PET, one of the following processes is almost certainly employed:

NGS Gene Panels

Sequencing using gene panels allows high-throughput focused sequencing on a specific portion of the genome, usually a set, or panel of genes with specific loci known to be involved in the disease phenotype.[112] Specific loci are enriched from genomic DNA using either capture probe sets or targeted amplification and then sequenced using high-throughput sequencing platforms. Gene panels are particularly useful in diagnostic testing as there is a step change in diagnostic utility compared to Sanger sequencing: rather than just one or a small number of relevant regions being sequenced at a time, which may require several exclusion tests to get to a diagnosis, or no diagnosis at all, NGS panels allow testing of all currently relevant areas, for a large number of patient samples, in one sequencing reaction. Panels are also customisable to allow new regions of interest to be added to the panel. There is a theoretical point in terms of technical sequencing capacity and read depth for diagnostic utility, with respect to increasing panel size at which point whole-exome sequencing (WES) is a more cost-effective diagnostic tool. As a diagnostic tool for the investigation of SIDS, a panel is likely to be large in terms of relevant genes required on the panel and WES using virtual panels may be the more viable option longer term. However, limiting any panel to only those loci of specific interest allows a relatively clear and therefore efficient analytical and interpretive pipeline, in order to maximise the clinical value of a test within a diagnostic timescale of a few weeks.

Whole-Exome Sequencing (WES)

WES is a targeted resequencing approach which deep sequences either all the exons of a genome (the essential protein coding sequences within a genome) or all the known clinically relevant exons of a genome. It is based on exome capture; the construction of DNA libraries enriched for the exonic fraction of the genome and then sequencing. Advantages of exome sequencing over NGS panel type analysis are that the whole of the protein coding regions are captured and using bioinformatics tools, a 'virtual' panel can be created pulling out only those regions of relevance in the investigation, although all the regions could be analysed if required. This means that a common WES protocol can be adopted for many diagnostic referrals of different aetiologies, utilising bioinformatic tools to select regions of interest post-sequencing. Additional regions of interest can be added to the virtual panel bioinformatically without having to re-engineer a diagnostic panel with additional primer sets. Compared to whole-genome sequencing (WGS), genomic variants are also restricted to functionally annotated regions of the genome which enables much more rapid interpretation and diagnostic utility. This is probably the optimal tool to use for investigation of SIDS longer term, balancing cost for a sequencing run requiring a large 'panel or virtual panel' of relevant genes, with diagnostic utility within a reasonable timescale of a few weeks.

Whole-Genome Sequencing

WGS sequences the whole genome which includes the intronic regions in addition to the exonic protein coding regions. It does not require prior knowledge of the genome in terms of which regions to target and selectively capture and therefore will detect variants throughout the genome. This is a powerful technique in terms of broad spectrum analysis of the variability across the genome and therefore for population studies to detect genomic loci associated with complex phenotypic traits. There are multiple studies being undertaken on a national and international basis for just this purpose. The limiting factors relate to cost; due to the capacity of sequencing required per patient,

limiting the number of samples per run per sequencing machine; and due to the huge raw volume of the data produced requiring additional computational and bioinformatics resource. There is the potential for detection of a vast number of variants which are currently not easy or necessarily possible to interpret as many are novel and currently unclassified. This limits the variant classification and interpretation which can be achieved within a diagnostic timescale and NGS gene panel or WES will remain much more attractive in terms of diagnostic investigation of SIDS.

Conclusion

Identification of gene susceptibility for SIDS, including underlying gene mutations and polymorphisms that may be responsible for imparting an intrinsic vulnerability to some infants, is a key step in understanding the mechanisms of death from SIDS. Routine molecular/genetic screening soon after birth may identify a subset of infants who may be at risk from dying from SIDS and may allow opportunities for specific genetic counselling for the parents to minimise exposure to environmental risk factors which may be potentially harmful for the infant, like bed-sharing, avoidance of the prone position, abstinence from smoking etc. It would also allow the health professionals to devise appropriate therapeutic strategies.[8]

It is widely acknowledged that SIDS is not a single disease entity but is a heterogeneous group of disorders with multifactorial aetiologies.[22] It is likely that in most cases SIDS may not simply be a result of a single gene defect but may represent a complex interplay of multiple genes and their interaction with the environmental risk factors.

References

SIDS: Introduction

1. Willinger M, James LS, Catz C. Defining the Sudden Infant Death Syndrome (SIDS): deliberations of an expert panel convened by the National Institute of Child Health and Human Development. *Pediatr Pathol*, 1991; **11**(5):677–84.

2. Krous HF, Beckwith JB, Byard RW, Rognum TO, Bajanowski T, Corey T, et al. Sudden Infant Death Syndrome and unclassified sudden infant deaths: a definitional and diagnostic approach. *Pediatrics*, 2004; **114**(1):234–8.

3. Beal SM, Baghurst P, Antoniou G. Sudden Infant Death Syndrome (SIDS) in South Australia 1968–97. Part 2: the epidemiology of non-prone and non-covered SIDS infants, *J Paediatr Child Health*, 2000; **36**(6):548–51.

4. Moon RY, Horne R S, Hauck FR. 'Sudden Infant Death Syndrome', *Lancet*, 2007; **370**(9598):1578–87.

5. Lullaby Trust website: https://www.lullabytrust.org.uk/safer-sleep-advice/what-is-sids/ (accessed 13 October 2018).

6. Mathews TJ, MacDorman MF. Infant mortality statistics from the 2004 period linked birth/infant death data set, *Natl Vital Stat Rep*, 2007; **55**(14):1–32.

7. Van Norstrand DW, Ackerman MJ. Genomic risk factors in Sudden Infant Death Syndrome, *Genome Med*, 2010; **2**(11):86.

8. Paterson DS. Serotonin gene variants are unlikely to play a significant role in the pathogenesis of the Sudden Infant Death Syndrome. *Respir Physiol Neurobiol*, 2013; **189**(2):301–14.

9. Hunt CE, Hauck FR. Sudden Infant Death Syndrome, *CMAJ*, 2006; **174**(13):1861–9.

10. Moon RY, Fu LY. Sudden Infant Death Syndrome. *Pediatr Rev*, 2007; **28**(6):209–14.

11. Guntheroth WG, Spiers PS The triple-risk hypotheses in Sudden Infant Death Syndrome, *Pediatrics*, 2002; **110**(5):e64.

12. Hauck FR, Herman SM, Donovan M, Iyasu S, Merrick Moore C, et al. Sleep environment and the risk of Sudden Infant Death Syndrome in an urban population: the Chicago Infant Mortality Study, *Pediatrics*, 2003; **111**(5 Pt 2):1207–14.

13. Tappin D, Brooke H, Ecob R. Bedsharing and Sudden Infant Death Syndrome (SIDS) in Scotland, UK, *Lancet*, 2004; **363**(9413):994.

14. Tappin, D., Ecob, R. and Brooke, H. Bedsharing, roomsharing, and Sudden Infant Death Syndrome in Scotland: a case-control study, *J Pediatr*, 2005; **147**(1):32–7.

15. Mitchell EA, Milerad J. Smoking and the Sudden Infant Death Syndrome, *Rev Environ Health*, 2006; **21**(2):81–103.

16. Vennemann MM, Bajanowski T, Brinkmann B, Jorch G, Sauerland C, et al. Sleep environment risk factors for Sudden Infant Death Syndrome: the German Sudden Infant Death Syndrome Study, *Pediatrics*, 2009; **123**(4):1162–70.

17. Trachtenberg FL, Haas EA, Kinney HC, Stanley C, Krous HF. Risk factor changes for Sudden Infant Death Syndrome after initiation of Back-to-Sleep campaign, *Pediatrics*, 2012; **129**(4):630–8.

18. Salomonis N. Systems-level perspective of Sudden Infant Death Syndrome. *Pediatr Res*, 2014; **76**(3):220–9.

19. Broadbelt KG, Paterson DS, Belliveau RA, Trachtenberg FL, Haas EA, et al. Decreased GABAA receptor binding in the medullary serotonergic system in the Sudden Infant Death Syndrome, *J Neuropathol Exp Neurol*, 2011; **70**(9):799–810.

20. Kinney HC, Broadbelt KG, Haynes RL, Rognum IJ, Paterson DS. The serotonergic anatomy of the developing human medulla oblongata: implications for pediatric disorders of homeostasis. *J Chem Neuroanat*, 2011; **41**(4):182–99.

21. Wong LC, Behr ER. Sudden unexplained death in infants and children: the role of undiagnosed inherited cardiac conditions. *Europace*, 2014; **16**(12):1706–13.

22. Weese-Mayer DE, Ackerman MJ, Marazita ML and Berry-Kravis EM Sudden Infant Death Syndrome: review of implicated genetic factors, *Am J Med Genet A*, 2007; **143A**(8):771–88.

23. Neubauer J, Lecca MR, Russo G, Bartsch C, Medeiros-Domingo A, Berger W, Haas C. Post-mortem whole-exome analysis in a large Sudden Infant Death Syndrome cohort with a focus on cardiovascular and metabolic genetic diseases. *Eur J Hum Genet*, 2017; **25**(4):404–9.

24. Carlin RF, Moon RY. Risk factors, protective factors, and current recommendations to reduce Sudden Infant Death Syndrome: a review. *JAMA Pediatr*, 2017; **171**(2):175–180.

Cardiac Defects

25. Tester DJ, Ackerman MJ. Cardiomyopathic and channelopathic causes of sudden unexplained death in infants and children. *Ann Rev Med*, 2009; **60**:69–84.

26. Hertz CL, Christiansen SL, Larsen MK, Dahl M, Ferrero-Miliani L, Weeke PE, et al. Genetic investigations of sudden unexpected deaths in infancy using next-generation sequencing of 100 genes associated with cardiac diseases. *Eur J Hum Genet*, 2016; **24**(6):817–22.

27. Campuzano O, Beltrán-Alvarez P, Iglesias A, Scornik F, Pérez G, Brugada R. Genetics and cardiac channelopathies. *Genet Med*, 2010; **12**(5):260–7.

28. Grant AO, Carboni MP, Neplioueva V, Starmer CF, Memmi M, Napolitano C, Priori S. Long QT syndrome, Brugada syndrome, and conduction system disease are linked to a single sodium channel mutation. *J Clin Invest*, 2002; **110**(8):1201–9.

29. Cerrone M, Napolitano C, Priori SG. Genetics of ion-channel disorders. *Curr Opin Cardiol*, 2012; **27**(3):242–52.

30. Chugh SS, Senashova O, Watts A, Tran PT, Zhou Z, Gong Q, et al. Postmortem molecular screening in unexplained sudden death. *J Am Coll Cardiol*, 2004; **43**(9):1625–9.

31. Skinner JR, Crawford J, Smith W, Aitken A, Heaven D, Evans CA, et al. Prospective, population-based long QT molecular autopsy study of postmortem negative sudden death in 1 to 40 year olds. *Heart Rhythm*, 2011; **8**(3):412–19.

32. Tester DJ, Ackerman MJ. The molecular autopsy: should the evaluation continue after the funeral? *Pediatr Cardiol*, 2012; **33**(3):461–70.

33. Tester DJ, Dura M, Carturan E, Reiken S, Wronska A, Marks AR, Ackerman MJ. A mechanism for Sudden Infant Death Syndrome (SIDS): stress-induced leak via ryanodine receptors. *Heart Rhythm*, 2007; **4**(6):733–9.

34. Winkel BG, Larsen MK, Berge KE, Leren TP, Nissen PH, Olesen MS, et al. The prevalence of mutations in KCNQ1, KCNH2, and SCN5A in an unselected national cohort of young sudden unexplained death cases. *J Cardiovasc Electrophysiol*, 2012; **23**(10):1092–8.

35. Wang D, Shah KR, Um SY, Eng LS, Zhou B, Lin Y, et al. Cardiac channelopathy testing in 274 ethnically diverse sudden unexplained deaths. *Forensic Sci Int*, 2014; **237**:90–9.

36. Cronk LB, Ye B, Kaku T, Tester DJ, Vatta M, Makielski JC, Ackerman MJ. Novel mechanism for Sudden Infant Death Syndrome: persistent late sodium current secondary to mutations in caveolin-3. *Heart Rhythm*, 2007; **4**(2):161–6.

37. Van Norstrand DW, Valdivia CR, Tester DJ, Ueda K, London B, Makielski JC, Ackerman MJ. Molecular and functional characterization of novel glycerol-3-phosphate dehydrogenase 1 like gene (GPD1-L) mutations in Sudden Infant Death Syndrome. *Circulation*, 2007; **116**(20):2253–9.

38. Cheng J, Norstrand DW, Medeiros-Domingo A, Tester DJ, Valdivia CR, Tan BH, et al. LQTS-associated mutation A257 G in α1-syntrophin interacts with the intragenic variant P74 L to modify its biophysical phenotype. *Cardiogenetics*, 2011; **1**(1): e13; https://www.pagepressjournals.org/index.php/cardiogen/article/view/cardiogenetics.2011.e13 (accessed 28 October 2018).

39. Cheng J, Van Norstrand DW, Medeiros-Domingo A, Valdivia C, Tan BH, Ye B, et al. Alpha1-syntrophin mutations identified in Sudden Infant Death Syndrome cause an increase in late cardiac sodium current. *Circ Arrhythm Electrophysiol*, 2009; **2**(6): 667–76.

40. Tan BH, Pundi KN, Van Norstrand DW, Valdivia CR, Tester DJ, Medeiros-Domingo A, et al. Sudden Infant Death Syndrome-associated mutations in the sodium channel beta subunits. *Heart Rhythm*, 2010; **7**(6):771–8.

41. Wang DW, Desai RR, Crotti L, Arnestad M, Insolia R, Pedrazzini M, et al. Cardiac sodium channel dysfunction in Sudden Infant Death Syndrome. *Circulation*, 2007; **115**(3):368–76.

42. Plant LD, Bowers PN, Liu Q, Morgan T, Zhang T, State MW, et al. A common cardiac sodium channel variant associated with sudden infant death in African Americans, SCN5A S1103Y. *J Clin Invest*, 2006; **116**(2): 430–5.

43. Van Norstrand DW, Tester DJ, Ackerman MJ. Overrepresentation of the proarrhythmic, sudden death predisposing sodium channel polymorphism S1103Y in a population-based cohort of African-American Sudden Infant Death Syndrome. *Heart Rhythm*, 2008; **5**(5):712–15.

44. Gando I, Morganstein J, Jana K, McDonald TV, Tang Y, Coetzee WA. Infant sudden death: mutations responsible for impaired Nav1.5 channel trafficking and function. *Pacing Clin Electrophysiol*, 2017; **40**(6): 703–12.

45. Tester DJ, Ackerman MJ. Cardiomyopathic and channelopathic causes of sudden unexplained death in infants and children. *Annu Rev Med*, 2009; **60**:69–84.

46. Hof T, Liu H, Sallé L, Schott JJ, Ducreux C, Millat G, et al. TRPM4 non-selective cation channel variants in long QT syndrome. *BMC Med Genet*, 2017; **18**(1):31.

47. Osawa M, Kimura R, Hasegawa I, Mukasa N, Satoh F. SNP association and sequence analysis of the NOS1AP gene in SIDS. *Leg Med (Tokyo)*, 2009; **11** Suppl 1:S307–8.

48. Eijgelsheim M, Aarnoudse AL, Rivadeneira F, Kors JA, Witteman JC, Hofman A, et al. Identification of a common variant at the NOS1AP locus strongly associated to QT-interval duration. *Hum Mol Genet*, 2009; **18**(2):347–57.

49. Eijgelsheim M, Newton-Cheh C, Aarnoudse AL, van Noord C, Witteman JC, Hofman A, et al. Genetic variation in NOS1AP is associated with sudden cardiac death: evidence from the Rotterdam Study. *Hum Mol Genet*, 2009; **18**(21):4213–18.

50. van Noord C, Aarnoudse AJ, Eijgelsheim M, Sturkenboom MC, Straus SM, Hofman A, et al. Calcium channel blockers, NOS1AP, and heart-rate-corrected QT prolongation. *Pharmacogenet Genomics*, 2009; **19**(4):260–6.

51. Arnestad M, Crotti L, Rognum TO, Insolia R, Pedrazzini M, Ferrandi C, et al. Prevalence of long-QT syndrome gene variants in Sudden Infant Death Syndrome. *Circulation*, 2007; **115**(3):361–7.

Central Nervous System Pathways

52. Haynes RL, Frelinger AL, Giles EK, Goldstein RD, Tran H, Kozakewich HP, et al. High serum serotonin in Sudden Infant Death Syndrome. *Proc Natl Acad Sci USA*, 2017; **114**(29):7695–700.

53. Kinney HC, Thach BT. The Sudden Infant Death Syndrome. *N Engl J Med*, 2009; **361**(8):795–805.

54. Hilaire G, Voituron N, Menuet C, Ichiyama RM, Subramanian HH, Dutschmann M. The role of serotonin in respiratory function and dysfunction. *Respir Physiol Neurobiol*, 2010; **174**(1–2):76–88.

55. Buchanan GF, Richerson GB. Central serotonin neurons are required for arousal to CO_2. *Proc Natl Acad Sci USA*, 2010; **107**(37):16354–9.

56. Narita N, Narita M, Takashima S, Nakayama M, Nagai T, Okado N. Serotonin transporter gene variation is a risk factor for Sudden Infant Death Syndrome in the Japanese population. *Pediatrics*, 2001; **107**(4):690–2.

57. Weese-Mayer DE, Berry-Kravis EM, Maher BS, Silvestri JM, Curran ME, Marazita ML. Sudden Infant Death Syndrome: association with a promoter polymorphism of the serotonin transporter gene. *Am J Med Genet A*, 2003; **117A**(3):268–74.

58. Weese-Mayer DE, Zhou L, Berry-Kravis EM, Maher BS, Silvestri JM, Marazita ML. Association of the serotonin transporter gene with Sudden Infant Death Syndrome: a haplotype analysis. *Am J Med Genet A*, 2003; **122A**(3):238–45.

59. Weese-Mayer DE, Ackerman MJ, Marazita ML, Berry-Kravis EM. Sudden Infant Death Syndrome: review of implicated genetic factors. *Am J Med Genet A*, 2007; **143A**(8):771–88.

60. Opdal SH, Vege A, Rognum TO. Serotonin transporter gene variation in Sudden Infant Death Syndrome. *Acta Paediatr*, 2008; **97**(7):861–5.

61. Filiano JJ, Kinney HC. A perspective on neuropathologic findings in victims of the Sudden Infant Death Syndrome: the triple-risk model. *Biol Neonate*, 1994; **65**(3–4):194–7.

62. Kinney HC, Filiano JJ, Sleeper LA, Mandell F, Valdes-Dapena M, White WF. Decreased muscarinic receptor binding in the arcuate nucleus in Sudden Infant Death Syndrome. *Science*, 1995; **269**(5229):1446–50.

63. Kinney HC. Brainstem mechanisms underlying the Sudden Infant Death Syndrome: evidence from human pathologic studies. *Dev Psychobiol*, 2009; **51**(3):223–33.

64. Lavezzi AM, Ferrero S, Roncati L, Matturri L, Pusiol T. Impaired orexin receptor expression in the Kölliker-Fuse nucleus in Sudden Infant Death Syndrome: possible involvement of this nucleus in arousal pathophysiology. *Neurol Res*, 2016; **38**(8):706–16.

65. Pattyn A, Goridis C, Brunet JF. Specification of the central noradrenergic phenotype by the homeobox gene Phox2b. *Mol Cell Neurosci*, 2000; **15**(3):235–43.

66. Pattyn A, Hirsch M, Goridis C, Brunet JF. Control of hindbrain motor neuron differentiation by the homeobox gene Phox2b. *Development*, 2000; **127**(7):1349–58.

67. Liebrechts-Akkerman G, Liu F, Lao O, Ooms AH, van Duijn K, Vermeulen M, et al. PHOX2B polyalanine repeat length is associated with Sudden Infant Death Syndrome and unclassified sudden infant death in the Dutch population. *Int J Legal Med*, 2014; **128**(4):621–9.

68. Wilson RJ, Cumming KJ. Pituitary adenylate-cyclase-activating polypeptide is vital for neonatal survival and the neuronal control of breathing. *Respir Physiol Neurobiol*, 2008; **164**(1–2):168–78.

69. Farnham MM, Pilowsky PM. The role of PACAP in central cardiorespiratory regulation. *Respir Physiol Neurobiol*, 2010; **174**(1–2):65–75.

70. Arata S, Nakamachi T, Onimaru H, Hashimoto H, Shioda S. Impaired response to hypoxia in the respiratory center is a major cause of neonatal death of the PACAP-knockout mouse. *Eur J Neurosci*, 2013; **37**(3):407–16.

71. Courts C, Grabmüller M, Madea B. Monoamine oxidase A gene polymorphism and the pathogenesis of Sudden Infant Death Syndrome. *J Pediatr*, 2013; **163**(1):89–93.

72. Gross M, Bajanowski T, Vennemann M, Poetsch M. Sudden Infant Death Syndrome (SIDS) and polymorphisms in monoamine oxidase A gene (MAOA): a revisit. *Int J Legal Med*, 2014; **128**(1):43–9.

73. Kijima K, Sasaki A, Niki T, Umetsu K, Osawa M, Matoba R, Hayasaka K. Sudden Infant Death Syndrome is not associated with the mutation of PHOX2B gene, a major causative gene of congenital central hypoventilation syndrome. *Tohoku J Exp Med*, 2004; **203**(1):65–8.

74. Li A, Emond L, Nattie E. Brainstem catecholaminergic neurons modulate both respiratory and cardiovascular function. *Adv Exp Med Biol*, 2008; **605**:371–6.

75. Klintschar M, Heimbold C. Association between a functional polymorphism in the MAOA gene and Sudden Infant Death Syndrome. *Pediatrics*, 2012; **129**(3):e756–61.

Immune Dysfunction

76. Opdal SH, Vege A, Stray-Pedersen A, Rognum TO. Aquaporin-4 gene variation and Sudden Infant Death Syndrome. *Pediatr Res*, 2010; **68**(1):48–51.

77. Blackwell CC, Moscovis SM, Gordon AE, Al Madani OM, Hall ST, Gleeson M, et al. Ethnicity, infection, and Sudden Infant Death Syndrome. *FEMS Immunol Med Microbiol*, 2004; **42**(1):53–65.

78. Blackwell CC, Moscovis SM, Gordon AE, Al Madani OM, Hall ST, Gleeson M, et al. Cytokine responses and Sudden Infant Death Syndrome:

genetic, developmental, and environmental risk factors. *J Leukoc Biol*, 2005; **78**(6):1242–54.

79. Gordon AE, MacKenzie DA, El Ahmer OR, Al Madani OM, Braun JM, Weir DM, et al. Evidence for a genetic component in Sudden Infant Death Syndrome. *Child Care Health Dev*, 2002; **28**(Suppl 1): 27–9.

80. Vege A, Rognum TO, Scott H, Aasen AO, Saugstad OD. SIDS cases have increased levels of interleukin-6 in cerebrospinal fluid. *Acta Paediatr*, 1995; **84**(2):193–6.

81. Arnestad M, Andersen M, Vege A, Rognum TO. Changes in the epidemiological pattern of Sudden Infant Death Syndrome in southeast Norway, 1984–1998: implications for future prevention and research. *Arch Dis Child*, 2001; **85**(2):108–15.

82. Moscovis SM, Gordon AE, Al Madani OM, Gleeson M, Scott RJ, Roberts-Thomson J, et al. Interleukin-10 and Sudden Infant Death Syndrome. *FEMS Immunol Med Microbiol*, 2004; **42**(1):130–8.

83. Moscovis SM, Gordon AE, Al Madani OM, Gleeson M, Scott RJ, Roberts-Thomson J, et al. IL6 G-174 C associated with Sudden Infant Death Syndrome in a caucasian Australian cohort. *Hum Immunol*, 2006; **67**(10):819–25.

84. Moscovis SM, Gordon AE, Al Madani OM, Gleeson M, Scott RJ, Hall ST, et al. Genetic and Environmental Factors Affecting TNF-α Responses in Relation to Sudden Infant Death Syndrome. *Front Immunol*, 2015; **6**:374.

85. Moscovis SM, Gordon AE, Al Madani OM, Gleeson M, Scott RJ, Hall ST, et al. Virus infections and sudden death in infancy: the role of interferon-γ. *Front Immunol*, 2015; **6**:107.

86. Summers AM, Summers CW, Drucker DB, Hajeer AH, Barson A, Hutchinson IV. Association of IL-10 genotype with Sudden Infant Death Syndrome. *Hum Immunol*, 2000; **61**(12):1270–3.

87. Ferrante L, Opdal SH. Sudden Infant Death Syndrome and the genetics of inflammation. *Front Immunol*, 2015; **6**:63.

88. Ferrante L, Opdal SH, Vege A, Rognum TO. IL-1 gene cluster polymorphisms and Sudden Infant Death Syndrome. *Hum Immunol*, 2010; **71**(4):402–6.

89. Arnestad M, Vege A, Rognum TO. Evaluation of diagnostic tools applied in the examination of sudden unexpected deaths in infancy and early childhood. *Forensic Sci Int*, 2002; **125**(2–3):262–8.

90. Rognum IJ, Haynes RL, Vege A, Yang M, Rognum TO, Kinney HC. Interleukin-6 and the serotonergic system of the medulla oblongata in the Sudden Infant Death Syndrome. *Acta Neuropathol*, 2009; **118**(4):519–30.

91. Schneider PM, Wendler C, Riepert T, Braun L, Schacker U, Horn M, et al. Possible association of sudden infant death with partial complement C4 deficiency revealed by post-mortem DNA typing of HLA class II and III genes. *Eur J Pediatr*, 1989; **149**(3): 170–4.

92. Weber MA, Klein NJ, Hartley JC, Lock PE, Malone M, Sebire NJ. Infection and sudden unexpected death in infancy: a systematic retrospective case review. *Lancet*, 2008; **371**(9627):1848–53.

93. Thach BT. Potential central nervous system involvement in sudden unexpected infant deaths and the Sudden Infant Death Syndrome. *Compr Physiol*, 2015; **5**(3):1061–8.

Inborn Errors of Metabolism

94. Côté A. Investigating sudden unexpected death in infancy and early childhood. *Paediatr Respir Rev*, 2010; **11**(4):219–25.

95. Lundemose JB, Kølvraa S, Gregersen N, Christensen E, Gregersen M. Fatty acid oxidation disorders as primary cause of sudden and unexpected death in infants and young children: an investigation performed on cultured fibroblasts from 79 children who died aged between 0–4 years. *Mol Pathol*, 1997; **50**(4):212–17.

96. Moczulski D, Majak I, Mamczur D. An overview of beta-oxidation disorders. *Postepy Hig Med Dosw* (online), 2009; **63**:266–77.

Nicotine Response

97. Adgent MA. Environmental tobacco smoke and Sudden Infant Death Syndrome: a review. *Birth Defects Res B Dev Reprod Toxicol*, 2006; **77**(1):69–85.

98. Poetsch M, Czerwinski M, Wingenfeld L, Vennemann M, Bajanowski T. A common FMO3 polymorphism may amplify the effect of nicotine exposure in Sudden Infant Death Syndrome (SIDS). *Int J Legal Med*, 2010; **124**(4):301–6.

99. Duncan JR, Paterson DS, Kinney HC. The development of nicotinic receptors in the human medulla oblongata: inter-relationship with the serotonergic system. *Auton Neurosci*, 2008; **144**(1–2):61–75.

100. Touiki K, Rat P, Molimard R, Chait A, de Beaurepaire R. Effects of tobacco and cigarette smoke extracts on serotonergic raphe neurons in the rat. *Neuroreport*, 2007; **18**(9):925–9.

101. Say M, Machaalani R, Waters KA. Changes in serotoninergic receptors 1A and 2A in the piglet brainstem after intermittent hypercapnic hypoxia (IHH) and nicotine. *Brain Res*, 2007; **1152**:17–26.

Inner-Ear Defects

102. Ramirez S, Allen T, Villagracia L, Chae Y, Ramirez JM, Rubens DD. Inner ear lesion and the differential roles of hypoxia and hypercarbia in triggering active movements: potential implication for the Sudden Infant Death Syndrome. *Neuroscience*, 2016; **337**:9–16.

103. Allen T, Garcia Iii AJ, Tang J, Ramirez JM, Rubens DD. Inner ear insult ablates the arousal response to hypoxia and hypercarbia. *Neuroscience*, 2013; **253**:283–91.

104. SIDS Research Guild website: https://www.lullabytrust.org.uk/safer-sleep-advice/what-is-sids/ (accessed 13 November 2017).

105. Rubens DD, Vohr BR, Tucker R, O'Neil CA, Chung W. Newborn oto-acoustic emission hearing screening tests: preliminary evidence for a marker of susceptibility to SIDS. *Early Hum Dev*, 2008; **84**(4): 225–9.

106. Rubens D, Sarnat HB. Sudden Infant Death Syndrome: an update and new perspectives of etiology. *Handb Clin Neurol*, 2013; **112**:867–74.

Genetic Analysis

107. Gardner JM, Sutherland GR, Shaffer LG. *Chromosome Abnormalities and Genetic Counseling.* 4th edn. Oxford Monographs on Medical Genetics. Oxford University Press, 2012.

108. Pinkel D, Segraves R, Sudar D, Clark S, Poole I, Kowbel D, et al. High resolution analysis of DNA copy number variation using comparative genomic hybridization to microarrays. *Nat Genet*, 1998; **20**(2): 207–11.

109. Miller DT, Adam MP, Aradhya S, Biesecker LG, Brothman AR, Carter NP, et al. Consensus statement: chromosomal microarray is a first-tier clinical diagnostic test for individuals with developmental disabilities or congenital anomalies. *Am J Hum Genet*, 2010; **86**(5):749–64.

110. Robson SC, Chitty LS, Morris S, et al. Evaluation of array comparative genomic hybridisation in prenatal diagnosis of fetal anomalies: a multicentre cohort study with cost analysis and assessment of patient, health professional, and commissioner preferences for array comparative genomic hybridisation. Efficacy and Mechanism Evaluation, 2017, 4(1):eme04010 https://www.ncbi.nlm.nih.gov/books/NBK423961/ (accessed 31 October 2018).

111. Stranneheim H, Lundeberg J. Stepping stones in DNA sequencing. *Biotechnol J*, 2012; 7(9):1063–73.

112. Chiara M, Pavesi G. Evaluation of quality assessment protocols for high throughput genome resequencing data. *Front Genet*, 2017; **8**:94.

Chapter 29

Cardiac Arrhythmias

Chris Miles and Elijah Behr

Introduction

SIDS may result from inherited cardiac conditions such as the primary arrhythmia syndromes, a heterogeneous group of genetic cardiac ion channelopathies that predispose to ventricular arrhythmia and sudden death in the setting of a structurally normal heart. This is very much in keeping with the normal autopsy findings expected in SIDS. The channelopathies are mainly inherited in an autosomal dominant manner and are often caused by mutations in genes encoding cardiac ion-channel subunits or channel-interacting proteins. They include long QT syndrome (LQTS), Brugada syndrome (BrS), and catecholaminergic polymorphic ventricular tachycardia (CPVT).

The relationship between cardiac channelopathies and SIDS has largely relied on post-mortem genetic studies, the 'molecular autopsy'. Causation has been proposed by the discovery of putative 'pathogenic' rare variants in candidate cardiac genes (see Figure 29.1 and Table 2.9). These variants either have established disease association or, more commonly, a presumed effect on disease expression backed up by *in vitro* experimental data and/or *in silico* tools for assessing pathogenicity. The accuracy of these methods is however variable.[1]

It is increasingly recognised that mutations in SIDS may arise *de novo* and are associated with a more malignant clinical phenotype, manifesting in early-onset disease in keeping with a number of severe paediatric neurodevelopment disorders.[2] While our understanding of the complexity of cardiac genetic susceptibility in SIDS continues to evolve, recent guidelines include post-mortem genetic testing alongside familial evaluation in cases where LQTS, BrS, or CPVT is suspected, usually due to a family history.[3,4]

Long QT Syndrome

LQTS was the first channelopathy to be associated with SIDS and has been proposed to account for

approximately 4–20% of cases.[5] It is characterised by prolongation of the QT interval on the electrocardiogram (ECG), indicative of delayed cardiac repolarisation, and an increased risk of sudden death due to the characteristic polymorphic ventricular arrhythmia, Torsades de Pointes.[3] Clinical diagnosis of LQTS was initially made using the 'Schwartz score', a criterion which tabulates individual symptoms, family history, and corrected QT values to inform likelihood of disease.[6] In the general population, the prevalence of LQTS is estimated to be 1:2000 of live births.[7]

In 1976, Maron reported that a significant proportion of first degree relatives of SIDS victims demonstrated QT prolongation on the ECG, a finding described in 11/42 (26%) sets of parents.[8] Subsequently, a prospective study of more than 30,000 infants indicated that QT prolongation in the first week of life was an important risk factor for sudden death.[9] The authors proposed two possible mechanisms: developmental alterations in cardiac sympathetic innervation triggering arrhythmia in electrically unstable hearts, and arrhythmias occurring in the context of a genetic LQTS vulnerability.

Over the last two decades, this genetic vulnerability has been investigated with hundreds of mutations identified in multiple genes mainly encoding the repolarising potassium currents and the sodium channel current (Nav1.5). In the majority of index cases (75%), three LQTS major genes are implicated: loss-of-function mutations in *KCNQ1* (LQT1, 35%) and *KCNH2* (LQT2, 35%); and gain-of-function mutations in the sodium channel gene *SCN5A* (LQT3, 5%).[10] Significantly, as the yield of genetic testing in LQTS is not 100%, molecular autopsy may underestimate the true contribution of the syndrome to the occurrence of arrhythmic death in SIDS. QT prolongation and arrhythmic risk in LQTS are thought to be mediated by decreased outward potassium current or increased inward sodium/calcium current, which prolong repolarisation within cardiac

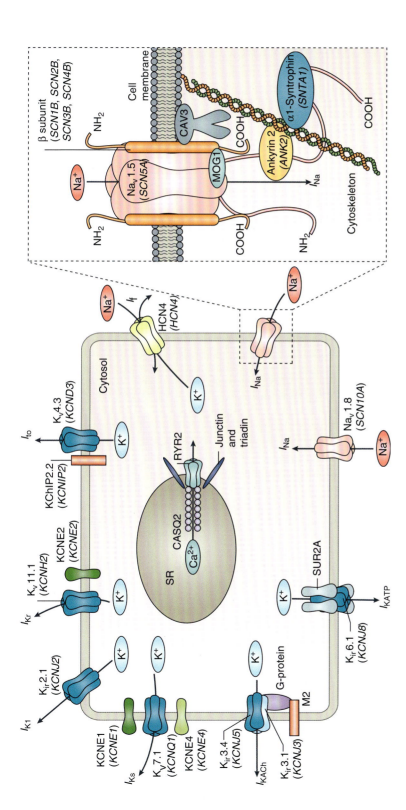

Figure 29.1 Main proteins involved in inherited arrhythmia syndromes. Mutations in the genes (in parenthesis) encoding ion-channel proteins, channel-interacting proteins, and Ca²⁺-handling proteins are associated with arrhythmia syndromes (Table 29.1). CASQ2, calsequentrin 2; CAV3, caveolin 3; I_f, hyperpolarisation-activated cyclic nucleotide-gated-mediated current; IK1, inward-rectifier K⁺ current; IK$_{ACh}$, acetylcholine-activated inward-rectifier K⁺ current; IK$_{ATP}$, ATP-dependent K⁺ current; IKr, rapid component of delayed-rectifier K⁺ current; IKs, slow component of delayed-rectifier K⁺ current; Ito, transient-outward K⁺ current; KCNE1, potassium voltage-gated channel subfamily E member 1; MOG1, Ran guanine nucleotide release factor; RYR2, ryanodine receptor 2; SR, sarcoplasmic reticulum. Reproduced by permission from Springer Nature: Baruteau et al.[12]

Table 29.1 | Main genes associated with inherited arrhythmia syndromes relevant to SIDS

Gene	Locus	Protein	Current	Disease (MIM)
K+ channels				
KCNQ1	11p15.5-p15.4	α-subunit of IKs channel (Kv7.1)	IKs	LQT1 (192500), JLN1 (220400), SQT2 (609621)
KCNH2	7q36.1	α-subunit of IKr channel (Kv11.1)	IKr	LQT2 (613688), SQT1 (609620), BrS20 (-)
KCNE1	21q22.12	MinK	IKs	LQT5 (613695), JLN2 (612347)
KCNE2	21q22.11	MiRP1	IKr	LQT6 (613693)
KCNJ2	17q24.3	Kir2.1	IK1	LQT7 (170390), SQT3 (609622)
KCNJ5	11q24.3	IK$_{ACh}$ channel, α subunit (Kir3.4)	IK$_{ACh}$	LQT13 (613485)
KCNJ8	12p12.1	α-subunit, KIR6.1 potassium channel	IK$_{ATP}$	BrS10 (-)
KCND3	1p13.2	α-subunit, KV4.3 potassium channel	Ito$_1$	BrS9 (616399)
Na+ channel				
SCN5A	3p22.2	α-subunit, Na$_v$1.5	I$_{Na}$	BrS1 (601144), LQT3 (603830)
SCN10A	3p22.2	α-subunit, Nav1.8	I$_{Na}$	BrS21 (-)
SCN1B	19q13.11	β-subunit, Navβ1	I$_{Na}$	BrS5 (612838)
SCN2B	11q23.3	β-subunit, Navβ2	I$_{Na}$	BrS16 (-)
SCN3B	11q24.1	β-subunit, Navβ3	I$_{Na}$	BrS7 (613120)
SCN4B	11q23.3	β subunit, Navβ4	I$_{Na}$	LQT10 (611819)
CAV3	3p25.3	Caveolin 3	I$_{Na}$	LQT9 (611818)
GPD1-L	3p22.3	Glycerol-3-phosphate dehydrogenase 1-like	I$_{Na}$	BrS2 (611877)
SNTA1	20q11.21	Syntrophin-α1	I$_{Na}$	LQT12 (612955)
Ca2+-related genes				
CALM1	14q32.11	Calmodulin 1	Ca^{2+} regulation	LQT14 (616247), CPVT4 (614916)
RyR2	1q43	Ryanodine receptor	Ca^{2+} regulation	CPVT1 (604772)
CASQ2	1p13.1	Calsequestrin 2	Ca^{2+} regulation	CPVT2 (611938)
TRPM4	19q13.33	Calcium-activated non-selective ion channel	TRPM4 current	BrS15 (-)
Other inherited arrhythmias				
ANK2	4q25-q26	Ankyrin-B	Na$^+$/K$^+$	LQT4 (600919)
HCN4	15q24.1	Hyperpolarisation-activated cyclic nucleotide-gated channel 4	I$_f$	BrS8 (613123)

BrS, Brugada syndrome; CPVT, catecholaminergic polymorphic ventricular tachycardia; I$_f$, hyperpolarisation-activated cyclic nucleotide-gated-mediated current; IK1, inward-rectifier K$^+$ current; IK$_{ACh}$, acetylcholine-activated inward-rectifier K$^+$ current; IK$_{ATP}$, ATP-dependent K$^+$ current; IKr, rapid component of delayed-rectifier K$^+$ current; IKs, slow component of delayed-rectifier K$^+$ current; I$_{Na}$, Na$^+$ current; Ito$_1$, transient-outward K$^+$ current; JLN, Jervell, and Lange–Nielsen syndrome; LQT, long QT syndrome; SQT, short QT syndrome

Adapted by permission from Springer Nature from Baruteau et al.[12].

cells and lead to early and delayed afterdepolarisations and triggered activity that may induce Torsades de Pointes.[11]

From a treatment perspective, the advent of genetic testing has identified individual genotype/phenotype correlations, enabling therapeutic strategies to be tailored according to underlying genotype. For example, beta-blocker therapy, the mainstay of treatment, carries greater efficacy among LQT1 patients when compared with LQT2 and LQT3. Distinct appearances to the morphology of the T-wave on the resting ECG are also seen across genotypes and LQT1 patients are more prone to arrhythmias in the context of sympathetic activation during exercise. Conversely, gain-of-function mutations in the sodium channel *SCN5A* gene (LQT3) confer greater risk of sudden death at times of rest (sleep) or high vagal tone.

Historical genetic studies in SIDS have identified a variable yield of LQTS-associated rare variants in varying sized cohorts relying on rarity of variants to support pathogenicity.[12] For example, Tester performed comprehensive mutational analysis of five candidate LQTS genes in a population-based cohort of 93 infants (KCNQ1, KCNH2, SCN5A, KCNE1, KCNE2). Putative disease-causing variants were identified in 5.1% of white infants, and 2.9% of black infants.[13] In addition, three novel rare variants were reported in the potassium channel genes KCNQ1, KCNH2 and KCNE2, and a fourth variant in KCNH2 was found in a separate analysis; however, pathogenicity is currently uncertain.

In a large Norwegian study of 201 expertly validated cases,[14] seven genes associated with LQTS were also evaluated, reporting putative mutations and rare genetic variants in 26 cases (12.9%). Among these, 11 variants (55%) were not identified in ethnically matched controls or previously reported control populations and were mostly comprised of missense mutations. Rare variants were most frequently described in the *SCN5A* gene, but were also reported in the potassium channel genes *KCNQ1, KCNH2*, and *KCNE2*, and the *CAV3* gene, which is thought to facilitate gain-of-function increase in late sodium current and prolongation of cardiac repolarisation. Based on assessment of available functional data, the variants in this cohort were thought to be causal in 9.5%.

Brugada Syndrome

Brugada syndrome (BrS) is diagnosed clinically by the finding of ≥2 mm of coved ST segment elevation with T-wave inversion in at least one of the standard or high lead right precordial ECG leads: the type 1 pattern. This pattern may be concealed and provoked by environmental factors such as fever or drugs that block cardiac sodium channels. If drug-induced then other clinical factors such as family history and/or symptoms are required.[3,4] In Asian countries, the prevalence of the type 1 ECG is approximately 0.15, compared with <0.02% in the Western population.[15] It may manifest with syncope and/or sudden death due to polymorphic ventricular tachycardia and ventricular fibrillation.

Over 200 mutations in the sodium channel gene *SCN5A* have been described, where pathogenic loss-of-function mutations are seen in approximately 20% of individuals.[16] The yield of genetic testing in BrS is significantly lower than LQTS and the genotype-phenotype relationship currently carries little clinical utility. Nevertheless, mutations in the *SCN5A* gene may overlap with other clinical syndromes including progressive cardiac conduction defect, sick sinus syndrome, and LQT3.[17]

To date, BrS has been implicated principally in a small number of case reports and genetic studies. In one report examining a family where five children had died suddenly (including two SIDS cases), the Brugada ECG phenotype was recorded in a child following admission to hospital after a cardiac arrest.[18] A pathogenic missense variant in the *SCN5A* gene was identified and later found to segregate in the family. In a large study of 292 SIDS cases, targeted mutational analysis of genes encoding cardiac sodium channel beta subunits (β1–4) identified three rare missense variants, representing 1% of the cohort.[19] These were proposed as consistent with BrS and/or LQT3, suggesting mutations in sodium channel beta subunits may play an important role in the dysregulation of $Na_V1.5$ channel current.

Other Channelopathies

Other channelopathies associated with SIDS include CPVT and short QT syndrome (SQTS). CPVT is characterised by adrenergically-mediated bidirectional ventricular tachycardia and/or polymorphic ventricular tachycardia which may cause syncope and/or sudden death. The prevalence of CPVT is estimated around 1:10,000 and the disorder principally arises due to rare variants in two genes: *RYR2* and *CASQ2*. The mechanism of arrhythmia is largely due to intracellular calcium mishandling, which results in uncontrolled calcium release from the sarcoplasmic reticulum during diastole, triggered activity, and onset of ventricular arrhythmias.[20]

The contribution of CPVT to SIDS has been determined from a limited selection of genetic studies. In 134 SIDS cases, 2 cases exhibited novel functionally significant rare variants in the *RYR2* gene, representing a small proportion (1–2%) of the overall cohort. [21] Further evaluation of the *RYR2* gene reported rare variants in 9.4% of 32 SIDS cases.[22] This was higher than previously reported and is probably explained by the presence of predominantly novel variants, absence of functional modelling, and lack of detailed family segregation analysis limiting the extent in which true pathogenicity could be ascribed.

SQTS is an extremely rare and genetically heterogeneous disease defined by a shortening of the QT interval due to abbreviated repolarisation.[3] Gain-of-function mutations in genes encoding potassium channels and loss-of-function calcium channel mutations may lead to shortening of the cardiac action potential and a predilection to sudden cardiac death. [23] In the aforementioned Norwegian SIDS study, one of the variants in *KCNQ1* had a gain-of function effect, suggestive of short QT phenotype.[14] However, the true prevalence and contribution of SQTS to sudden cardiac death is yet to be determined and its relationship with SIDS is speculative, currently limited to isolated reports in the literature.

SIDS and the Molecular Autopsy

The molecular autopsy, or post-mortem genetic testing, involves the collection of tissue suitable for DNA extraction at autopsy and mutation analysis for a specified group of genes for diagnostic purposes. In adult sudden arrhythmic death, putative 'disease-causing' rare variants in inherited cardiac conditions genes have been estimated to be present in up to 35% of cases.[24] However, with more robust assessment of pathogenicity it appears that yields are as low as 13%.[25] In SIDS, when combining all available data, the overall diagnostic yield of putative 'disease-causing' rare variants is 14%. [12] It is likely however that the true yield of pathogenic and likely pathogenic variants is lower.

This problem of variant interpretation is compounded by the rapid development of NGS technology which has demonstrated an abundance of rare genetic variation in affected and healthy individuals. This has made determination of variant pathogenicity problematic, especially where functional assessment is lacking: the variant of unknown significance

(VUS).[26] Moreover, there is an increased likelihood of identifying novel sporadic genetic disease in SIDS, requiring parental genetic analysis to make sense of findings.[12] The use of NGS has expanded the range of genes that can be examined such that a recent study identified a 7% yield in cardiomyopathy genes of 'potentially causative' rare variants.[27] However, as the role for structural diseases such as cardiomyopathy in autopsy negative infant death seems questionable, these findings may at least in part represent the background genetic variation in these genes and may not have functional significance. Until more robust data are available comparing the burden of genetic variation in cardiac genes in large case and control cohorts, then the significance of inherited cardiac conditions in SIDS remains unclear. It is also feasible that SIDS may result from interaction of common genetic variation with functional effects on the cardiac action potential, suggesting a polygenic model. This has yet to be explored comprehensively in any large genome-wide association study but candidate studies have suggested roles in specific ethnic groups: for example, the *SCN5A* S1103Y variant in the African-American population.[28]

Current guidelines recommend the use of molecular autopsy in selected cases of SIDS, especially where family history, and the characteristics and circumstances of death may suggest a diagnosis of LQTS or CPVT.[3] The identification of rare genetic variants known to be 'disease-causing' may then assist in determining cause of death and allow cascade genetic evaluation of at-risk blood relatives. Thus, when a rare variant is identified by molecular autopsy, cascade genetic evaluation should initially focus on the parents to determine whether the variant is *de novo* or potentially inherited.[12] There is, however, a paucity of evidence supporting familial evaluation in the absence of informative post-mortem genetic data and research is required to establish its utility. Currently it may only be useful when a family history of sudden or other SIDS deaths is present.

References

1. Eilbeck K, Quinlan A, Yandell M. Settling the score: variant prioritization and Mendelian disease. *Nat Rev Genet*, 2017; **18**(10):599–612.

2. McRae JF, et al. Deciphering developmental disorder study. Prevalence and architecture of de novo mutations in developmental disorders. *Nature*, 2017; **542** (7642):433–8.

3. Priori SG, Wilde AA, Horie M, Cho Y, Behr ER, Berul C, et al. HRS/EHRA/APHRS expert consensus statement on the diagnosis and management of patients with inherited primary arrhythmia syndromes: document endorsed by HRS, EHRA, and APHRS in May 2013 and by ACCF, AHA, PACES, and AEPC in June 2013. *Heart Rhythm*, 2013; **10**(12):1932–63.

4. Priori SG, Blomstrom-Lundqvist C. European Society of Cardiology guidelines for the management of patients with ventricular arrhythmias and the prevention of sudden cardiac death summarized by co-chairs. *Eur Heart J*, 2015; **36**(41):2757–9.

5. Ioakeimidis NS, Papamitsou T, Meditskou S, Iakovidou-Kritsi Z. Sudden Infant Death Syndrome due to long QT syndrome: a brief review of the genetic substrate and prevalence. *J Biol Res (Thessalon)*, 2017; **24**:6; https://www.ncbi.nlm.nih.gov/pmc/articles/PMC5348737/ (accessed 31 October 2018).

6. Schwartz PJ, Moss AJ, Vincent GM, Crampton RS. Diagnostic criteria for the long QT syndrome. An update. *Circulation*, 1993; **88**(2):782.

7. Schwartz PJ, Stramba-Badiale M, Crotti L, Pedrazzini M, Besana A, Bosi G, et al. Prevalence of the congenital long QT Syndrome. *Circulation*, 2009; **120**(18):1761–7.

8. Maron BJ, Clark CE, Goldstein RE, Epstein SE. Potential role of QT interval prolongation in Sudden Infant Death Syndrome. *Circulation*, 1976; **54**(3):423–30.

9. Schwartz PJ, Stramba-Badiale M, Segantini A, Austoni P, Bosi G, Giorgetti R, et al. Prolongation of the QT interval and the Sudden Infant Death Syndrome. *N Engl J Med*, 1998; **338**(24):1709–14.

10. Mizusawa Y, Horie M Wilde AM, Wilde AA. Genetic and clinical advances in congenital long QT syndrome. *Circ J*, 2014; **78**(12):2827–33.

11. Weiss JN, Garfinkel A, Karagueuzian HS, Chen P, Qu Z. Early afterdepolarizations and cardiac arrhythmias. *Heart Rhythm*, 2010; **7**(12):1891–9.

12. Baruteau A-E, Tester DJ, Kapplinger JD, Ackerman MJ, Behr ER. Sudden Infant Death Syndrome and inherited cardiac conditions. *Nat Rev Cardiol*, 2017; **14** (12):715–26.

13. Tester DJ, Ackerman MJ. Sudden Infant Death Syndrome: how significant are the cardiac channelopathies? *Cardiovasc Res*, 2005; **67**(3):388–96.

14. Arnestad M, Crotti L, Rognum TO, Insolia RF, Pedrazzini MF, Ferrandi CF, et al. Prevalence of long-QT syndrome gene variants in Sudden Infant Death Syndrome. *Circulation*, 2007;**115**(3):361–7.

15. Kamakura S. Epidemiology of Brugada syndrome in Japan and rest of the world. *J Arrhythmia; Special Issue: Brugada Syndrome from Bench to Bedside*, 2013; **29** (2):52–5.

16. Kapplinger JD, Tester DJ, Alders MF, Benito BF, Berthet MF, Brugada JF, et al. An international compendium of mutations in the SCN5A-encoded cardiac sodium channel in patients referred for Brugada syndrome genetic testing. *Heart Rhythm*, 2010; **7**(1):33–46.

17. Remme CA. Cardiac sodium channelopathy associated with SCN5A mutations: electrophysiological, molecular, and genetic aspects. *J Physiol (Lond)*, 2013; **591**:4099–116.

18. Priori SG, Napolitano C, Giordano U, Collisani G, Memmi M. Brugada syndrome and sudden cardiac death in children. *Lancet*, 2000; **355**(9206):808–9.

19. Tan BH, Pundi KN, Van Norstrand DW, Valdivia CR, Tester DJ, Medeiros-Domingo A, et al. Sudden Infant Death Syndrome-associated mutations in the sodium channel beta subunits. *Heart Rhythm*, 2010; **7** (6):771–8.

20. Landstrom AP, Dobrev D, Wehrens XHT. Calcium signaling and cardiac arrhythmias. *Circ Res*, 2017; **120** (12):1969.

21. Tester DJ, Dura M, Carturan E, Reiken S, Wronska A, Marks AR, et al. A mechanism for Sudden Infant Death Syndrome (SIDS): stress-induced leak via ryanodine receptors. *Heart Rhythm*, 2007; **4**(6):733–9.

22. Larsen MK, Berge KE, Leren TP, Nissen PH, Hansen J, Kristensen IB, et al. Postmortem genetic testing of the ryanodine receptor 2 (RYR2) gene in a cohort of sudden unexplained death cases. *Int J Legal Med*, 2013; **127**(1):139–44.

23. Patel C, Yan G, Antzelevitch C. Short QT syndrome: from bench to bedside. *Circ Arrhythm Electrophysiol*, 2010; **3**(4):401–8.

24. Miles CJ, Behr ER. The role of genetic testing in unexplained sudden death. *Transl Res*, 2016; **168**:59–73.

25. Lahrouchi N, Raju H, Lodder EM, Papatheodorou E, Ware JS, Papadakis M, et al. Utility of post-mortem genetic testing in cases of Sudden Arrhythmic Death Syndrome. *J Am Coll Cardiol*, 2017; **69**(17):2134–45.

26. Ackerman MJ. Genetic purgatory and the cardiac channelopathies: exposing the variants of uncertain/unknown significance issue. *Heart Rhythm*, 2015; **12** (11):2325–31.

27. Neubauer J, Lecca MR, Russo G, Bartsch C, Medeiros-Domingo A, Berger W, et al. Post-mortem whole-exome analysis in a large Sudden Infant Death Syndrome cohort with a focus on cardiovascular and metabolic genetic diseases. *Eur J Hum Gen*, 2017; **25**(4):404–9.

28. Plant LD, Bowers PN, Liu Q, Morgan T, Zhang T, State MW, et al. A common cardiac sodium channel variant associated with sudden infant death in African Americans, SCN5A S1103Y. *J Clin Invest*, 2005; **116** (2):430–5.

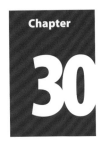

Chapter

30

Sudden Infant Death Syndrome from the Brainstem Perspective

Jan-Marino Ramirez and Christopher G. Wilson

Introduction

Sudden Infant Death Syndrome (SIDS) continues to be a major tragedy for young families. Significant advances in understanding the causes of SIDS came from the discovery of critical risk factors such as a prone sleeping position or smoking.[1–6] Campaigns, such as the 'back-to-sleep', or the smoking cessation campaigns[7,8] have significantly reduced infant mortality due to SIDS.[5,9] But, epidemiological and pathological studies continue to identify more risk factors including various genetic predispositions.[10–13] The identification of multiple risk factors has pointed towards one particular hypothesis for explaining the causes of SIDS: i.e. the failure to arouse to both hypoxic and hypercapnic stimuli (Figure 30.1). However, failure to arouse can be caused by many other predisposing risk factors and conditions. Thus, while this mechanism provides an important conceptual framework for understanding the causes of SIDS, there are, likely, many causes, which is one of the reasons SIDS continues to be both sudden and unexpected.

The causes and risk factors leading to the failure to arouse need to be seen within the context of the triple-risk hypothesis[14] as it is becoming increasingly evident that SIDS is typically the result of an accumulation of several risk factors and conditions that must converge to lead to an arousal failure and, ultimately, sudden death. The three principle factors that have been identified are first, a vulnerable infant, second, a critical period of ontogenetic development, and third, an exogenous stressor.[14,15] The combination of these risk factors can explain why SIDS occurs during a specific developmental time window, why an exogenous stressor does not always lead to SIDS, and why many different predispositions can ultimately culminate in a tragic downward spiral of events that results in sudden death.

Because we do not yet have comprehensive knowledge of the underlying mechanisms that result in

SIDS, further research efforts are critical to better understand the conditions that render a child vulnerable and prevent exposure of a vulnerable child to exogenous stressors. It is also critical to define the developmental conditions during which SIDS occurs. It is very likely that this developmental time window is not defined by one particular mechanism, but rather by several changes occurring during each child's development, including development of the brain and other organ systems. Many changes in the brain, the vasculature, and the heart occur during the first year of development, and – if not temporally coordinated – can lead to dysregulation of these key systems that ultimately may be fatal. Here we will discuss how the pathophysiological changes during development can result in failure to arouse. We will discuss how changing behavioural state (i.e. sleep/wake cycles), the regulation of breathing, the neuronal mechanisms underlying cardiorespiratory control and how dysregulation in these domains can result in the sudden death. We will focus in particular on brainstem mechanisms that seem to be critical for understanding how endogenous and exogenous mechanisms contribute to SIDS.

A Stereotypic Response to Life-threatening Events

Children develop protective responses to prepare them against the conditions that can lead to SIDS, and these protective mechanisms are located within the brainstem. Interestingly, the protective response seems to begin with a sigh (Figure 30.1). Exposure to hypoxia, or even in case of spontaneous arousals, often result in the generation of sighs which are subsequently followed by increased somatic activity, a characteristic heart-rate change, and sleep state transitions or transition into wakefulness.[16–22] Insight into the arousal response has come from controlled experiments on healthy, sleeping infants which all seem to suggest that arousal from a variety of stimuli begins with a sigh, followed by

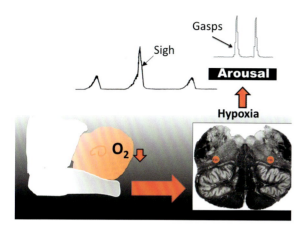

Figure 30.1 The child develops a stereotypic arousal response to hypoxia (decrease in oxygen), which involves the activation of neurons in the pre-Bötzinger complex (preBötC; inset: transverse section of the medulla of a human). The preBötC generates sighs and gasps that play a critical role in the generation of sighs (see integrated phrenic nerve recording) and gasps (2 gasps shown as integrated phrenic nerve recordings).

the occurrence of hand and leg movements, eye opening, and importantly, repositioning of the head. Heroic prospective studies by Andre Kahn have demonstrated that SIDS victims exhibited a lower frequency of sighs during sleep compared to age-matched controls.[23] Mechanistically the link to sighs is explained by the finding that the generation of sighs is activated by subtle changes in blood gases, particularly hypoxia.[24–28] This central hypoxic sensitivity seems to be rooted in brainstem neurons of the so-called pre-Bötzinger complex (Figures 30.1–3).[28–30] This brainstem region is essential for breathing and thought to generate in particular the inspiratory phase of breathing.[31] This region also generates specifically the sigh,[26] and a hypoxic response in vitro that shows an augmentation and generation of sighs, followed by a depression associated with a reconfiguration from 'fictive eupneic activity' to 'fictive gasping'[26] (Figure 30.3). The link between sighs and arousal is best explained by a close interaction between neurons or glia responsible for the generation of the sigh and the noradrenergic C1-neurons that are known to mediate arousal and changes in cortical states.[32] The connection between sighs and C1 neurons thus provides an important clue into the mechanisms that ultimately lead to SIDS. It is also consistent with the observation that spontaneous and induced arousals from sleep are significantly reduced in children that died of SIDS.[33–38]

There is however, a third important determinant of the arousal response – i.e. the integration between breathing and heart-rate control. In response to hypoxia, there is an initial increase in the heart rate.[39–43] The heart rate, however, shows a characteristic modulation with breathing known as sinus arrhythmia. Specifically, the heart-rate increases during inspiration and therefore also during the inspiratory phase of the sigh. The heart rate phasically decreases during the so-called 'post-sigh apnoea'.[20,44–47] An important clue towards understanding SIDS came from studies by Thach and colleagues who described that arousal depended on the heart-rate change associated with the sigh: larger heart-rate changes were associated with the arousal of the child.[21,48] Moreover, decreased heart-rate variability during the sigh was also described for infants that later died of SIDS[23,49,50] and more recent work using multiparametric heart-rate analysis may provide early warning and the possibility of intervention.[51] Whether the association between sigh, arousal and heart-rate change can also be attributed to the activation of the C1 neurons is an open, yet likely explanation for understanding how failure in these important brainstem mechanisms leads to SIDS.

Yet, the protective response to hypoxia does not end with the generation of a sigh, increased heart rate, and subsequent arousal. Rather, as hypoxic conditions become increasingly severe, a second, important phase in the arousal response follows. This second phase, also called 'secondary depression', is associated with the activation of gasps which, like sighs, are linked to heart-rate changes and arousal of the healthy child.[52] During this phase there is also a general heart-rate decrease (bradycardia) which is only interrupted by a transient period of tachycardia that coincides with the generation of the gasps.[53–55] Thus, while the sigh can be considered the initial defence response, gasping is the last chance to arouse.[53–55] Mechanistically gasps are characterised by rapid decrementing inspiratory efforts.[54–57] An important study on SIDS victims showed that children that died of SIDS, had either a very limited number of gasps or showed gasping that was not adequately associated with heart-rate changes. These gasps were ineffective in triggering autoresuscitation[55] and this pattern has been replicated in a mouse model of SIDS.[58]

Again, in this context it will be important to better understand how the activation of C1 neurons and the

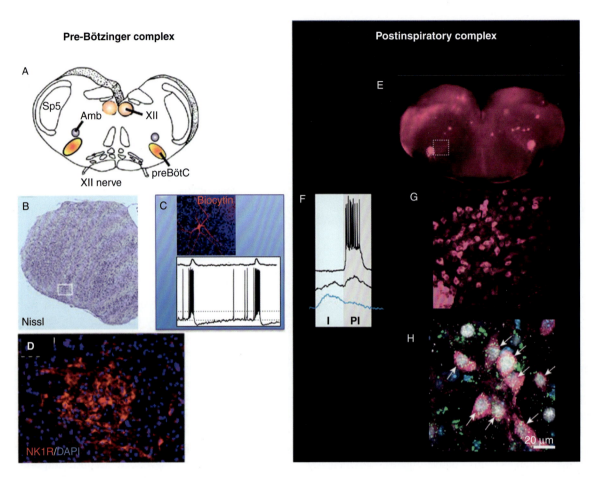

Figure 30.2 Characterisation of two regions critical for the generation of inspiration (preBötC, A-D) and Postinspiration (post-inspiratory complex (PiCo), E-H). A: schematic cross section through the medulla of a mouse showing the location of the *Nucleus ambiguus* (AMB), preBötC, hypoglossus (XII), and trigeminal nucleus (Sp5). B: Nissl staining of a transverse slice containing the preBötC. The white box indicates the location of the anatomical region showing NK1receptor and DAPI staining (D). C: Intracellular recording (lower trace) and integrated population activity (upper trace) of an inspiratory neuron shown as biocytin staining. E: Transverse slice of the mouse medulla located more rostral to the preBötC. The ChAT staining shows clearly the location of the *Nucleus ambiguus*, which is magnified in G and further magnified in H. Note the cholinergic neurons dorsal and medial of the *Nucleus ambiguus* that are characterised as belonging to PiCo. F: intracellular recording from a post-inspiratory neuron located in PiCo (upper trace), recorded simultaneously with an integrated population recording from PiCo which is in phase with Postinspiration (PI; middle trace) and the preBötC which is in phase with inspiration (I; lower trace).

A–D reproduced with permission of Society For Neuroscience from Koch et al.[131]; permission conveyed through Copyright Clearance Center, Inc. E–H reproduced from Anderson et al.[61]. See sources for full details.

respiratory neurons in the pre-Bötzinger complex or the wider respiratory network contribute to failed autoresuscitation. This core circuitry will also reveal how exogenous stressors may contribute to SIDS. For example, it is known that increased ambient temperature is an important risk factor for SIDS as this is known to decrease oxygen saturation, increase arousal threshold, and decrease gasping.[49,50,59] If the child fails to arouse from sighing and subsequently from gasping, an irreversible spiral begins which is caused

by severe hypoxic-ischaemic damage in the brain, and the failure to generate an appropriate cardiac response, ultimately cumulating in the death of the child. Thus, a child exposed to an exogenous stressor – such as hypoxia – needs to mount a stereotypic arousal response to survive (Figure 30.1). This response begins with sighs and the initiation of movements away from the hypoxic stimulus with concomitant cortical arousal. If this first stage fails, gasping becomes the last chance to autoresuscitate, before

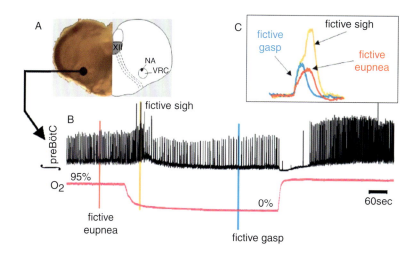

Figure 30.3 The pre-Bötzinger complex is a critical region for sensing oxygen within the CNS. Even upon isolation this network generates different forms of respiratory activities and responds dynamically to hypoxia and deoxygenation.

Inset: Recording traces: Red trace indicates fictive eupnea which is generated under well-oxygenated conditions; yellow trace indicates fictive sighs that are facilitated by hypoxia, and the blue trace indicates the activity generated during gasping.

Reproduced from Garcia et al.[132] with permission of Elsevier.

severe hypoxic damage results in a death spiral that leads to the irreversible terminal apnoea and ultimately cardiorespiratory collapse.

The Brainstem Circuitry Controlling the Heart and Breathing

The cardiorespiratory control system is located in specific brainstem regions within the ventrolateral medulla. Each of these brainstem regions has very specific roles in controlling different aspects of breathing and modulation of the heartbeat. Each of these networks or microcircuits is characterised by synaptic and intrinsic membrane properties that are responsible for the generation of the different aspects of cardiorespiratory control.[60] Three separate but interconnected networks have been identified, each generating one phase of normal breathing: The best understood circuit is the pre-Bötzinger complex, which controls inspiration.[29] The recently discovered post-inspiratory complex that controls post-inspiratory activity, also referred to as 'passive expiration' or the 'brake of breathing' (Figure 30.2),[61] and finally the so-called parafacial respiratory group (pFRG) controlling active expiration.[62,63] This latter group is also referred to as the retrotrapezoid nucleus or RTN, which seems to have extensive overlap with the neurons responsible for central chemosensitivity.[64–68] Other regions, including the nucleus ambiguus (NA), which gives rise to the cardiac

vagal neurons that are responsible for the parasympathetic control of the heart are crucial to control of heart rate. Indeed, it is likely that an important aspect of cardiorespiratory coupling is dependent on the interaction between the pre-Bötzinger complex and the nucleus ambiguus as both areas are very closely localised.[69,70] A reasonable hypothesis is that, during each inspiratory burst, inhibitory inspiratory neurons within the pre-Bötzinger complex inhibit cardiac vagal neurons in the nucleus ambiguus, which then causes disinhibition of the heart, resulting in an inspiratory-related heart-rate increase. As mentioned above, this is a key component of autoresuscitation and vitally important within the context of SIDS. We specifically hypothesise that a vulnerable child can be characterised by the disturbance of this core circuitry.[71,72] One could test this hypothesis by quantifying and cross-correlating these rhythms to assess the degree of disturbance of the rhythms generated by these oscillators.

The aforementioned retrotrapezoid nucleus (RTN) also plays a potential role in SIDS. This region contains Phox-2B neurons that are not only critical for sensing CO_2 but also exert sympathetic control over the heart.[64–68] The raphe nuclei are important for the control of CO_2 sensing and contain GABAergic and serotonergic neurons.[73,74] Closely associated with these brainstem networks, the nucleus tractus solitarius (nTS) is a brainstem nucleus, the first order point of integration of visceral afferent signals.

181

The nTS integrates critical peripheral afferent information from the carotid bodies – chemosensory organs that are exquisitely sensitive to changes in arterial blood oxygen levels.[75–78]

As we have already discussed, it is also important to consider the noradrenergic nuclei, such as the C1 region, and their role in behavioural state. These areas play a critical role in the arousal response, sleep-wake cycling, and the neural control of breathing. They are critically involved in airway-defensive reflexes, such as sighs, and gasping, but also contribute phasic input crucial to stabilising normal, eupneic activity. A disturbance in any of these nuclei and areas responsible for cardiorespiratory control can contribute to SIDS, which explains why SIDS can be caused via numerous avenues, each of which could result in a state of dysautonomia leading to failure to arouse. Importantly, many other important structures influence these networks, which explains why breathing, and cardiac control are among the most tightly integrated and coordinated behaviours. These regions include networks in the cerebellum, neocortex, hippocampus, amygdala, the hypothalamus and the periaqueductal grey (PAG).[79–85] Each of these areas influences breathing and the synergy of cardiac and respiratory control. Thus, not surprisingly, the cerebellum and hippocampus have also been implicated in SIDS, and more recently, in the context of Sudden Unexplained Death in Childhood.[15,86–90] So, dysregulation of adrenergic inputs to cardiorespiratory control centres in the brainstem may be key contributors to failure to resuscitate.

The pre-Bötzinger Complex and its Control of Inspiration and Neuromodulation

The pre-Bötzinger complex (preBötC) has long been known for its critical role in the generation of inspiration (Figures 30.1–3).[29,30,91] PreBötC lesions have been associated with pronounced disruption and the cessation of breathing.[31,92–94] Moreover, an elegant study by Schwarzacher and colleagues linked a variety of pathologies associated with breathing abnormalities to disturbances in the preBötC, including *Multiple Systems Atrophy* (MSA).[30] Moreover, astrogliosis in SIDS victims has been discovered in areas that co-localise with the preBötC.[95]

Several anatomical markers define the preBötC, including the neurokinin receptor NK1, a receptor

that is targeted by endogenously released substance P,[96] or receptors for the peptide somatostatin.[97] More recently, neurons in the preBötC were defined by a developmentally expressed transcription factor: Dbx1.[98,99] These Dbx1 neurons are glutamatergic and critical for inspiratory rhythm generation.[99,100] Interestingly Dbx1 neurons define not only the preBötC but also extend more dorsally to include the premotor neurons innervating the hypoglossal (XII) nucleus[100,101] as elegantly demonstrated using a variety of imaging techniques[102,103]). However, the Dbx1 neurons are only a subpopulation and the preBötC also contains inhibitory neurons that seem to be critical in mediating afferent information from the lungs to the inspiratory rhythm-generating network in the preBötC.[104,105]

The preBötC also generates the different forms of breathing, such as the sighs, gasps, and the normal breathing as demonstrated first by Lieske et al.[28] Mice in which sigh generation is prevented by a calcium channel mutation die, suggesting important implications for SIDS.[106] Sighs and normal breathing are differentially modulated by a variety of neurotransmitters and neuromodulators, including norepinephrine, serotonin, and acetylcholine,[107–109] a disturbance in any of these modulatory systems could contribute to a failure to sigh or gasp and these modulatory systems are certainly key for understanding the causes leading to SIDS.

A modulatory system that has been directly linked to SIDS arises from the raphe nuclei. These regions contain serotonergic neurons which release serotonin (5-HT), and substance P (SP) which act on 5-HT2A and NK1 receptors within the preBötC.[110] One of the earliest proposed mouse models for SIDS exhibited a loss of up to 80% of 5-HT neurons and showed pronounced breathing pattern variability with many more respiratory pauses than seen in wild-type mice[111] and a developmental phenotype that mimics that seen in SIDS. Models of 5-HT loss have repeatedly shown that serotonin is a key neuromodulator necessary for eupneic breathing, healthy cardiovascular control, and appropriate chemosensory responses.[112–114] This body of evidence suggests that the loss of serotonergic drive could lead to the loss of activity in autorhythmic neurons that depend on the persistent sodium current (I_{NaP}) and are known to be critical for the generation of gasping and sighing.[52,115] Recent transcriptomic work has suggested a role for inward-rectifying potassium channels as a substrate for pH sensitivity in serotonergic neurons[116] as well. In the context of the arousal response, as discussed above, a disturbance in the neuromodulatory drive to neurons driving inspiratory rhythm could partly explain why a disturbance in a modulatory circuitry could contribute to SIDS.

Dysregulation of the raphe suggests a highly complex perturbation of the brainstem circuitry driving respiratory and cardiac rhythm, since any disturbance in the expression of serotonin receptor subtypes or the aminergic transport system can impair the arousal response. In this context it is important to also consider the 5-HT1A receptor subtype which serves as an autoreceptor within the raphe and which could be responsible for decreased serotonergic release. Thus, from the perspective of human pathology, it is conceivable, and indeed likely that different types of serotonergic abnormalities can be associated with SIDS. Moreover, the raphe also contains substance P, which as already mentioned also plays a critical role within the preBötC. Other modulators include the already mentioned noradrenaline,[117,118] acetylcholine,[107] orexin, and bombesin.[119,120] All of these neuromodulators control sighs and are associated with changes in the sleep-and-wake cycle.

The Role of Inflammation in Altering Brainstem Breathing Control

Finally, within the context of the triple-risk model, exogenous stressors like cigarette smoke or airway and lung inflammation can contribute to perturbation of breathing that ultimately results in SIDS. The first few weeks-to-months of life are a critical window for susceptibility to infection in infants.[121] There are dramatic differences in both inflammatory responses[122] and patterns of cytokine up-regulation in newborns when compared to adults. In newborns, the time course of inflammatory up-regulation and cytokine release can occur quickly after exposure to the pathogen, i.e. minutes to hours.[123,124] The complexity of the response makes it difficult to determine when to intervene with anti-inflammatory drugs (indomethacin, ibuprofen, aspirin, etc.) and whether that would even be appropriate in the case of SIDS. So, treatment of inflammation in infants may or may not reduce the likelihood of sudden cardiorespiratory failure on top of the background of the other factors in the triple-risk model. Our laboratories.[125,126] and others[127] have shown that LPS-induced inflammation alters breathing control

and plasticity – primarily by altering the response to hypoxia.[128] The mechanism by which this occurs is prostaglandin E2 dependent and likely mediated by EP3 receptors that blunt excitability of neurons in the brainstem.[129,130] Thus, our understanding of the role that neuroinflammation plays in altering excitability in cardiorespiratory circuits of the brainstem is nascent and will require further investigation; research focused on the role of neuroinflammation in mouse models of SIDS is key for understanding the mechanisms of autoresuscitative failure and applying this knowledge to clinical assessment and prophylactic therapy.

Acknowledgements:

This study was supported by grants from the National Institute of Health (PO1HL090554; R01 HL 126523–01) and LLU GRASP Innovative Research Program.

References

1. Chiodini BA, Thach BT. Impaired ventilation in infants sleeping facedown: potential significance for Sudden Infant Death Syndrome. *J Pediatr*, 1993; **123**:686–92.

2. de Jonge GA, Engelberts AC, Koomen-Liefting AJ, Kostense PJ. Cot death and prone sleeping position in the Netherlands. *BMJ*, 1989; **298**:722.

3. Kemp JS, Kowalski RM, Burch PM, Graham MA, Thach BT. Unintentional suffocation by rebreathing: a death scene and physiologic investigation of a possible cause of sudden infant death. *J Pediatr*, 1993; **122**:874–80.

4. McGlashan ND. Sudden infant deaths in Tasmania, 1980–1986: a seven-year prospective study. *Soc Sci Med*, 1989; **29**:1015–26.

5. Trachtenberg FL, Haas EA, Kinney HC, Stanley C, Krous HF. Risk factor changes for Sudden Infant Death Syndrome after initiation of Back-to-Sleep campaign. *Pediatrics*, 2012; **129**:630–8.

6. Cerpa VJ, Aylwin ML Beltrán-Castillo S, Bravo EU, Llona IS et al. The alteration of neonatal raphe neurons by prenatal–perinatal nicotine meaning for Sudden Infant Death Syndrome. *Am J Respir Cell Mol Biol*, 2015; **53**:489–99.

7. Leung CG, Mason P. Physiological properties of raphe magnus neurons during sleep and waking. *J Neurophysiol*, 1999; **81**:584–95.

8. Bérard A, Zhao JP, Sheehy O. Success of smoking cessation interventions during pregnancy. *Am J Obstet Gynecol*, 2016; **215**:611.

9. Mage DT, Donner M. A unifying theory for SIDS. *Int J Pediatr*, 2009: **9**:368270.

10. Paterson DS, Thompson EG, Kinney HC. Serotonergic and glutamatergic neurons at the ventral medullary surface of the human infant: Observations relevant to central chemosensitivity in early human life. *Auton Neurosci*, 2006a; **124**:112–24.

11. Paterson DS, Trachtenberg FL, Thompson EG, Belliveau RA, Beggs AH, Darnall R, et al. Multiple serotonergic brainstem abnormalities in Sudden Infant Death Syndrome. *JAMA*, 2006b; **296**:2124–32.

12. Carlin RF, Moon RY. Risk factors, protective factors, and current recommendations to reduce Sudden Infant Death Syndrome: a review. *JAMA Pediatr*, 2017; **171**, 175–80.

13. Van Norstrand DW, Ackerman MJ. Genomic risk factors in Sudden Infant Death Syndrome. *Genome Med*, 2010; **2**:86.

14. Filiano JJ, Kinney HC. A perspective on neuropathologic findings in victims of the Sudden Infant Death Syndrome: the triple-risk model. *Biol Neonate*, 1994; **65**:194–7.

15. Kinney HC, Thach BT. The Sudden Infant Death Syndrome. *N Engl J Med*, 2009; **361**:795–805.

16. Glogowska M, Richardson PS, Widdicombe JG, Winning AJ. The role of the vagus nerves, peripheral chemoreceptors, and other afferent pathways in the genesis of augmented breaths in cats and rabbits. *Respir Physiol*, 1972; **16**:179–96.

17. McGinty DJ, London MS, Baker TL, Stevenson M, Hoppenbrouwers T, Harper RM, et al. Sleep apnea in normal kittens. *Sleep*, 1979; **1**:393–412.

18. Orem J, Trotter RH. Medullary respiratory neuronal activity during augmented breaths in intact unanesthetized cats. *J Appl Physiol (1985)*, 1993; **74**:761–9.

19. Lijowska AS, Reed NW, Chiodini BA, Thach BT. Sequential arousal and airway-defensive behavior of infants in asphyxial sleep environments. *J Appl Physiol (1985)*, 1997; **83**:219–28.

20. McNamara F, Wulbrand H, Thach BT. Characteristics of the infant arousal response. *J Appl Physiol (1985)*, 1998; **85**:2314–21.

21. Thach BT, Lijowska A. Arousals in infants. *Sleep*, 1996; **19**:S271–3.

22. Anderson CA, Dick TE, Orem J. Respiratory responses to tracheobronchial stimulation during sleep and wakefulness in the adult cat. *Sleep*, 1996; **19**:472–8.

23. Kahn A, Blum D, Rebuffat E, Sottiaux M, Levitt J, Bochner A, et al. Polysomnographic studies of infants who subsequently died of Sudden Infant Death Syndrome. *Pediatrics*, 1988; **82**:721–7.

24. Bartlett D. Origin and regulation of spontaneous deep breaths. *Respir Physiol*, 1971; **12**:230–8.

25. Bell HJ, Haouzi P. Acetazolamide suppresses the prevalence of augmented breaths during exposure to hypoxia. *Am J Physiol Regul Integr Comp Physiol*, 2009; **297**:R370–81.

26. Cherniack NS, von Euler C, Glogowska M, Homma I. Characteristics and rate of occurrence of spontaneous and provoked augmented breaths. *Acta Physiol Scand*, 1981; **111**:349–60.

27. Hill AA, Garcia AJ, Zanella S, Upadhyaya R, Ramirez JM. Graded reductions in oxygenation evoke graded reconfiguration of the isolated respiratory network. *J Neurophysiol*, 2011: **105**:625–39.

28. Lieske SP, Thoby-Brisson M, Telgkamp P, Ramirez JM. Reconfiguration of the neural network controlling multiple breathing patterns: eupnea, sighs and gasps. *Nat Neurosci*, 2000; **3**:600–7.

29. Smith JC, Ellenberger HH, Ballanyi K, Richter DW, Feldman JL. Pre-Bötzinger complex: a brainstem region that may generate respiratory rhythm in mammals. *Science*, 1991; **254**:726–9.

30. Schwarzacher SW, Rub U, Deller T. Neuroanatomical characteristics of the human pre-Bötzinger complex and its involvement in neurodegenerative brainstem diseases. *Brain*, 2011; **134**:24–35.

31. Tan W, Janczewski WA, Yang P, Shao XM, Callaway EM, Feldman JL. Silencing preBötzinger complex somatostatin-expressing neurons induces persistent apnea in awake rat. *Nat Neurosci*, 2008; **11**:538–40.

32. Burke PG, Abbott SB, Coates MB, Viar KE, Stornetta RL, Guyenet PG. Optogenetic stimulation of adrenergic C1 neurons causes sleep state-dependent cardiorespiratory stimulation and arousal with sighs in rats. *Am J Respir Crit Care Med*, 2014; **190**:1301–10.

33. Dunne KP, Fox GP, O'Regan M, Matthews TG. Arousal responses in babies at risk of Sudden Infant Death Syndrome at different postnatal ages. *Ir Med J*, 1992; **85**:19–22.

34. Kahn A, Groswasser J, Rebuffat E, Sottiaux M, Blum D, Foerster M, et al. Sleep and cardiorespiratory characteristics of infant victims of sudden death: a prospective case-control study. *Sleep*, 1992; **15**:287–92.

35. Kato I, Scaillet S, Groswasser J, Montemitro E, Togari H, Lin JS, et al. Spontaneous arousability in prone and supine position in healthy infants. *Sleep*, 2006; **29**:785–90.

36. McCulloch K, Brouillette RT, Guzzetta AJ, Hunt CE. Arousal responses in near-miss Sudden Infant Death Syndrome and in normal infants. *J Pediatr*, 1982; **101**:911–17.

37. Sawaguchi T, Kato I, Franco P, Sottiaux M, Kadhim H, Shimizu S, et al. Apnea, glial apoptosis, and neuronal plasticity in the arousal pathway of victims of SIDS. *Forensic Sci Int*, 2005; **149**:205–17.

38. Schechtman VL, Harper RM, Wilson AJ, Southall DP. Sleep state organization in normal infants and victims of the Sudden Infant Death Syndrome. *Pediatrics*, 1992; **89**:865–70.

39. Bamford OS, Schuen JN, Carroll JL. Effect of nicotine exposure on postnatal ventilatory responses to hypoxia and hypercapnia. *Respir Physiol*, 1996; **106**:1–11.

40. Horne RS, Sly DJ, Cranage SM, Chau B, Adamson TM. Effects of prematurity on arousal from sleep in the newborn infant. *Pediatr Res*, 2000; **47**:468–74.

41. Nock ML, Difiore JM, Arko MK, Martin RJ. Relationship of the ventilatory response to hypoxia with neonatal apnea in preterm infants. *J Pediatr*, 2004; **144**:291–5.

42. Hehre DA, Devia CJ, Bancalari E, Suguihara C. Brainstem amino acid neurotransmitters and ventilatory response to hypoxia in piglets. *Pediatr Res*, 2008; **63**:46–50.

43. Horne RS, Parslow PM, Harding R. Postnatal development of ventilatory and arousal responses to hypoxia in human infants. *Respir Physiol Neurobiol*, 2005; **149**:257–71.

44. Haupt ME, Goodman DM, Sheldon SH. Sleep-related expiratory obstructive apnea in children. *J Clin Sleep Med*, 2012; **8**:673–9.

45. Porges WL, Hennessy EJ, Quail AW, Cottee DB, Moore PG, McIlveen SA, et al. Heart-lung interactions: the sigh and autonomic control in the bronchial and coronary circulations. *Clin Exp Pharmacol Physiol*, 2000; **27**:1022–7.

46. Weese-Mayer DE, Kenny AS, Bennett HL, Ramirez JM, Leurgans SE. Familial dysautonomia: frequent, prolonged, and severe hypoxemia during wakefulness and sleep. *Pediatr Pulmonol*, 2008; **43**:251–60.

47. Wulbrand H, McNamara F, Thach BT. The role of arousal related brainstem reflexes in causing recovery from upper airway occlusion in infants. *Sleep*, 2008; **31**:833–40.

48. Thach BT. Graded arousal responses in infants: advantages and disadvantages of a low threshold for arousal. *Sleep Med*, 2002; **3**(Suppl 2):S37-40.

49. Franco P, Szliwowski H, Dramaix M, Kahn A. Polysomnographic study of the autonomic nervous system in potential victims of Sudden Infant Death Syndrome. *Clin Auton Res*, 1998; **8**:243–9.

50. Franco P, Verheulpen D, Valente F, Kelmanson I, de Broca A, Scaillet S, et al. Autonomic responses to sighs in healthy infants and in victims of sudden infant death. *Sleep Med*, 2003; **4**:569–77.

51. Lucchini M, Signorini MG, Fifer WP, Sahni R Multi-parametric heart rate analysis in premature babies exposed to Sudden Infant Death Syndrome. *Conf Proc IEEE Eng Med Biol Soc*, 2014; **2014**:6389–92; https://www.ncbi.nlm.nih.gov/pubmed/25571458 (accessed 31 October 2018).

52. Pena F, Parkis MA, Tryba AK, Ramirez JM. Differential contribution of pacemaker properties to the generation of respiratory rhythms during normoxia and hypoxia. *Neuron*, 2004; **43**:105–17.

53. Harper RM, Kinney HC, Fleming PJ, Thach BT. Sleep influences on homeostatic functions: implications for Sudden Infant Death Syndrome. *Respir Physiol*, 2000; **119**:123–32.

54. Hunt CE. The cardiorespiratory control hypothesis for Sudden Infant Death Syndrome. *Clin Perinatol*, 1992; **19**:757–71.

55. Poets CF, Meny RG, Chobanian MR, Bonofiglo RE. Gasping and other cardiorespiratory patterns during sudden infant deaths. *Pediatr Res*, 1999; **45**:350–4.

56. Cherniack NS, Edelman NH, Lahiri S. The effect of hypoxia and hypercapnia on respiratory neuron activity and cerebral aerobic metabolism. *Chest*, 1971; **59**(Suppl):29S.

57. Pena F, Aguileta MA. Effects of riluzole and flufenamic acid on eupnea and gasping of neonatal mice in vivo. *Neurosci Lett*, 2007; **415**:288–93.

58. Erickson JT, Sposato BC Autoresuscitation responses to hypoxia-induced apnea are delayed in newborn 5-HT-deficient Pet-1 homozygous mice. *J Appl Physiol (1985)*. 2009; **106**(6):1785–92.

59. Serdarevich C, Fewell JE. Influence of core temperature on autoresuscitation during repeated exposure to hypoxia in normal rat pups. *J Appl Physiol (1985)*, 1999; **87**:1346–53.

60. Ramirez JM, Dashevskiy T, Marlin IA, Baertsch N. Microcircuits in respiratory rhythm generation: commonalities with other rhythm generating networks and evolutionary perspectives. *Curr Opin Neurobiol*, 2016; **41**:53–61.

61. Anderson TM, Garcia AJ, Baertsch NA, Pollak J, Bloom JC, Wei AD, et al. A novel excitatory network for the control of breathing. *Nature*, 2016; **536**:76–80.

62. Janczewski WA, Feldman JL. Distinct rhythm generators for inspiration and expiration in the juvenile rat. *J Physiol*, 2006; **570**:407–20.

63. Pagliardini S, Janczewski WA, Tan W, Dickson CT, Deisseroth K, Feldman JL. Active expiration induced by excitation of ventral medulla in adult anesthetized rats. *J Neurosci*, 2011; **31**:2895–905.

64. Guyenet PG. Regulation of breathing and autonomic outflows by chemoreceptors. *Compr Physiol*, 2014; **4**:1511–62.

65. Guyenet PG, Bayliss DA. Neural control of breathing and CO2 homeostasis. *Neuron*, 2015; **87**:946–61.

66. Kumar NN, Velic A, Soliz J, Shi Y, Li K, Wang S, et al. PHYSIOLOGY. Regulation of breathing by CO(2) requires the proton-activated receptor GPR4 in retrotrapezoid nucleus neurons. *Science*, 2015; **348**:1255–60.

67. Ramanantsoa N, Hirsch MR, Thoby-Brisson M, Dubreuil V, Bouvier J, Ruffault PL et al. Breathing without CO(2) chemosensitivity in conditional Phox2b mutants. *J Neurosci*, 2011; **31**:12880–8.

68. Ruffault PL, D'Autreaux F, Hayes JA, Nomaksteinsky M, Autran S, Fujiyama T et al. The retrotrapezoid nucleus neurons expressing Atoh1 and Phox2b are essential for the respiratory response to CO(2). *eLife*, 2015; **4**:e07051; https://www .ncbi.nlm.nih.gov/pmc/articles/PMC4429526/ (accessed 31 October 2018).

69. Mendelowitz D. Advances in parasympathetic control of heart rate and cardiac function. *News Physiol Sci*, 1999; **14**:155–61.

70. Neff RA, Simmens SJ, Evans C, Mendelowitz D. Prenatal nicotine exposure alters central cardiorespiratory responses to hypoxia in rats: implications for Sudden Infant Death Syndrome. *J Neurosci*, 2004; **24**:9261–8.

71. Carroll MS, Kenny AS, Patwari PP, Ramirez JM, Weese-Mayer DE. Respiratory and cardiovascular indicators of autonomic nervous system dysregulation in familial dysautonomia. *Pediatr Pulmonol*, 2012; **47**:682–91.

72. Garcia AJ, Koschnitzky JE, Dashevskiy T, Ramirez JM. Cardiorespiratory coupling in health and disease. *Auton Neurosci*, 2013; **175**:26–37.

73. Fu W, Le Maitre E, Fabre V, Bernard JF,David Xu ZQ, Hokfelt T. Chemical neuroanatomy of the dorsal raphe nucleus and adjacent structures of the mouse brain. *J Comp Neurol*, 2010 **518**: 3464–94.

74. Stornetta RL, Rosin DL, Simmons JR, McQuiston TJ, Vujovic N, Weston MC, Guyenet PG. Coexpression of vesicular glutamate transporter-3 and gamma-aminobutyric acidergic markers in rat rostral medullary raphe and intermediolateral cell column. *J Comp Neurol*, 2005; **492**:477–94.

75. Accorsi-Mendonca D, Castania JA, Bonagamba LG, Machado BH, Leao RM. Synaptic profile of nucleus tractus solitarius neurons involved with the peripheral chemoreflex pathways. *Neuroscience*, 2011; **197**:107–20.

76. Chitravanshi VC, Sapru HN. Chemoreceptor-sensitive neurons in commissural subnucleus of nucleus tractus solitarius of the rat. *Am J Physiol*, 1995; **268**: R851–8.

77. Machado BH. Neurotransmission of the cardiovascular reflexes in the nucleus tractus solitarii of awake rats. *Ann N Y Acad Sci*, 2001; **940**:179–96.

78. Mifflin SW. Arterial chemoreceptor input to nucleus tractus solitarius. *Am J Physiol*, 1992; **263**:R368–75.

79. Brannan S, Liotti M, Egan G, Shade R, Madden L, Robillard R, et al. Neuroimaging of cerebral activations and deactivations associated with hypercapnia and hunger for air. *Proc Natl Acad Sci USA*, 2001; **98**:2029–34.

80. Burdakov D, Karnani MM, Gonzalez A. Lateral hypothalamus as a sensor-regulator in respiratory and metabolic control. *Physiol Behav*, 2013; **121**:117–24.

81. Chamberlin NL, Saper CB. Topographic organization of respiratory responses to glutamate microstimulation of the parabrachial nucleus in the rat. *J Neurosci*, 1994; **14**: 6500–10.

82. Masaoka Y, Sugiyama H, Katayama A, Kashiwagi M, Homma I. Slow breathing and emotions associated with odor-induced autobiographical memories. *Chem Senses*, 2012; **37**:379–88.

83. Nattie E, Li A. Respiration and autonomic regulation and orexin. *Prog Brain Res*, 2012; **198**:25–46.

84. Ramirez JM, Doi A, Garcia AJ, Elsen FP, Koch H, Wei AD. The cellular building blocks of breathing. *Compr Physiol*, 2012; **2**:2683–731.

85. Subramanian HH, Holstege G. Stimulation of the midbrain periaqueductal gray modulates preinspiratory neurons in the ventrolateral medulla in the rat in vivo. *J Comp Neurol*, 2013; **521**:3083–98.

86. Cruz-Sanchez FF, Lucena J, Ascaso C, Tolosa E, Quinto L, Rossi ML. Cerebellar cortex delayed maturation in Sudden Infant Death Syndrome. *J Neuropathol Exp Neurol*, 1997; **56**, 340–6.

87. Lavezzi AM, Ottaviani G, Mauri M, Matturri L. Alterations of biological features of the cerebellum in sudden perinatal and infant death. *Curr Mol Med*, 2006; **6**:429–35.

88. Calton MA, Howard JR, Harper RM, Goldowitz D, Mittleman G. The cerebellum and SIDS: disordered breathing in a mouse model of developmental cerebellar Purkinje cell loss during recovery from hypercarbia. *Front Neurol*, 2016; **7**:78.

89. Kinney HC, Cryan JB, Haynes RL, Paterson DS, Haas EA, Mena OJ, et al. Dentate gyrus abnormalities in sudden unexplained death in infants: morphological marker of underlying brain vulnerability. *Acta Neuropathol*, 2015; **129**:65–80.

90. Hefti MM, Kinney HC, Cryan JB, Haas EA, Chadwick AE, Crandall LA, et al. Sudden unexpected death in early childhood: general observations in a series of 151 cases: Part 1 of the investigations of the

San Diego SUDC Research Project. *Forensic Sci Med Pathol*, 2016; **12**:4–13.

91. Ramirez JM. The human pre-Bötzinger complex identified. *Brain*, 2011; **134**:8–10.

92. McKay LC, Janczewski WA, Feldman JL. Sleep-disordered breathing after targeted ablation of preBötzinger complex neurons. *Nat Neurosci*, 2005; **8**:1142–4.

93. Ramirez JM, Schwarzacher SW, Pierrefiche O, Olivera BM, Richter DW. Selective lesioning of the cat pre-Bötzinger complex in vivo eliminates breathing but not gasping. *J Physiol*, 1998; **507**(Pt 3):895–907.

94. Wenninger JM, Pan LG, Klum L, Leekley T, Bastastic J, Hodges MR, et al. Large lesions in the pre-Bötzinger complex area eliminate eupneic respiratory rhythm in awake goats. *J Appl Physiol (1985)*, 2004; **97**: 1629–36.

95. Naeye RL, Ladis B, Drage JS. Sudden Infant Death Syndrome. A prospective study.*Am J Dis Child*, 1976; **130**:1207–10.

96. Gray PA, Rekling JC, Bocchiaro CM, Feldman JL. Modulation of respiratory frequency by peptidergic input to rhythmogenic neurons in the preBötzinger complex. *Science*, 1999; **286**:1566–8.

97. Stornetta RL, Rosin DL, Wang H, Sevigny CP, Weston MC, Guyenet PG. A group of glutamatergic interneurons expressing high levels of both neurokinin-1 receptors and somatostatin identifies the region of the pre-Bötzinger complex. *J Comp Neurol*, 2003; **455**:499–512.

98. Bouvier J, Thoby-Brisson M, Renier N, Dubreuil V, Ericson J, Champagnat J, et al. Hindbrain interneurons and axon guidance signaling critical for breathing. *Nat Neurosci*, 2010; **13**:1066–74

99. Gray PA, Hayes JA, Ling GY, Llona I, Tupal S, Picardo MC, et al. Developmental origin of preBötzinger complex respiratory neurons. *J Neurosci*, 2010; **30**:14883–95.

100. Wang X, Hayes JA, Revill AL, Song H, Kottick A, Vann NC, et al. Laser ablation of Dbx1 neurons in the pre-Bötzinger complex stops inspiratory rhythm and impairs output in neonatal mice. *eLife*, 2014; 3:e03427.

101. Revill AL, Vann NC, Akins VT, Kottick A, Gray PA, Del Negro CA, Funk GD. Dbx1 precursor cells are a source of inspiratory XII premotoneurons. *eLife*, 2015; **4**:e12301; https://www.ncbi.nlm.nih.gov/pmc/a rticles/PMC4764567/; (accessed 31 October 2018).

102. Koizumi H, Mosher B, Tariq MF, Zhang R, Koshiya N, Smith JC. Voltage-dependent rhythmogenic property of respiratory pre-Bötzinger complex glutamatergic, Dbx1-derived, and somatostatin-expressing neuron populations revealed

by graded optogenetic inhibition. *eNeuro*, 2016; **3**(3); https://doi.org/10.1523/ENEURO.0081-16.2016 (accessed 31 October 2018).

103. Vann NC, Pham FD, Hayes JA, Kottick A, Del Negro CA. Transient suppression of Dbx1 preBötzinger interneurons disrupts breathing in adult mice. *PLoS One*, 2016; **11**:e0162418; https://www.ncbi.nlm.nih.gov/pmc/articles/PMC5017730/ (accessed 31 October 2018).

104. Sherman D, Worrell JW, Cui Y, Feldman JL. Optogenetic perturbation of preBötzinger complex inhibitory neurons modulates respiratory pattern. *Nat Neurosci*, 2015; **18**:408–14.

105. Winter SM, Fresemann J, Schnell C, Oku Y, Hirrlinger J, Hulsmann S. Glycinergic interneurons are functionally integrated into the inspiratory network of mouse medullary slices. *Pflugers Arch*, 2009; **458**:459–69.

106. Koch H, Caughie C, Elsen FP, Doi A, Garcia AJ, Zanella S, Ramirez JM. Prostaglandin E2 differentially modulates the central control of eupnoea, sighs, and gasping in mice. *J Physiol*, 2015; **593**:305–19

107. Tryba AK, Pena F, Lieske SP, Viemari JC, Thoby-Brisson M, Ramirez JM. Differential modulation of neural network and pacemaker activity underlying eupnea and sigh-breathing activities. *J Neurophysiol*, 2008; **99**:2114–25

108. Doi A, Ramirez JM. State-dependent interactions between excitatory neuromodulators in the neuronal control of breathing. *J Neurosci*, 2010; **30**:8251–62.

109. Pena F, Ramirez JM. Substance P-mediated modulation of pacemaker properties in the mammalian respiratory network. *J Neurosci*, 2004; **24**:7549–56.

110. Pena F, Ramirez JM. Endogenous activation of serotonin-2A receptors is required for respiratory rhythm generation in vitro. *J Neurosci*, 2002; **22**:11055–64.

111. Erickson JT, Shafer G, Rossetti MD, Wilson CG, Deneris ES. Arrest of 5-HT neuron differentiation delays respiratory maturation and impairs neonatal homeostatic responses to environmental challenges. *Respir Physiol Neurobiol*. 2007; **159**(1):85–101.

112. Cummings KJ, Hewitt JC, Li A, Daubenspeck JA, Nattie EE. Postnatal loss of brainstem serotonin neurones compromises the ability of neonatal rats to survive episodic severe hypoxia. *J Physiol*. 2011; **589**(21):5247–56.

113. Buchanan GF, Richerson GB. Central serotonin neurons are required for arousal to CO2. *Proc Natl Acad Sci USA*, 2010; **107**(37):16354–9.

114. Hodges MR, Wehner M, Aungst J, Smith JC, Richerson GB. Transgenic mice lacking serotonin

neurons have severe apnea and high mortality during development. *J Neurosci.* 2009; **29**(33):10341–9.

115. Tryba AK, Pena F, Ramirez JM. Gasping activity in vitro: a rhythm dependent on 5-HT2A receptors. *J Neurosci*, 2006; **26**:2623–34.

116. Puissant MM, Mouradian GC, Liu P, Hodges MR. Identifying candidate genes that underlie cellular pH sensitivity in serotonin neurons using transcriptomics: a potential role for Kir5.1 channels. *Front Cell Neurosci*, 2017; **11**:34; https://www.ncbi.nlm.nih.gov/pmc/articles/PMC5318415/ (accessed 31 October 2018).

117. Viemari JC, Garcia AJ, Doi A, Elsen G, Ramirez JM. beta-Noradrenergic receptor activation specifically modulates the generation of sighs in vivo and in vitro. *Front Neural Circuits*, 2013; **7**:179.

118. Viemari JC, Garcia AJ, Doi A, Ramirez JM. Activation of alpha-2 noradrenergic receptors is critical for the generation of fictive eupnea and fictive gasping inspiratory activities in mammals in vitro. *Eur J Neurosci*, 2011; **33**:2228–37.

119. Li A, Nattie E. Antagonism of rat orexin receptors by almorexant attenuates central chemoreception in wakefulness in the active period of the diurnal cycle. *J Physiol*, 2010; **588**:2935–44.

120. Li P, Janczewski WA, Yackle K, Kam K, Pagliardini S, Krasnow MA, Feldman JL. The peptidergic control circuit for sighing. *Nature*, 2016; **530**:293–7.

121. Levy O. Innate immunity of the newborn: basic mechanisms and clinical correlates. *Nat Rev Immunol*, 2007; **7**(5):379–90.

122. Walker JC, Smolders MAJC, Gemen EFA, Antonius TAJ, Leuvenink J, de Vries E. Development of lymphocyte subpopulations in preterm infants. *Scand J Immunol*, 2011; **73**(1):53–8.

123. An G, Nieman G, Vodovotz Y. Toward computational identification of multiscale 'tipping points' in acute inflammation and multiple organ failure. *Ann Biomed Eng*, 2012; **40**(11):2414–24.

124. Mi Q, Constantine G, Ziraldo C, Solovyev A, Torres A, Namas R, Bentley T, et al. A dynamic view of trauma/hemorrhage-induced inflammation in mice: principal drivers and networks. *PLoS One*, 2011; **6**(5):e19424.

125. Balan KV, Kc P, Hoxha Z, Mayer CA, Wilson CG, Martin RJ. Vagal afferents modulate cytokine-mediated respiratory control at the neonatal medulla oblongata. *Respir Physiol Neurobiol*, 2011; **178**(3):458–64.

126. Gresham K, Boyer B, Mayer CA, Foglyano R, Martin R, Wilson CG. Airway inflammation and central respiratory control: results from in vivo and in vitro neonatal rat. *Respir Physiol Neurobiol*, 2011; **178**(3):414–21.

127. Huxtable AG, Vinit S, Windelborn JA, Crader SM, Guenther CG, Watters JJ, Mitchell GS. Systemic inflammation impairs respiratory chemoreflexes and plasticity. *Respir Physiol Neurobiol*, 2011; **178**(3):482–9.

128. Vinit S, Windelborn JA, Mitchell GS. Lipopolysaccharide attenuates phrenic long-term facilitation following acute intermittent hypoxia. *Respir Physiol Neurobiol*, 2011; **176**(3):130–5.

129. Olsson A, Kayhan G, Lagercrantz H, Herlenius E. IL-1 beta depresses respiration and anoxic survival via a prostaglandin-dependent pathway in neonatal rats. *Pediatr Res*, 2003; **54**(3):326–31.

130. Hofstetter AO, Saha S, Siljehav V, Jakobsson P, Herlenius E. The induced prostaglandin e2 pathway is a key regulator of the respiratory response to infection and hypoxia in neonates. *Proc Natl Acad Sci USA*, 2007; **104**(23):9894–9.

Chapter 31

Arousal and Risk Factors for SIDS

Robert A. Darnall

Introduction

The ability to wake up from sleep when challenged with hypoxia, hypercapnia or asphyxia could be considered the most important response, and arousal failure has been implicated in the pathogenesis of SIDS for at least three decades. Importantly, dysfunction in brainstem and forebrain regions responsible for sleep and arousal has been reported in up to 70% of SIDS victims.[1]

Definition of Arousal

The usual definition of 'arousal' or 'awakening' from sleep includes a constellation of physiologic responses including increases in heart rate (HR), blood pressure (BP) and muscle tone, a sustained inspiratory effort or breathing pause, and activation of the EEG. In potentially asphyxiating environments, arousals are often associated with 'thrashing' movements that may serve to move the infant out of a potentially dangerous situation.[2] Autonomic or subcortical components of the arousal response involving changes in HR, BP, and upper airway control may serve to provide cardiovascular support to a full cortical arousal or maintain airway patency, particularly during obstructive apnoea, without fully disrupting sleep.

Arousal in Response to Hypoxia, Hypercapnia, or Their Combination (Asphyxia)

Although spontaneous arousals occur without an apparent stimulus, arousal in response to hypoxia, hypercapnia and/or asphyxia, and/or airway obstruction is likely the most important contributor to the pathogenesis of SIDS. In one popular scenario, failure of arousal to an asphyxiating environment leads to hypoxic coma, bradycardia, and gasping and

ultimately a failure of autoresuscitation.[3] It has become clear that the ability to arouse either spontaneously or in response to a stimulus is affected by sleep state. In human infants, the *probability* of arousing to hypoxia is very high during active sleep (AS) and is low during quiet sleep (QS) and arousal *latencies* are shorter during AS compared to QS. In contrast to findings in human infants, where arousal is blunted during QS, newborn, young, and adult animals exhibit delayed or impaired arousal during AS. In more altricial species, including mice and rats, pups transition rapidly between QS, AS, and wakefulness and there is no state related electro-cortical activity discernible before postnatal day 11 (P11). Thus, it is not possible to study hypoxia-related arousal separately during QS and AS before P11. In human infants, arousal to wakefulness in response to hypercapnia appears to be more robust than to hypoxia and does not seem to be affected by age. at least from 1 to 13 weeks postnatal age. In P15 rat pups, during putative QS, we found that arousal latency in response to 8% CO_2 in room air was 34.7 ± 2.3 sec and the CO_2 arousal threshold was $4.4 \pm 0.3\%$.

Intermittent Hypoxia, Arousal Habituation, and SIDS

Both premature and full-term newborn infants and children with obstructive sleep apnoea (OBS), are frequently exposed to intermittent hypoxia and re-oxygenation which adversely affects executive function and cognition. Importantly, intermittent hypoxia associated with apnoea and periodic breathing in preterm infants may contribute to the relative poor neurodevelopmental outcome in this population.[4] In animal studies, exposure to intermittent hypoxia in the neonatal period results in long-lasting adverse effects on a number of physiological systems, including cardiorespiratory control, neuropathologic, and neurocognitive deficits, neuronal integrity, and apoptosis. Several lines of evidence suggest that underlying hypoxia contributes to the pathogenesis of SIDS[5] and it is thought that many infants who die of SIDS experience clusters of apnoea, hypoxia, and bradycardia in the weeks and months prior to death. Others have hypothesised that repeated exposure to intermittent hypoxia may blunt arousal responses, increasing the risk for sudden death. It is thought that the process of habituation serves to allow the elimination of non-essential responses to biologically relevant stimuli. Habituation to repeated hypoxia, however, does not seem to be a good strategy, as the lack of an arousal response could be fatal. Nevertheless, a decrement of arousal in response to intermittent hypoxia has been well documented. Using a rat pup model, we have shown that habituation in response to repeated exposures to hypoxia is highly dependent on the presence of $GABA_A$ receptors in the medullary raphe[6] and is modulated by serotonergic mechanisms (see below).

Role of Brainstem Serotonergic Mechanisms in Arousal to Hypoxia and Hypercapnia: Brainstem Mechanisms

An important subset of SIDS infants have decreased binding to serotonin (5-HT) 1A receptors, increased numbers of immature 5-HT neurons and decreased medullary levels of TPH2, the rate-limiting enzyme for 5-HT production.[1] We have used two approaches to examine the role of serotonin in arousal and arousal habituation. The first involved direct injection, into the medullary raphe, of 5,7-DHT a neuronal toxin, specific for 5-HT neurons (when noradrenergic uptake is blocked with desipramine). Two-day-old (P2) rat pups were injected with 5,7-DHT into the cisterna magnum, which generally results in an 80% reduction in medullary 5-HT neurons, and then studied at P5, P15, and P25. Compared to pups injected with artificial CSF, or those injected with 5,7-DHT but that had limited neuronal destruction (i.e., ineffective administration), pups effectively injected with 5,7-DHT had significant medullary neuronal destruction at all three ages, had longer arousal latencies, and had a reduced respiratory rate response to hypoxia. Thus, destruction of medullary 5-HT neurons resulted in a generalised blunting of arousal with little or no effect on arousal habituation. Figure 31.1 shows arousal latencies in pups with significant 5-HT neuronal destruction compared with controls.[7]

Our second approach involved examining mice lacking ~70% of 5-HT neurons (*Pet-1*$^{-/-}$). Pups were exposed at P6-P10 to four episodes of hypoxia during sleep to elicit an arousal response. Arousal, HR, and respiratory rate (RR) responses of *Pet-1*$^{-/-}$ mice pups were compared to responses of null (WT + HET) pups. The time to arousal from the onset of hypoxia (latency) was measured during four hypoxia exposures, while HR, RR, and chamber oxygen concentration were continuously monitored. Arousal latencies in *Pet-1*$^{-/-}$ pups were significantly longer and arousal habituation was more robust compared to the latencies and habituation in the null pups. In addition, *Pet-1*$^{-/-}$ pups had lower metabolic rates, HR, and RR compared to null pups. Figure 31.2 shows arousal latencies in PET$^{-/-}$ compared to controls over 4 trials of hypoxia. Taken together, the results of these two approaches indicate that 5-HT neurons modulate arousal and perhaps arousal habituation in response to hypoxia.[8]

In adult mice, arousal to CO_2 appears to be dependent on the presence of 5-HT neurons, which have been shown to be chemosensitive after P12. Mice hemizygous for ePet1-Cre and homozygous for floxed Lmx1b (Lmx1b$^{f/f/P}$), which have no 5-HT neurons, fail to arouse to CO_2, but seem to arouse normally to hypoxia, sound, and an air puff.[9] These mice were only tested during NREM sleep, however. It is unknown whether 5-HT neurons play such a role during REM sleep, since they are normally silent during this state. In addition, these findings are in contrast to our findings in rat pups that either destruction of medullary 5-HT neurons or a genetically engineered lack of 5-HT neurons decrease the ability to arouse in response to repeated exposures to hypoxia.[7,8] The reason for this discrepancy is unclear, but it may be that the newborn and young pups rely more on serotonergic input to arousal during hypoxia than does the adult.

The carotid body and central chemoreceptors contribute heavily to arousal in response to hypoxia and hypercapnia. Whether the carotid body and/or central chemoreceptor stimulation directly stimulates arousal networks or whether this is done indirectly through respiratory networks remains unclear, but some combination is likely. An attractive hypothesis is that medullary raphe, arousal, and respiratory networks are connected and overlapping in that all of these networks are activated in the arousal process. The parabrachial nucleus appears to be an essential

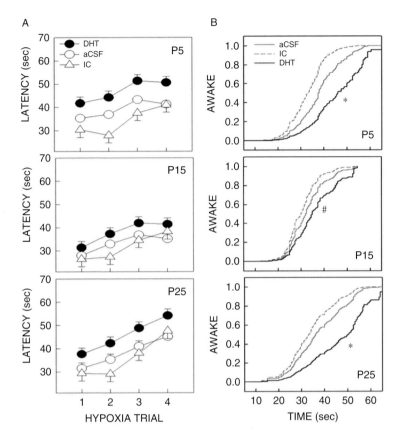

Figure 31.1 a): arousal latencies across four repeated hypoxia trials at P5, P15, and P25 after 80% reduction of medullary 5-HT neurons. Pups were exposed to four episodes of hypoxia (10% O_2) begun in quiet sleep and the latency to subsequent behavioural arousal determined. Latencies of pups with loss of 5-HT neurons after DHT administration (closed circles) were compared with those in pups injected with aCSF (open circles) and those injected with DHT but without a significant reduction of medullary 5-HT neurons (open triangles). Latency increased with successive trials (habituation) in all treatment groups ($P < 0.001$). The mean arousal latency was greatest in the DHT pups at P5 and P25. Values are expressed as the mean ± SEM. b): Cox regression analysis showing the proportion of pups awake at various times after the onset of hypoxia. For any given time, the probability of being awake was lower in the DHT groups compared with the controls at all ages. For example, at P25, 40 s after the onset of hypoxia, 60–75% of the control pups had aroused but only 33% of the DHT-treated pups. Consistent with our mixed model analysis, the effects of DHT were more prominent at P5 (*$P < 0.001$) and P25 (*$P < 0.001$) compared with P15 pups (#$P = 0.039$). Adapted from Darnall, et al., 2016.[7]

component of the arousal pathway and neurons in this region project to the basal forebrain, amygdala, periaqueductal grey, and cerebral cortex. In addition, the retrotrapezoid nucleus (RTN) appears be both an important central chemoreceptor and a convergence point for a number of arousal and respiratory related inputs, including the medullary raphe.[10,11]

Arousal and Epidemiological Risk Factors for SIDS

Smoking during pregnancy is a major preventable risk factor for SIDS;[12] 5–6-month-old infants born to mothers who smoke have longer arousal latencies in

response to breathing 15% oxygen compared to infants born to non-smoking mothers. Nicotine, a well-characterised component in cigarette smoke, has been largely used in animal experiments. Nicotine exposure during pregnancy alters nicotine receptor (nAChR) expression and receptor binding in the fetal and infant medullae. In newborn lambs, arousal to 10% oxygen is delayed and occurs at a lower SaO_2 after a short-term IV infusion of nicotine compared to lambs treated similarly after an infusion of normal saline.[12] We recently examined arousal and arousal habituation during acute intermittent hypoxia (AIH) in rat pups continuously exposed prenatally to nicotine (PNE) and a tryptophan deficient diet (TD),

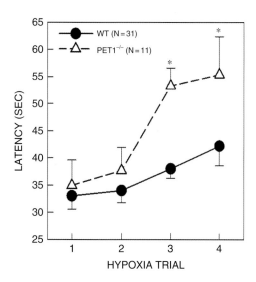

Figure 31.2 A comparison of arousal latencies during four exposures to 10% oxygen in PET$^{-/-}$ and control mice. Pups were exposed at P6-P10 to four episodes of hypoxia during sleep to illicit an arousal response. The time to arousal from the onset of hypoxia (latency) was measured during four hypoxia exposures. Arousal latencies in *Pet-1$^{-/-}$* pups (open triangles), dashed lines) were significantly longer compared to the latencies in the null pups (closed circles, solid lines) and arousal habituation was more apparent in the *Pet-1$^{-/-}$* pups. Values are expressed as means ± SEM. Overall, there was a main effect of group (P=0.032) and Trial (P<0.001). Latencies were significantly longer during trials 3 and 4 (asterisk). Adapted from Darnall et al.[8]

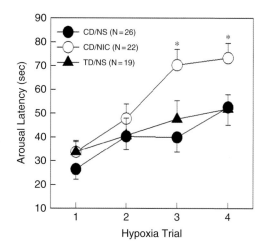

Figure 31.3 The effects of prenatal nicotine exposure (NIC) and a mild 5-HT deficiency induced with a reduced tryptophan diet (TD) on arousal to repeated exposures to hypoxia. Pups were fed either a control diet (CD) or a TD diet in combination with either normal saline (NS) or NIC delivered by osmotic pump. Pups were exposed either at P7 or P13 to four episodes of hypoxia (3 minutes of 10% oxygen alternating with 7 minutes of normoxia) to determine the latency to arousal and the degree of arousal habituation. The closed symbols represent the responses of pups with a CD + NS infusion (closed circles) or pups with a TD + NS infusion (closed triangles). There were no differences between the groups indicating that the mild 5-HT deficiency did not affect arousal in response to hypoxia. In contrast pups that received a CD + NIC infusion had latencies that were significantly longer (P<0.05) and more robust habituation. Pups that received a TD + NIC (data not shown) had latencies that were intermediate between the CD/NIC and the CD or TD/NS groups that were not different from the three groups shown in the graph. We concluded that prenatal nicotine exposure significantly impaired arousal but that arousal was not affected by a mild 5-HT deficiency.

which results in a mild serotonergic deficiency in the pups. Pregnant dams from gestation day 4 (E4) to 10 days after delivery given a normal control diet (CD) or a TD also received either normal saline (NS) or nicotine (NIC) (6 mg/kg/day) continuously delivered by a subcutaneously implanted osmotic pump. The NIC dose corresponded to about 0.5–1 pack of cigarettes a day in human smokers. Four groups of litters were studied: CD/NS (N=26), CD/NIC (N=22), TD/NS (N=19) and TD/NIC (N=22). P7 and p13 pups from each litter were evaluated for arousal and arousal habituation in response to AIH. At P13, but not at P7, arousal latencies were longer in the CD/NIC pups compared to the CD/NS and TD/NS pups. Arousal latencies for the TD/NIC pups fell between those of the CD/NIC and the CD/NS pups but were not significantly different from the other three groups. We concluded that pregnancy nicotine exposure (PNE) impairs arousal in response to hypoxia whereas arousal is not affected by a mild 5-HT deficiency, compared to a more severe 5-HT deficiency (see above). There were no effects of either

prenatal nicotine or a mild 5-HT deficiency on arousal habituation. Figure 31.3 illustrates the effect of PNE on arousal and arousal habituation.[13]

Prenatal alcohol (ETOH) exposure (PAE) increases the risk for SIDS.[12] In human infants, PAE during the first trimester is associated with sleep and arousal disturbances in infants but there is little information about arousal or arousal habituation in response to hypoxia after PAE. We recently examined the effects of PAE in rat pups on arousal and arousal habituation in response to hypoxia. Since arousal and arousal habituation are modulated by GABAergic and serotonergic mechanisms we also wanted to examine whether any effects of PAE were enhanced or inhibited by manipulating brainstem GABAergic neurons by direct medullary injections of aCSF, nipecotic acid (NIP), and gabazine (GABA$_A$ receptor antagonist). Finally, we wanted to determine

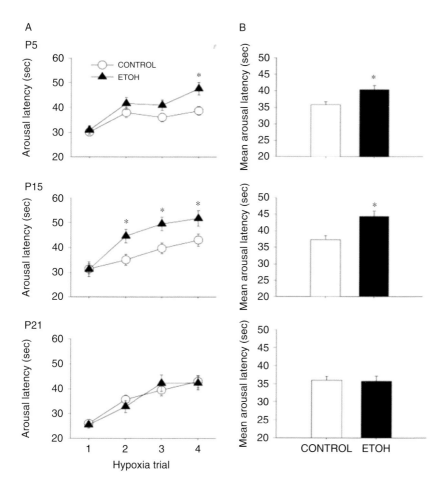

Figure 31.4 The effect of prenatal alcohol exposure on arousal in response to 4 exposures to 10% oxygen (AIH) compared to those that received either a liquid isocaloric or a standard chow diet at three different ages. Pregnant dams were fed either a liquid alcohol diet in a binge pattern or a liquid isocaloric diet or a standard chow diet during pregnancy. The isocaloric liquid diet and chow diets were combined for analysis and considered a control diet. Pups were removed at P5, P15, and P25, and exposed to AIH. a): Arousal latencies of P5, P15 and P25 pups exposed to prenatal alcohol (closed triangles) and controls (open circles) during 4 trials of hypoxia. b): The mean arousal latencies (averaged over the 4 trials of hypoxia) of pups exposed to prenatal alcohol (black bars) compared to controls (open bars). Values are expressed as means ± SEM and asterisks indicate significance at least at P<0.05. Reproduced from Sirieix et al under CC by 4.0 license (https:creativecommons.org/licenses/by/4.0/).[14]

whether PAE altered brainstem concentrations of various neurotransmitters, including 5-HT, and GABA. Pregnant dams were fed either an alcohol containing diet (ETOH), a calorically matched non-alcohol containing liquid diet (PF) or a standard chow diet (CHOW). Our main finding was that compared to control pups (PF and CHOW combined) arousal latency was increased at P15 and P21 and brainstem GABA concentrations were elevated at P21. NIP injections into control animals resulted in arousal latencies similar in magnitude to those in ETOH pups after aCSF injections. NIP injected ETOH pups had no further increases in arousal latencies. We concluded that PAE impairs arousal but does

not affect arousal habituation and this is mediated or modulated by GABAergic mechanisms. Arousal results after PAE are shown in Figure 31.4.[14]

Summary

Arousal from sleep is a major defence mechanism in infants against hypoxia and/or hypercapnia during rebreathing, airway obstruction, and apnoea. The combination of subcortical and cortical arousal allows the infant to move out of a dangerous situation and mount an appropriate physiological response. Decades of research suggests that arousal failure may be an important contributor to SIDS. Areas of the brainstem that have found to be abnormal in a majority of SIDS infants are involved in the arousal process. Arousal is influenced by medullary 5-HT mechanisms and repeated exposure to hypoxia causes a progressive blunting of arousal (arousal habituation) that involves medullary raphe GABAergic mechanisms. That the medullary raphe contributes to the process of arousal in response to hypoxia has important implications for the Sudden Infant Death Syndrome. Up to 70% of these infants have decreased medullary raphe serotonin and TPH2 levels which may result in a loss or decrease in an important excitatory input to the arousal process. Medullary GABAergic mechanisms are involved in arousal habituation that may increase vulnerability when exposed to repeated exposures to hypoxia that might occur in asphyxiating sleeping environments and importantly, preventable risk factors for SIDS, including prenatal nicotine, and alcohol exposure significantly impair arousal in animal models.

References

1. Kinney HC, Richerson GB, Dymecki SM, Darnall RA, Nattie EE. The brainstem and serotonin in the Sudden Infant Death Syndrome. *Ann Rev Pathol*, 2009: 4:517–50; https://www.ncbi.nlm.nih.gov/pmc/articles/PMC3268259/pdf/nihms347951.pdf (accessed 31 October 2018).

2. Lijowska AS, Reed, NW, Mertins Chiodini BA, Thach BT. Sequential arousal and airway-defensive behavior of infants in asphyxial sleep environments. *J Appl Physiol*, 1997; 83(1):219–28.

3. Kinney HC, Thach BT. The Sudden Infant Death Syndrome. *N Engl J Med*, 2009; 361(8): 795–805.

4. Hunt CE, Corwin MJ, Baird T, et al. Cardiorespiratory events detected by home memory monitoring and one-year neurodevelopmental outcome. *J Pediatr*, 2004; 145(4):465–71.

5. Naeye RL. Hypoxemia and the Sudden Infant Death Syndrome. *Science*, 1974; 186(4166):837–8.

6. Darnall RA, Schneider RW, Tobia CM, Zemel, BM. Arousal from sleep in response to intermittent hypoxia in rat pups is modulated by medullary raphe GABAergic mechanisms. *Am J Physiol Regul Integr Comp Physiol*, 2012; 302(5):R551-60.

7. Darnall RA, Schneider RW, Tobia CM, Commons KG. Eliminating medullary 5-HT neurons delays arousal and decreases the respiratory response to repeated episodes of hypoxia in neonatal rat pups. *J Appl Physiol (1985)*, 2016; 120(5):514–25.

8. Darnall RA, Schneider RW, Tobia CM, et al., PET1 knockout mouse pups have impaired arousal in response to intermittent hypoxia: Implications for the Sudden Infant Death Syndrome (SIDS). Abstract presented at the Society for Neuroscience. 2011, Washington, DC; http://www.abstractsonline.com/Plan/SSResults.aspx (accessed 28 October 2018).

9. Buchanan GF, Richerson GB. Central serotonin neurons are required for arousal to CO2. *Proc Natl Acad Sci USA*, 2010; 107(37):16354–9.

10. Darnall RA, The carotid body and arousal in the fetus and neonate. *Respir Physiol Neurobiol*, 2013;185(1): 132–43.

11. Guyenet PG, Abbott SB. Chemoreception, and asphyxia-induced arousal. *Respir Physiol Neurobiol*, 2013;188(3):333–43.

12. Moon RY, Moon S. SIDS, and other sleep-related infant deaths: evidence base for 2016 updated recommendations for a safer infant sleeping environment. *Pediatrics*, 2016;138(5):e 20162940; http://pediatrics.aappublications.org/content/pediatrics/138/5/e20162940.full.pdf (accessed 31 October 2018).

13. Sirieix CM, Lee S, Darnall RA. Effect of prenatal nicotine exposure and serotonin deficiency on arousal to hypoxia in rat pups. *FASEB J*, 2015;29:861.3.

14. Sirieix CM, Tobia CM, Schneider RW, Darnall RA. Impaired arousal in rat pups with prenatal alcohol exposure is modulated by GABAergic mechanisms. *Physiol Rep*, 2015;3(6):e12424.

Chapter 32

Serotonin Abnormalities in the Brainstem of Sudden Infant Death Syndrome

Robin L. Haynes

Introduction

Serotonin (5-hydroxytryptamine, 5-HT) is a neurotransmitter produced from the essential amino acid tryptophan which mediates a large variety of functions both peripherally and centrally. Within the central nervous system, 5-HT is produced in the brainstem and acts to modulate arousal, chemoreception, autonomic function, upper airway reflexes, and thermoregulation. Over the last two decades, research has provided direct evidence in the human infant supporting a role for 5-HT and abnormalities of the 5-HT system in the pathology of Sudden Infant Death Syndrome (SIDS). This evidence of central 5-HT abnormalities in SIDS supports a hypothesis of brainstem-mediated homeostatic dysfunction as an underlying vulnerability in a subset of SIDS infants who face homeostatic challenges such as hypoxia resulting from a face-down sleeping position. While much of the research to date supporting this hypothesis has focused on biochemical abnormalities within the brainstem, genetic abnormalities of 5-HT metabolism have also been reported, suggesting a potential genetic basis for the 5-HT-related pathology. This chapter begins with a brief discussion of the anatomy of the brainstem 5-HT system, specifically the 5-HT system of the medulla oblongata, and the animal studies supporting the role of this system in homeostasis. It is followed by a discussion of the enzymes and receptors involved in 5-HT neurotransmission and of 5-HT abnormalities reported in the brainstem of SIDS infants. Lastly it highlights hypotheses yet to be addressed in SIDS research related to the role of 5-HT in the pathogenesis of SIDS.

The Serotonergic System of the Medulla Oblongata: Anatomy and Function

Within the central nervous system, 5-HT synthesis is restricted to specific nuclei of the brainstem, including the pons and midbrain (the 'rostral' 5-HT system) and the medulla oblongata (the 'caudal' 5-HT system) (Figure 32.1). The rostral 5-HT system projects to the cortex, thalamus, hypothalamus, basal ganglia, hippocampus, and amygdala, and plays a significant role in cognition, waking, and mood. The caudal 5-HT system projects to sites within the brainstem and spinal cord and plays a significant role in respiratory and autonomic regulation, including regulation of upper airway control, autoresuscitation, central chemoreceptor responses to hypercapnia and hypoxia, cardiovascular control, and thermoregulation. Rostral and caudal 5-HT systems have generally been considered distinct in terms of anatomy, development, and function but with the existence of neuroanatomic interconnections and functional overlap between the two systems (reviewed in [1]). In recent work in the mouse, however, the combined use of genetic fate mapping and genome-wide RNA sequencing has allowed a much finer resolution of the 5-HT systems yielding evidence of molecularly defined 5-HT neuronal subtypes organised by a combination of developmental rhombomere-derived lineage and anatomy.[2] The molecular work in combination with electrophysiology, subtype-specific neuron silencing, and conditional gene knockout methodology have yielded additional evidence that the molecularly defined 5-HT neurons are also functionally distinct.[2] Below we summarise the 5-HT deficits in the human in SIDS focusing predominately on 5-HT deficits within the medulla, given that it is the caudal 5-HT system which has been most implicated in SIDS pathology. While these caudal medullary deficits have yet to be mapped to a molecularly defined 5-HT subtype, the potential for this work is significant and will allow better understanding of the functional consequences of specific deficits in SIDS infants.

Within the medulla, 5-HT synthesis occurs within 5-HT neurons in the following key nuclei; raphe (raphe obscurus, raphe magnus, and raphe pallidus), extra-

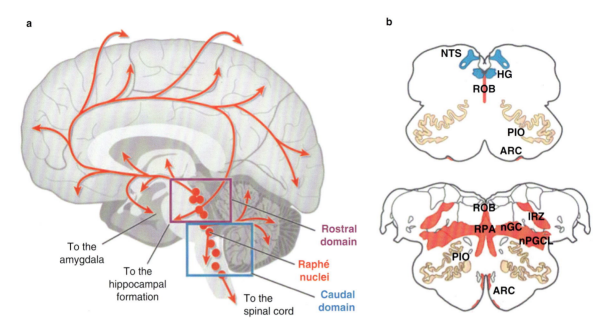

Figure 32.1 The 5-HT system of the human brainstem © by *Annual Reviews*.

a). Sagittal view of the whole human brain with the site of 5-HT neuronal cell bodies (red circles) and their projections (red lines) superimposed. The purple box highlights 5-HT neurons of the rostral domain within the rostral pons and midbrain. These neurons project rostrally to the cerebral cortex, thalamus, hypothalamus, hippocampus, and basal ganglia. The blue box highlights 5-HT neurons of the caudal domain within the medulla. These neurons project caudally to other brainstem regions, cerebellum, and spinal cord. The caudal domain is postulated to regulate homeostatic function (see text for details). b) Diagrams of the medullary 5-HT system at mid-medullary level (top) and rostral medullary level (bottom). The nuclei in red are sites of 5-HT cell bodies and nuclei in blue are major target sites of 5-HT projections. Abbreviations: ARC, arcuate nucleus; IRZ, intermediate reticular zone; nGC, nucleus gigantocellularis; nPGCL, nucleus paragigantocellularis; ROB, raphe obscurus; RPA, raphe pallidus. This figure has been reproduced with permission by *Annual Reviews* from Kinney et al.[3]

raphe (gigantocellularis, paragigantocellularis lateralis, intermediate reticular zone, lateral reticular nucleus, and nucleus subtrigeminalis), and ventral surface (arcuate nucleus)[1] (Figure 32.1). These 5-HT neurons project to and innervate the effector nuclei of respiration, including (1) the phrenic nucleus in the cervical spinal cord (drive to the diaphragm) (2) the hypoglossal nucleus (upper airway patency), and (3) the pre-Bötzinger complex, the site of central rhythm generation for breathing (reviewed in [3]). As determined in animal models during critical periods of development, medullary 5-HT neurons are also involved in the following mechanisms critical in the response to homeostatic challenges such as hypoxia, hypercapnia, or thermal stress: first, autoresuscitation and the initiation of gasping, processes that result in spontaneous recovery from hypoxia-induced apnoea and bradycardia;[4–7] second, chemoreception with responses to hypercapnia and hypoxia (reviewed in [3,8,9]); third, arousal leading to head-lifting or

turning (reviewed in [3,10]) and fourth, thermoregulation involving the modulation of sympathetic control of brown adipose tissue thermogenesis and thermoregulatory skin vasoconstriction (reviewed in [3,11,12]). Implicated in the pathogenesis of some SIDS cases is the laryngeal chemoreflex (LCR), a response commonly occurring during the newborn period elicited by liquids (including aspirated gastric content) in the lumen of the larynx and resulting in apnoea and swallowing.[13,14] In infants, a prolonged LCR can potentially result in prolonged and potentially lethal apnoea. 5-HT in the nucleus of the solitary tract (NTS) (a target for 5-HT projections) has been shown to shorten the LCR in neonatal rats.[15]

Mediators of 5-HT Neurochemistry Within the Brain

Within the brainstem, 5-HT neurons synthesise 5-HT via a two-step synthesis from the amino acid tryptophan, which is transported from the blood into the brain across the blood brain barrier. In the first step of synthesis, tryptophan is converted to 5-hydroxytryptophan by tryptophan hydroxylase 2 (TPH2), the rate-limiting step in the production of 5-HT in the brain. 5-hydroxytryptophan is subsequently converted to 5-HT by aromatic L-amino acid decarboxylase (AADC). Within the brain, the de-amination of 5-HT into 5-hydroxyindolacetic acid (5-HIAA) is catalysed primarily by monoamine oxidase A (MAOA), which is most abundantly expressed in noradrenergic neurons and moderately expressed in 5-HT neurons.[16] In the developing mouse, MAOA is coexpressed with another isoform MAOB in the 5-HT neurons of the raphe from E12 to P7 with a decline in MAOA postnatally.[16]

5-HT neurotransmission is mediated by the interaction of 5-HT with 5-HT receptors on the surface of neuronal elements including the soma, dendrites, and synapses. Within the brain, seventeen different subtypes of 5-HT receptors within seven different families are expressed with receptor subtypes divided according to distribution, molecular structure, cell response, and function. With the exception of $5-HT_3$, a ligand-gated ion channel, each of the subtypes functions through G-proteins and second messenger signalling. In terms of function, two of the families, $5-HT_1$, and $5-HT_5$ are inhibitory in nature, while the others are excitatory (reviewed in [17]). In SIDS, multiple studies have examined the role of $5-HT_{1A}$ in the pathogenesis of SIDS (see below). $5-HT_{1A}$, an autoreceptor, is located on the soma of 5-HT neurons and functions in a negative feedback loop that inhibits 5-HT release and signalling. $5-HT_{1A}$ receptors are also located on postsynaptic non-5-HT neurons to mediate 5-HT signalling (reviewed in [17]). Also of interest in regard to SIDS pathogenesis is the $5-HT_{2A}$ receptor which is required in rodents for the respiratory rhythm generator, localised in the pre-Bötzinger complex within the medulla[18] and the $5-HT_3$ receptor which plays a role in central cardiorespiratory responses to hypoxia[19] and in the shortening of the LCR.[20]

Critical to the control of 5-HT levels within the extracellular space is the 5-HT transporter (5-HTT), which is expressed on 5-HT cell bodies and projections and transports 5-HT into the cell, thus regulating synaptic 5-HT levels. Following reuptake into the cell by 5-HTT, 5-HT is degraded by MAOA (see above) or packaged into vesicles by vesicular monoamine transporter 2 (VMAT2) (reviewed in [21])

Medullary 5-HT Abnormalities in SIDS

Experimental Datasets and Findings

The hypothesis of brainstem 5-HT dysfunction in SIDS has now been examined in multiple, independent studies with unique databases. Below we describe the results of six of these studies. In four of the six studies, quantitative receptor autoradiography in frozen tissue was utilised to examine potential abnormalities in 5-HT receptor number and/or receptor binding affinity.[22–25] In two of the studies, immunocytochemistry was utilised to confirm reduced 5-HT receptor expression in SIDS.[26,27] In one of the six studies, immunocytochemistry and cell counting were used to examine 5-HT cell number and morphology in SIDS.[24] In one of the studies, high performance liquid chromatography (HPLC) was utilised to examine 5-HT content.[25] In this same study, western blot analysis was used to examine expression levels of TPH2.[25] Together these studies provide evidence of multiple deficiencies in the 5-HT system within the brainstem of a subset of SIDS infants. These studies support the hypothesis that the pathogenesis of SIDS in this subset relates to brainstem dysfunction in a neurotransmitter system that participates in the regulation of normal autonomic responses and in responses to homeostatic stressors (see above). Each of these studies is described with results summarised in Table 32.1 below.

One of the first studies examining the 5-HT system in SIDS involved quantitative autoradiography utilising the radioligand ^{3}H-lysergic acid diethylamide (^{3}H-LSD), a broad 5-HT ligand with affinity to multiple 5-HT receptor subtypes, including all 13 serotonergic subtypes that function as G-protein-coupled receptors (see above). The dataset utilised in this study was collected from 1985–97, primarily in a period of time before the national Back-To-Sleep campaign.[22] Cases were collected in the medical examiners systems of Boston (Massachusetts), Providence (Rhode Island), and San Diego (California) and in the Departments of Pathology, Boston Children's Hospital, and San Diego Children's Hospital. Binding was measured in 19 nuclei of the medulla and was found to be significantly reduced in SIDS (n=52) compared to acute controls (n=15) and chronic controls with oxygenation disorders (n=17) in 6 nuclei including nuclei containing 5-HT neurons (arcuate nucleus, raphe obscurus, paragigantocellularis lateralis, intermediate reticular zone, and gigantocellularis) and a nucleus containing 5-HT projections (inferior olive) (Table 32.1).[22] This 5-HT reduction was reported in a dataset previously used to show no deficits in opioid[28] and a2-adrenergic receptors,[29] thus supporting the specificity of a 5-HT deficit in SIDS.

The deficiency in ^{3}H-LSD binding described above was replicated in a second, independent study by Kinney et al., this time in a cohort of American Indians studied in the Aberdeen Area Infant Mortality Study (AAIMS).[23] This population was found by the AAIMS to have a SIDS rate 5.7 times the national rate for white infants during the period of the study. In this study, ^{3}H-LSD binding was examined in 23 SIDS cases and 6 controls cases who died suddenly, but with a determined cause of death. Mean binding, adjusted for age, was reduced in the arcuate nucleus, as previously described.[22] Abnormalities of other 5-HT containing nuclei in the medulla (gigantocellularis, paragigatocellularis lateralis, and intermediate reticular zone) were also significant compared to controls but when examining the effect of age on binding levels (diagnosis versus age interaction); that is, binding in these nuclei in SIDS cases were initially elevated in the SIDS cases but declined to lower values with increasing postconceptional age, whereas binding levels did not change with age in the control cases. Analysis within the raphe dorsalis, a pontine, and midbrain nucleus, similarly showed a significant diagnosis versus age interaction. The study using the AAIMS dataset is significant in that it independently confirmed the first ^{3}H-LSD study described above and it linked 5-HT abnormalities with exposure to adverse prenatal exposures, cigarette smoking, and alcohol, during the periconceptional period or throughout pregnancy (see below).

The third and fourth studies both utilised independent cohorts of cases from the San Diego medical examiners and both focused specifically on the 5-HT$_{1A}$ receptor rather than the multiple 5-HT receptor subtypes examined with ^{3}H-LSD, the ligand utilised in previous studies. The first of these studies by Paterson et al., examined cases from the period of 1997–2005, including 31 SIDS cases and 10 controls.[24] Significant 5-HT$_{1A}$

receptor binding deficiencies were confirmed in 5 of the medullary nuclei containing 5-HT neurons and previously shown to be deficient in ^{3}H-LSD binding (raphe obscurus, gigantocellularis, paragigantocellular lateralis, intermediate reticular zone, and arcuate nucleus) (p=0.001 to 0.006), as well as 3 of the 5-HT projection nuclei (medial accessory olive, nucleus of the solitary tract, and hypoglossal nucleus) (p= <0.001 to 0.03)(Table 1). In addition to decreased 5-HT$_{1A}$ binding, Paterson et al. reported a significantly higher number of 5-HT cells and 5-HT cell density in SIDS compared to controls in the rostral medulla in the raphe, the nuclei lateral to the raphe (i.e, the extra raphe), and the ventral surface region (i.e, the arcuate nucleus) (p≤0.002). This increase in cell number and density in SIDS was accounted for by an increase in 5-HT morphology. Given that the morphology of granular neurons is consistent with immature neurons, whereas pyramidal neurons are consistent with neurons of a mature nature, the altered ratio in SIDS favouring increased immature neurons suggests a developmental abnormality involving 5-HT neuronal production and maturation. Of note, the finding of increased 5-HT cell number and density was replicated using an Australian cohort of SIDS (n=41) and controls (n=28).[30] Paterson et al. also measured binding of the 5-HT transporter (5-HTT) by receptor autoradiography. While there was no difference in overall 5-HTT binding in SIDS compared to controls, there was a significantly lower ratio of 5-HTT binding density to 5-HT neuronal count in the SIDS cases compared to controls (p=0.001).

The fourth study by Duncan et al., also using a cohort of cases from the San Diego medical examiners system, examined 41 SIDS cases, and 7 control cases dying from acute causes, all collected from 2004–8.[25] As in the previous study by Paterson, Duncan et al. analysed 5-HT$_{1A}$ receptor binding and confirmed abnormalities in binding in SIDS compared to acute controls within nuclei of the medulla containing either 5-HT cell bodies or 5-HT projections (Table 32.1). The abnormalities reported in SIDS were either absolute reductions in 5-HT$_{1A}$ binding and/or significant diagnosis versus age interactions, as had been reported previously[23] (Table 32.1). In addition to 5-HT$_{1A}$ binding, Duncan et al. reported significantly lower levels of TPH2 protein expression in the raphe obscurus of SIDS compared to controls (p=0.03), and lower levels of 5-HT itself in the raphe obscurus (p=0.05) and paragigan-tocellularis (p=0.04)[25] (Table 32.1). In addition to acute controls, Duncan also analysed 5 hospitalised infants with chronic hypoxia-ischaemia in the analy-sis of 5-HT levels and TPH2 expression and found a significant decrease in SIDS compared to hospital-ised controls in 5-HT levels but a significant increase in SIDS compared to hospitalised controls in TPH2 expression (Table 32.1).[25]

In support of the work described above, there have been additional studies using immunocytochemical methods that have confirmed abnormalities in the medullary 5-HT system in SIDS. Machaalani et al.[27] examined the 5-HT$_{1A}$ receptor by quantitative immu-nocytochemistry in the medulla of 67 SIDS and 25 controls and found significant decreases in 5-HT$_{1A}$ immunoreactivity in 6 medullary nuclei, including nuclei reported previously to be deficient in 5-HT$_{1A}$ binding (Table 32.1). In a study of 31 SIDS and 25 controls, Ozawa et al. used 5-HT$_{1A}$ immunocytochem-istry to show a decrease in 5-HT$_{1A}$ immunoreactivity in the dorsal motor nucleus of the vagus and the nucleus of the solitary tract.[26] In addition to 5-HT$_{1A}$, Ozawa also used immunocytochemistry to examine 5-HT$_{2A}$ and found decreased 5-HT$_{2A}$ immunostaining in the same medullary nuclei.[26] Interestingly, Ozawa found a significant increase in immunostaining for 5-HT$_{1A}$ and 5-HT$_{2A}$ in the periaqueductal grey matter of the midbrain in SIDS infants.[26]

Association of 5-HT Deficits with Risk Factors for SIDS

General. SIDS is associated with a number of risk factors which have been considered in regard to def-icits in medullary 5-HT in SIDS infants. These risk factors are classified as intrinsic risk factors, which are biological factors that affect the underlying vulner-ability of the infant (i.e., male sex, race, premature birth, adverse exposures to prenatal alcohol, and smoking) and extrinsic risk factors, which are the environmental stressors that would challenge an infant's homeostatic responses (i.e, prone sleep, bed sharing, and mild infections) (reviewed in [31]). Several studies have looked at the relationship between 5-HT abnormalities and risk factors present in SIDS infants to address the question as to whether the subgroups of SIDS with 5-HT abnormalities can be associated with any particular SIDS risk factor.

In reports by Paterson and Duncan, 95–100% of SIDS cases had at least one intrinsic risk factor and 90–93% had at least one extrinsic risk factor.[24,25] Duncan et al. reported that infants with SIDS but without known extrinsic risk factors have significantly lower 5-HT$_{1A}$ receptor binding compared to SIDS with extrinsic risk factors, thus suggesting that the presence of multiple risk factors is necessary to pre-cipitate death when the 5-HT$_{1A}$ binding is not or is only minimally compromised. The association of risk factors with 5-HT abnormalities in SIDS varied between studies and between 5-HT measures. Consistently found were associations between the presence of different risk factors and 5-HT$_{1A}$ recep-tors (binding or immunoreactivity). Within the dif-ferent SIDS groups, deficits in 5-HT$_{1A}$ were found to be associated with male sex,[24,27] prone sleep position,[25,27] and sleeping in an adult bed.[25] Also found were associations of 5-HT$_{1A}$ deficits with adverse prenatal exposures (see below). TPH2 levels were lower in SIDS infants with recent illnesses com-pared to those SIDS infants without illness.[25] There were no associations between risk factors and 5-HT tissue levels as determined by HPLC.[25] There was no association of 5-HT abnormalities with polymorph-isms in the promoter region (5-HTTLPR) of the 5-HTT gene (*SLC6A4*) (see below).[24]

Prenatal adverse exposure.

There have been several studies in which 5-HT deficits in SIDS have been associated with prenatal exposures to smoking and alcohol. The AAIMS study of the Northern Plains American Indians (described above) utilised exposure information provided by the mothers to examine the incidence of adverse prenatal exposure and SIDS risk and the association of adverse prenatal exposure with 5-HT$_{1A}$ receptor binding. While a higher percentage of SIDS mothers reported using alcohol during the three months prior to preg-nancy and during each trimester, the difference in the percentage using alcohol was statistically significant in the first trimester only.[32] Binge drinking in the first trimester was significantly increased in SIDS compared to controls and was associated with a six-fold increased risk for SIDS.[32] There was no statis-tical difference in the incidence of reported prenatal smoking or in the number of cigarettes per day. When analysing 5-HT receptor deficits (as measured by ^{3}H-LSD binding) in association with adverse prenatal exposures, Kinney et al. reported a significantly lower

Table 32.1 Experimental data in human tissue supporting 5-HT abnormalities within the medulla

Study Year (ref)	SIDS	Controls	3H-LSD Ligand binding	5-HT1A Ligand binding	5-HT1A ICC	5-HT neuronal cell count	5-HTT ligand binding	5-HT levels	TPH2 expression
Panigrahy 2000 (22)	52	15 Acute 17 Chronic oxygenation disorders	↓ in SIDS 3 group p-value (p=0.0001–0.003) ARC†* 68% Rob†* 58% IO†* 37% PGCL‡* 39% ↓ in SIDS SIDS vs Acute (p=0.048,0.022) IRZ 24% GC 31%						
Ozawa 2002 (26)	31	25			↓ in SIDS 5HT1A staining (p=0.01) DMX NTS VLM				
Kinney 2003 (23)	23	6	↓ in SIDS (p=0.003) ARC* 46% Diagnosis x age interaction (p=0.01–0.04) GC PGCL IRZ						
Paterson 2006 (24)	16–30	6–7		↓ in SIDS (p<0.001 – 0.03) ARC* 56% Rob* 56% GC* 41% PGCL* 45% IRZ* 42% MAO* 67% NTS* 52% HG* 38%		↑ in SIDS in rostral and mid medulla, 104%,75% respectively* (p<0.001) ↑ granular (immature) neurons in SIDS; ↓ multipolar neurons (mature) in SIDS	No 5-HT difference ↓ ratio of 5-HTT / 5-HT cell count* (p=0.001) 64%		

Study	n	n	n	

Machaalani 2009 (27) — 67, 25

↓ in SIDS (5-HT$_{1A}^+$ neurons) (p=<0.001–0.05)

IO	23%
DMX*	17%
NTS	26%
CUN	18%
VEST	34%

Duncan 2010 (25) — 41, 7 Acute, 5 Hospitalized (Hospital)

↓ in SIDS vs. acute controls (p=0.004–0.02)

HG*	38%
DMX*	45%
NTS*	29%

Diagnosis x age interaction (p=0.007–0.05)
GC
PGCL
IRZ
DAO

↓ in SIDS vs Acute (p=0.04,0.05)

PGCL*	21%
ROb*	27%

↓ in SIDS vs Acute (p=0.03)

ROb*	22%

↓ in SIDS vs Hospital (p=0.002,0.02)

PGCL*	56%
ROb*	35%

↑ in SIDS vs Hospital (p=0.04)

ROb*	47%

Legend: Percent differences were determined from the data reported in the articles. * The means used to determine % difference are age-adjusted. ‡ The percent differences shown are between SIDS and acute controls.

Abbreviations: ARC, arcuate nucleus; CUN, cuneate nucleus; DAO, dorsal accessory olive; DMX, dorsal motor nucleus of the vagus; GC, gigantocellularis; HG, hypoglossal nucleus; IO, inferior olive; IRZ, intermediate reticular zone; MAO, medial accessory olive; PGCL, paragigantocellularis lateralis; ROb, raphé obscurus; NTS, nucleus of the solitary tract; VEST, vestibular nucleus; VLM, ventrolateral medulla.

(p=0.011) mean binding in the arcuate nucleus of infants (SIDS and controls combined) of mothers who smoked before or during pregnancy compared to infants (SIDS and controls combined) of mothers who did not report smoking.[23] Marginally lowered binding was reported in the arcuate nucleus of infants whose mothers drank prior to or during pregnancy (p=0.075) and in infants whose mothers engaged in binge drinking 3 months prior to or during pregnancy (p=0.080).[23] Also reported from the AAIMS study was a case report of a full-term infant whose mother reported drinking and smoking prior to pregnancy and during the second trimester with no drinking or smoking during the first and third trimesters. This infant died at 2 postnatal weeks but had previous physiological assessments on the second day of life showing abnormal cardiorespiratory indices that suggested an altered ratio of parasympathetic to sympathetic tone during active sleep (higher than normal) and during quiet sleep (lower than normal).[33] This infant showed ^{3}H-LSD binding values below the level of other SIDS infants in medullary nuclei including the arcuate nucleus, gigantocellularis, paragigantocellularis, inferior olivary nucleus, and intermediate reticular zone. The case report substantiates not only the role of 5-HT deficits in autonomic and respiratory regulation but also the impact of adverse prenatal exposures on the medullary 5-HT system.[33] Adverse effects of cigarette smoke were further substantiated by Machaalani et al. with decreased 5-HT$_{1A}$ immunoreactivity in several medullary nuclei of infants whose mothers reported smoking during pregnancy.[27]

5-HT Genetic Susceptibility.

There have been a number of studies suggesting the role of genetic factors related to 5-HT in the pathogenesis of SIDS. These studies mostly involve candidate gene studies focusing on single nucleotide polymorphisms (SNP) or small insertion/deletion polymorphisms in genes related to 5-HT neurotransmission. Genes of interest that have been reported on in SIDS include the following: (1) Fifth Ewing Variant (FEV), the human homologue of the PET-1, which plays a critical role in differentiation and maintenance of 5-HT neuronal phenotype; (2) TPH2, the rate-limiting enzyme for synthesis of 5-HT in the brain; (3) 5-HT$_{1A}$ receptors, the somato-dendritic autoreceptor; (4) 5-HT$_{2A}$ receptors, a postsynaptic heteroreceptor; (5) 5-HTT, the serotonin transporter

controlling synaptic 5-HT levels and availability; and (6) monoamine oxidase A (MAOA), the mitochondrial enzyme primarily responsible for the intracellular degradation of 5-HT (see above). The studies examining each of these genes in SIDS are variable with results both supporting and refuting their role in SIDS. The details of these genetic studies are beyond the scope of this chapter but have been reviewed elsewhere.[34,35] In regard to genetic factors and 5-HT deficits in SIDS infants, Paterson report data from small cohorts of cases that had both measures of 5-HT neurotransmission and genotype data on 5-HTT polymorphisms (5-HTTLPR promotor region polymorphism and intron 2 polymorphism) and on MAOA polymorphisms (VNTR polymorphism in the promoter region).[34] Based on these data, Paterson concludes the unlikeliness that SIDS risk is conferred by these specific polymorphisms. Interpretation, however, was limited due to the small sample size.[34]

Significance of Brainstem 5-HT Abnormalities in SIDS

The implications of the brainstem abnormalities reported in SIDS infants centre upon the critical role that 5-HT plays in autonomic and respiratory regulation and maintenance of homeostasis when an infant is challenged due to an environmental stress (i.e., prone sleep position) (see above). The 5-HT abnormalities described in SIDS are reported in the medullary nuclei involved in these regulatory and homeostatic functions including nuclei containing 5-HT neurons and 5-HT projections. These nuclei interact together as a network and in concert with other neurotransmitters to maintain these functions. If we view SIDS pathogenesis according to the triple-risk model proposed by Filiano and Kinney,[36] the 5-HT deficiency defines one biological vulnerability putting an infant at risk for SIDS during a critical developmental window when the 5-HT network is still maturing. When these infants pass through the critical developmental period and face an exogenous stressor, the deficient 5-HT system fails to respond to homeostatic stressors and death occurs. In each of the studies described above, overlap exists between control, and SIDS infants suggesting that not every SIDS infant displays 5-HT deficits. Rather, the 5-HT deficits are represented within a single subgroup of infants with multiple 5-HT deficits or possibly different subgroups, each with deficits in different 5-HT indices. The finding of distinct subgroups of SIDS infants underscores the likelihood that SIDS is a heterogenous disorder with different pathogenic mechanisms underlying the death.

The question remains as to whether 5-HT abnormalities in SIDS are developmental in nature, acquired in utero as brain circuitry is being formed, or if they are acquired after birth, in the perinatal period. Supporting a developmental origin are the 5-HT abnormalities found in the arcuate nucleus which lies along the ventral medullary surface and contains 5-HT neurons as well as 5-HT fibres and receptors. Decreased 5-HT receptor binding was shown in the arcuate nucleus of SIDS compared to controls.[22–24] The arcuate nucleus is postulated to be homologous to known chemosensitive 5-HT neurons on the ventral surface of the rat medulla.[37,38] The decreased binding in the arcuate nucleus is consistent with findings of hypoplasia of the arcuate nucleus in 5% to 50% of SIDS cases,[39,40] and supports a developmental abnormality of this structure with embryonic origins. Also supporting a developmental origin, is evidence of increased immature 5-HT neurons in the medulla of SIDS infants.[24,30] 5-HT neurons can be detected in the human as early as 5 weeks gestation with adult-like topography by 20 weeks gestation.[41] Evidence of an increased number of 5-HT neurons with an increased ratio of immature to mature phenotype in SIDS suggests a potential overproduction of 5-HT neurons in the developmental period and/or a decrease in 5-HT neuronal maturation. Also supporting the idea that 5-HT deficits originate during development is the association of 5-HT abnormalities with adverse maternal drinking and smoking. Animal studies of prenatal exposures report postnatal deficiencies in 5-HT neurotransmission.[42–44]

Another possibility is that the 5-HT abnormalities seen in SIDS infants originate during the postnatal period in response to postnatal insults. It has been postulated that 5-HT deficits are a result of chronic intermittent hypoxia resulting from multiple episodes of unsafe sleep practices (reviewed in [3]). These reoccurring insults potentially affect 5-HT indices over time until the infant reaches a critical threshold beyond which the infant cannot respond to the final episode and dies. In the report by Duncan et al., 5-HT indices in SIDS were compared with those in hospitalised infants whose death was associated with chronic hypoxia (i.e, severe congenital heart disease). 5-HT deficiencies in SIDS were distinct from those in the hospitalised

infants.[25] While this suggests that the primary mechanism underlying 5-HT abnormalities in SIDS is not mediated by chronic hypoxia-ischaemia, it does not negate the possibility that intermittent episodes of hypoxia play a role. Other factors that potentially affect the postnatal 5-HT medullary system include postnatal environmental socio-economic stressors (i.e, poverty, maternal separation) (reviewed in [45–47]) or postnatal exposure to alcohol and cigarette smoke that may induce epigenetic changes influencing the function of 5-HT-related genes in early life. Given the increasingly appreciated role of the gut microbiome in brain development and function, including 5-HT development and function (reviewed in [48]), postnatal colonisation of gut microbiota must also be considered. Neither epigenetic changes in 5-HT genes or altered microbiome influences on brain 5-HT have been reported in SIDS infants.

Summary and Future Directions

In summary, the findings of brainstem abnormalities in a subset of SIDS infants have, to date, been reproducible between independent datasets and investigators. Currently unknown are the mechanisms (pre and/or postnatal) by which the specific 5-HT indices have been affected and how these mechanisms relate to each other. Does a developmental increase in 5-HT neurons result in a compensatory downregulation of 5-HT$_{1A}$ receptors? Are deficits in 5-HT$_{1A}$ receptor binding a result of decreases in 5-HT$_{1A}$ expression, originating either at the transcriptional or protein level or are they a function of reduced ability to bind to 5-HT due to alterations in receptor structure or cellular membrane (lipid) environment? Do the abnormal 5-HT neurons in SIDS represent a distinct phenotype of 5-HT neurons with distinct embryonic origin and function, as has been identified in cross intersectional mouse studies?[2] Addressing these questions through human pathology and animal modelling will allow us to better understand the pathogenic mechanisms defining the 5-HT related subset of SIDS infants. In addition, evidence of brainstem 5-HT abnormalities in a subset of SIDS infants provides testable hypotheses from which preventative strategies can be developed. For preventative strategies to be utilised in infants, however, infants at risk must be identified early in postnatal life. Currently there are no clinical or biochemical biomarkers available to identify infants at risk and/or to identify infants with abnormal brainstem 5-HT. While a recent study identified a significant increase in post-mortem serum 5-HT in 31% of SIDS infants,[49] it is currently unknown how this post-mortem marker relates to serum 5-HT in the postnatal living infant at risk for SIDS. The relationship of the increased serum 5-HT to the brainstem abnormalities in SIDS infants is also unknown and represents an important future direction for SIDS research. Another area of interest and future direction is the relationship between brainstem 5-HT deficiencies and hippocampal abnormalities reported in approximately 40% of SIDS cases.[50] Whether these 2 entities exist in the same infant or whether they represent different subgroups of SIDS with different lesions is currently unknown.

In summary, we postulate that abnormalities in the 5-HT system define one underlying vulnerability in a subset of SIDS infants that puts those infants at risk when faced with a homeostatic challenge. Increased knowledge of this vulnerability and its origin(s) will provide necessary insight on the means by which sudden unexpected death in this subset can be prevented.

Acknowledgments

The author thanks Dr Hannah C. Kinney for critical readings of this chapter.

References

1. Kinney HC, Broadbelt KG, Haynes RL, et al. The serotonergic anatomy of the developing human medulla oblongata: implications for pediatric disorders of homeostasis. *J. Chem. Neuroanat*, 2011; **41**:182–99.

2. Okaty BW, Freret ME, Rood BD, et al. Multi-scale molecular deconstruction of the serotonin neuron system. *Neuron*, 2015; **88**:774–91.

3. Kinney HC, Richerson GB, Dymecki SM et al. The brainstem and serotonin in the Sudden Infant Death Syndrome. *Annu Rev Path*, 2009; **4**:517–50.

4. Erickson JT, Sposato BC. Autoresuscitation responses to hypoxia-induced apnea are delayed in newborn 5-HT-deficient Pet-1 homozygous mice. *J Appl Physiol*, 2009; **106**:1785–92.

5. Cummings KJ, Commons KG, Hewitt JC, et al. Failed heart rate recovery at a critical age in 5-HT-deficient mice exposed to episodic anoxia: implications for SIDS. *J Appl Physiol*, 2011; **111**:825–33.

6. Chen J, Magnusson J, Karsenty G, Cummings KJ. Time- and age-dependent effects of serotonin on gasping and autoresuscitation in neonatal mice. *J Appl Physiol*, 2013; **114**:1668–76.

7. Barrett KT, Dosumu-Johnson RT, Daubenspeck JA, et al. Partial raphe dysfunction in neurotransmission is sufficient to increase mortality after anoxic exposures in mice at a critical period in postnatal development. *J Neurosci*, 2016; **36**:3943–53.

8. Hodges MR, Richerson GB. Medullary serotonin neurons and their roles in central respiratory chemoreception. *Respir Physiol Neurobiol*, 2010; **173**:256–63.

9. Cerpa VJ, Wu Y, Bravo E, et al. Medullary 5-HT neurons: switch from tonic respiratory drive to chemoreception during postnatal development. *Neuroscience*, 2017; **344**:1–14.

10. Darnall RA, Schneider RW, Tobia CM, Commons KG. Eliminating medullary 5-HT neurons delays arousal and decreases the respiratory response to repeated episodes of hypoxia in neonatal rat pups. *J Appl Physiol*, 2016; **120**:514–25.

11. Cerpa V, Gonzalez A, Richerson GB. Diphtheria toxin treatment of Pet-1-Cre floxed diphtheria toxin receptor mice disrupts thermoregulation without affecting respiratory chemoreception. *Neuroscience*, 2014; **279**:65–76.

12. Hodges MR, Best S, Richerson GB. Altered ventilatory and thermoregulatory control in male and female adult Pet-1 null mice. *Respir Physiol Neurobiol*, 2011; **177**:133–40.

13. Downing SE, Lee JC. Laryngeal chemosensitivity: a possible mechanism for sudden infant death. *Pediatrics*, 1975; **55**:640–9.

14. Van Der Velde L, Curran AK, Filiano JJ, et al. Prolongation of the laryngeal chemoreflex after inhibition of the rostral ventral medulla in piglets: a role in SIDS? *J Appl Physiol*, 2003; **94**:1883–95.

15. Donnelly WT, Bartlett D, Jr, Leiter JC. Serotonin in the solitary tract nucleus shortens the laryngeal chemoreflex in anaesthetized neonatal rats. *Exp Physiol*, 2016; **101**:946–61.

16. Vitalis T, Fouquet C, Alvarez C, et al. Developmental expression of monoamine oxidases A and B in the central and peripheral nervous systems of the mouse. *J Comp Neurol*, 2002; **442**:331–47.

17. Svob Strac D, Pivac N, Muck-Seler D. The serotonergic system and cognitive function. *Transl Neurosci*, 2016; **7**:35–49.

18. Pena F, Ramirez JM. Endogenous activation of serotonin-2A receptors is required for respiratory rhythm generation in vitro. *J Neurosci*, 2002; **22**:11055–64.

19. Dergacheva O, Kamendi H, Wang X, et al. The role of 5-HT3 and other excitatory receptors in central

cardiorespiratory responses to hypoxia: implications for Sudden Infant Death Syndrome. *Pediatr Res*, 2009; **65**:625–30.

20. Donnelly WT, Xia L, Bartlett D, Leiter JC. Activation of serotonergic neurons in the medullary caudal raphe shortens the laryngeal chemoreflex in anaesthetized neonatal rats. *Exp Physiol*, 2017; **102**:1007–18.

21. Charnay Y, Leger L. Brain serotonergic circuitries. *Dialogues Clin Neurosci*, 2010; **12**:471–87.

22. Panigrahy A, Filiano J, Sleeper LA, et al. Decreased serotonergic receptor binding in rhombic lip-derived regions of the medulla oblongata in the Sudden Infant Death Syndrome. *J Neuropathol Exp Neuro*, 2000; **59**:377–84.

23. Kinney HC, Randall LL, Sleeper LA, et al. Serotonergic brainstem abnormalities in Northern Plains Indians with the Sudden Infant Death Syndrome. *J Neuropathol Exp Neuro*, 2003; **62**:1178–91.

24. Paterson DS, Trachtenberg FL, Thompson EG, et al. Multiple serotonergic brainstem abnormalities in Sudden Infant Death Syndrome. *JAMA*, 2006; **296**: 2124–32.

25. Duncan JR, Paterson DS, Hoffman JM, et al. Brainstem serotonergic deficiency in Sudden Infant Death Syndrome. *JAMA*, 2010; **303**:430–7.

26. Ozawa Y, Okado N. Alteration of serotonergic receptors in the brain stems of human patients with respiratory disorders. *Neuropediatrics*, 2002; **33**:142–9.

27. Machaalani R, Say M, Waters KA. Serotoninergic receptor 1A in the Sudden Infant Death Syndrome brainstem medulla and associations with clinical risk factors. *Acta Neuropathol*, 2009; **117**:257–65.

28. Kinney HC, Filiano JJ, Assmann SF, et al. Tritiated-naloxone binding to brainstem opioid receptors in the Sudden Infant Death Syndrome. *Auton Neurosci*, 1998; **69**:156–63.

29. Mansouri J, Panigrahy A, Assmann SF, Kinney HC. Distribution of alpha 2-adrenergic receptor binding in the developing human brain stem. *Pediatr Dev Pathol*, 2001; **4**:222–36.

30. Bright FM, Byard RW, Vink R, Paterson DS. Medullary serotonin neuron abnormalities in an Australian cohort of Sudden Infant Death Syndrome. *J Neuropathol Exp Neuro*, 2017; **76**:864–73.

31. Kinney HC, Thach BT. The Sudden Infant Death Syndrome. *N Engl J Med*, 2009; **361**:795–805.

32. Iyasu S, Randall LL, Welty TK, et al. Risk factors for Sudden Infant Death Syndrome among Northern Plains Indians. *JAMA*, 2002; **288**:2717–23.

33. Kinney HC, Myers MM, Belliveau RA, et al. Subtle autonomic and respiratory dysfunction in Sudden

Infant Death Syndrome associated with serotonergic brainstem abnormalities: a case report. *J Neuropathol Exp Neuro*, 2005; **64**:689–94.

34. Paterson DS. Serotonin gene variants are unlikely to play a significant role in the pathogenesis of the Sudden Infant Death Syndrome. *Respir Physiol Neurobiol*, 2013; **189**:301–14.

35. Weese-Mayer DE, Ackerman MJ, Marazita ML, Berry-Kravis EM. Sudden Infant Death Syndrome: review of implicated genetic factors. *Am J Med Genet A*, 2007; **143A**:771–88.

36. Filiano JJ, Kinney HC. A perspective on neuropathologic findings in victims of the Sudden Infant Death Syndrome: the triple-risk model. *Biol Neonate*, 1994; **65**:194–7.

37. Bradley SR, Pieribone VA, Wang W, et al. Chemosensitive serotonergic neurons are closely associated with large medullary arteries. *Nat. Neurosci*, 2002; **5**:401–2.

38. Filiano JJ, Choi JC, Kinney HC. Candidate cell populations for respiratory chemosensitive fields in the human infant medulla. *J Comp Neurol*, 1990; **293**: 448–65.

39. Filiano JJ, Kinney HC. Arcuate nucleus hypoplasia in the Sudden Infant Death Syndrome. *J Neuropathol Exp Neuro*, 1992; **51**:394–403.

40. Matturri L, Biondo B, Mercurio P, Rossi L. Severe hypoplasia of medullary arcuate nucleus: quantitative analysis in Sudden Infant Death Syndrome. *Acta Neuropathol*, 2000; **99**:371–5.

41. Kinney HC, Belliveau RA, Trachtenberg FL, et al. The development of the medullary serotonergic system in early human life. *Auton Neurosci*, 2007; **132**:81–102.

42. Sari Y, Zhou FC. Prenatal alcohol exposure causes long-term serotonin neuron deficit in mice. *Alcohol Clin Exp Res*, 2004; **28**:941–8.

43. Slotkin TA, Skavicus S, Card J, et al. Developmental neurotoxicity of tobacco smoke directed toward cholinergic and serotonergic systems: more than just nicotine. *Toxicol Sci*, 2015; **147**:178–89.

44. Cerpa VJ, Aylwin Mde L, Beltrán-Castillo S, et al. The alteration of neonatal raphe neurons by prenatal–perinatal nicotine: meaning for Sudden Infant Death Syndrome. *Am J Respir Cell and Mol Biol*, 2015; **53**: 489–99.

45. Houwing DJ, Buwalda B, van der Zee EA, et al. The serotonin transporter and early life stress: translational perspectives. *Front Cell Neurosci*, 2017; **11**:117.

46. Iurescia S, Seripa D, Rinaldi M. Looking beyond the 5-HTTLPR polymorphism: genetic and epigenetic

layers of regulation affecting the serotonin transporter gene expression. *Mol Neurobiol*, 2017; **54:** 8386–403.

47. Provenzi L, Giorda R, Beri S, Montirosso R. SLC6A4 methylation as an epigenetic marker of life adversity exposures in humans: A systematic review of literature. *Neurosci Biobehav Rev*, 2016;**71**:7–20.

48. O'Mahony SM, Clarke G, Borre YE, et al. Serotonin, tryptophan metabolism, and the brain-gut-microbiome axis. *Behav Brain Res*, 2015;**277**:32–48.

49. Haynes RL, Frelinger AL, Giles EK, et al. High serum serotonin in Sudden Infant Death Syndrome. *Proc Natl Acad Sci*, 2017; **114**:7695–700.

50. Kinney HC, Cryan JB, Haynes RL, et al. Dentate gyrus abnormalities in sudden unexplained death in infants: morphological marker of underlying brain vulnerability. *Acta Neuropathol*, 2015;**129**:65–80.

Chapter 33

Inner-Ear Abnormalities in SIDS

Daniel D. Rubens and Sanja Ramirez

Introduction

Sudden Infant Death Syndrome (SIDS) is defined as the unexpected, unexplained sudden death of an infant less than 1 year of age.[1] By definition, SIDS implies that no cause of death has been identified after a thorough death scene investigation and complete autopsy. We explore here a novel avenue of research that offers new clues to understanding the inexplicable death of these seemingly healthy infants.

In 2008 a retrospective study compared the newborn hearing screening tests of 31 SIDS infants to those of a matched group of 31 control infants.[2] The study illustrated that the transient evoked otoacoustic emission (TEOAE) newborn hearing screens of SIDS infants portrayed reduced signal to noise ratios at 2000, 3000, and 4000 hz as compared to controls. The hearing depression was significant only in the right ear. This study was the first indicator of a possible correlation between inner-ear dysfunction and the incidences of SIDS. It was also the first study to identify any alteration in SIDS cases on a newborn screening test, well before the fatal event.

In a follow-up study, Rubens and coworkers created a mouse model to emulate the inner-ear dysfunction seen in the SIDS infants using intratympanic gentamicin (IT-Gent) injections.[3] The IT-Gent animals were exposed to a noxious gas environment (hypoxia and/or hypercarbia) under light anaesthesia four days after the IT-Gent injections. The ventilatory and body movement arousal responses were examined and compared to control animals. The study identified a significant suppression of the arousal movements in the IT-Gent mice compared to their age-matched control groups in response to the noxious gas mixtures: the arousal movement responses in animals that received IT-Gent injections displayed stunted movements on exposure to a combined 5% CO_2 anoxia gas mixture. While control animals exhibited a vigorous movement response (> 4 cm), IT-Gent injected mice displayed virtually no response.

The study also demonstrated that there was no significant difference in mice that received unilateral IT-Gent vs. bilateral injections (Figure 33.1).

The animal model contributed preliminary evidence for a connection between inner-ear damage and suppression of a primary arousal response that could be related to SIDS fatality. A subsequent study analysed the arousal response of the animals to the separate gas mixtures in order to tease apart the respective roles of hypoxia and hypercarbia in the movement response.[4] Surprisingly, the study identified that neither control nor IT-Gent mice displayed an arousal response to 5% C02. However, controls consistently instigated a vigorous response to anoxia alone.

To address the criticism that light anaesthesia might contribute to suppression of the arousal response, the next phase of experiments was conducted under natural sleep conditions.[4] Just as with the experiments under light anaesthesia, the mice exposed to hypercarbia under natural sleeping conditions did not display the vigorous movements seen in response to anoxia alone.

The study did however identify an unanticipated phenomenon during natural sleep that was not observed under light anaesthesia. Both controls and IT-Gent animals displayed 'mini-arousals'- small adjustment movements that occurred spontaneously during natural sleep. No significant difference was identified between the controls and IT-Gent animals and there was also no difference when animals were exposed to air or 5% CO_2 (Figure 33.2). This confirms the original finding, that anoxia rather than hypercarbia appears to be the potent stimulus for arousal survival movement during sleep.

To summarise, our findings suggest that there is a correlation between inner-ear dysfunction and failed arousal to hypoxia as it applies to SIDS cases.[5] The inner-ear dysfunction appears to suppress the survival body movements that could remove

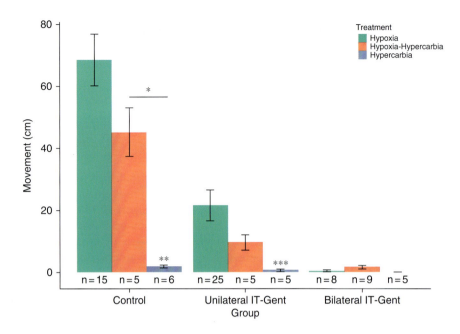

Figure 33.1 Comparison of body arousal movements for control and test groups under gas conditions of hypoxia, hypoxia-hypercarbia, and hypercarbia. Columns display the group medians and quartiles for each gas condition. Within the control groups, the hypercarbia treatment (Mdn = 2, IQR = 2–3, range = 0–3) displayed significantly suppressed arousal movements compared to hypoxia (Mdn = 57, IQR = 47.5–79, range = 29–134) and hypoxia-hypercarbia (Mdn = 45, IQR = 32–45, range = 0–2) ($p = 0.0015$ and $p = 0.0198$, respectively). Within the unilateral IT-Gent group, hypercarbia treatment (Mdn = 0, IQR = 0–1, range = 0–2) displayed significantly suppressed movements compared to hypoxia-hypercarbia (Mdn = 9, IQR = 6–9, range = 5–19, $p = 0.033$). Bilateral IT-Gent animals displayed little movement in response to any of the gas conditions ($p > 0.05$). * specifies $p < 0.05$ and ** specifies $p < 0.01$.

the animal or infant from the environment in which they cannot survive. We also identified that of the two noxious gas stimuli that a SIDS infant is likely to be faced with (too much C02/ too little O2), it appears to be the lack of 02 which triggers the arousal, and not the excess of C02.

While the field has yet to study the mechanism behind why the inner ear is causing this arousal suppression, we can hypothesise as to why this could be the case:

Previous studies have identified the vestibular organ as playing a major role in respiratory control as well as autonomic and cardiovascular regulation.[6–13] Thus, damage to the inner ear could precipitate dramatic suppression of autonomic responses to a severe hypoxic environment. While the field has not studied specific neuronal activity, it is recognised that vestibular hair cells are integrally involved in triggering balance adjustments.[14,15] They do so by depolarising the side towards which the head is turning while the opposite side is hyperpolarising. We thus speculate that severe hypoxia could elicit a unified depolarisation response in vestibular afferents on both sides since

anoxia will precipitate ischaemia of vestibular neurons (as well as cochlear neurons) irrespective of laterality.

The Potential Role of the Diving Reflex in Combination with Inner-Ear Dysfunction in SIDS

The diving reflex is a powerful oxygen-conserving reflex that is observed in 100% of infants between 2 and 6 months of age and 90% of infants between 6 months and one year of age.[16] The diving reflex response to hypoxia triggers bradycardia, apnoea, vocal cord closure, and suppression of metabolism.[17]

The diving reflex is initiated by any cause of hypoxia, although its primordial origin is to protect the healthy infant from drowning.[17] On submersion underwater, the infant is removed from its oxygen source. There is a consistent atmospheric pressure increase on submersion versus being at the surface. Evidence supports that there is a barometric pressure sensor located in the inner ear.[18,19] Previous studies have also identified inner-ear dysfunction with inflammation and swelling in SIDS infants.[20]

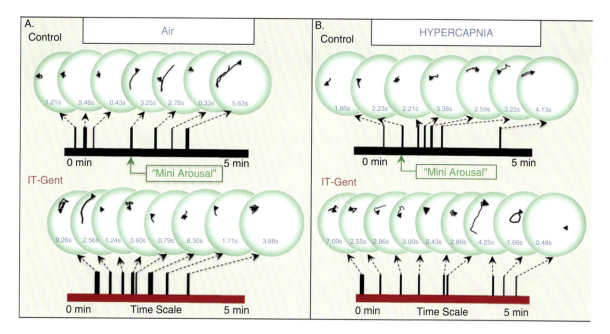

Figure 33.2 Representative figure portraying mini-arousal pattern during a five-minute period of natural sleep in air, tracking the movement phenotypes observed in control and unilateral IT-Gent mice.

We hypothesise that in the SIDS infant, on exposure to a hypoxic stimulus, increased swelling (and thus pressure) in the inner ear leads the system to respond as if the infant were submerged and therefore it goes into the diving reflex.

At some point, the infant without inner-ear swelling will break the reflex in order to appropriately access fresh air. We hypothesise that by contrast, SIDS infants with inner-ear swelling are perpetually exposed to increased pressure and therefore never break the diving reflex.

In summary, we propose that inner-ear dysfunction in SIDS cases suppresses the ability of these infants to appropriately break the diving reflex once instigated. The infant may be observed to make respiratory efforts, however this is likely to be against a closed glottis. Finally, the vocal cords open and the infant may gasp when the O2 has reached fatally low levels in plasma.

Thus, the inner-ear dysfunction which is present at birth affords the infant a specific underlying susceptibility to SIDS. We are currently investigating this hypothesis to understand the potential link between the inner ear and the diving reflex. Evidence supporting this line of research comes from the consistent finding on autopsy of intrathoracic petechiae in 85–90% of SIDS cases.[21] The finding of intrathoracic petechiae on the external surface of the organs is consistent with increased intrathoracic pressure due to internal airway obstruction from vocal cord closure rather than external upper airway obstruction.[21]

References

1. Hauck FR, Tanabe KO. International trends in Sudden Infant Death Syndrome: stabilization of rates requires further action. *Pediatrics*, 2008; **122**(3):660–6.

2. Rubens DD, Vohr BR, Tucker R, O'Neil CA, Chung W. Newborn oto-acoustic emission hearing screening tests: preliminary evidence for a marker of susceptibility to SIDS. *Early Hum Dev*, 2008; **84**(4):225–9.

3. Allen T, Garcia III AJ, Tang J, Ramirez JM, Rubens DD. Inner ear insult ablates the arousal response to hypoxia and hypercarbia. *Neuroscience*, 2013; **253**:283–91.

4. Ramirez S, Allen T, Villagracia L, Chae Y, Ramirez JM, Rubens DD. Inner ear lesion and the differential roles of hypoxia and hypercarbia in triggering active movements: potential implication for the Sudden Infant Death Syndrome. *Neuroscience*, 2016; **337**:9–16.

5. Kinney HC. Brainstem mechanisms underlying the Sudden Infant Death Syndrome: evidence from human pathologic studies. *Dev Psychobiol*, 2009; **51**(3):223–33.

6. Morinaka S, Nakamura H. Arterial blood gas abnormalities in patients with dizziness. *Ann Otol Rhinol Laryngol*, 1998; **107**(1):6–9.

7. Monahan KD, Sharpe MK, Drury D, Ertl AC, Ray CA. Influence of vestibular activation on respiration in humans. *Am J Physiol Regul Integr Comp Physiol*, 2002; **282**:R689–R694.

8. Thurrell A, Jáuregui-Renaud K, Gresty MA, Bronstein AM. Vestibular influence on the cardiorespiratory responses to whole-body oscillation after standing. *Exp Brain Res*, 2003; **150**(3):325–31.

9. Miyamura M, Ishida K, Katayama K, Shima N, Matsuo H, Sato K. Ventilatory and heart rate responses at the onset of chair rotation in man. *Jpn J Physiol*, 2004; **54**(5): 499–503.

10. Jauregui-Renaud K, Villanueva PL, del Castillo MS. Influence of acute unilateral vestibular lesions on the respiratory rhythm after acute change in posture in human subjects. *J Vestib Res*, 2005; **15**(1): 41–8.

11. Arshian M, Holtje RJ, Cotter LA, Rice CD, Cass SP, Yates BJ. Consequences of postural changes and removal of vestibular inputs on the movement of air in and out of the lungs of conscious felines. *J Appl Physiol*, 2007; **103**(1): 347–52.

12. Jian BJ, Acernese AW, Lorenzo J, Card JP, Yates BJ. Afferent pathways to the region of the vestibular nuclei that participates in cardiovascular and respiratory control. *Brain Res*, 2005; **1044**(2): 241–50.

13. Yates BJ, Bronstein AM. The effects of vestibular system lesions on autonomic regulation: observations, mechanisms, and clinical implications. *J Vestib Res*, 2005; **15**(3): 119–29.

14. Ganong WF. *Review of Medical Physiology*. 19th edn. Stamford: Appleton and Lange. 1999.

15. Purves D, Augustine GJ, Fitzpatrick D, et al., eds. *Neuroscience*. 2nd edn. Sunderland, MA: Sinauer Associates; 2001.

16. Pedroso FS, Riesgo RS, Gatiboni T, Rotta NT. The diving reflex in healthy infants in the first year of life. *J Child Neurol*, 2012; **27**(2):168–71.

17. Goksör E, Rosengren L, Wennergren G. Bradycardic response during submersion in infant swimming. *Acta Pædiatrica*, 2002; **91**:307–12

18. Funakubo M, Sato J, Honda T, Mizumura K. The inner ear is involved in the aggravation of nociceptive behavior induced by lowering barometric pressure of nerve injured rats. *Eur J Pain*, 2010; **14**(1):32–9.

19. Duong Dinh TA, Haasler T, Homann G, Jüngling E, Westhofen M, Lückhoff A. Potassium currents induced by hydrostatic pressure modulate membrane potential and transmitter release in vestibular type II hair cells. *Pflugers Arch*, 2009; **458**(2): 379–87.

20. Josset P, Lecomte D, Omur M, Chabolle F, Hannoun L, Chouard CH. Anatomo-pathologic study of the temporal bone in our 4 cases of sudden infant death. *Ann Otolaryngol Chir Cervicofac*, 1985; **102**(6): 425–32.

21. Krous HF, Haas EA, Chadwick AE et al. *Forensic Sci Med Pathol*, 2008; **4**:234.

Chapter 34

Inherited Metabolic Disease and Sudden Unexplained Death in Infancy and Childhood: Pathophysiology

Simon E. Olpin

Introduction

Garrod in 1909 used the term *Inborn Errors of Metabolism* in defining a spectrum of genetically inherited disorders characterised by blocks in the metabolic pathway.[1] Garrod described only four disorders which were known at the time but our current knowledge of the human genome has expanded exponentially since then. Given the advancement in second-generation sequencing, the number of newly defined disorders continues to increase, so that at present there are a wide and expanding list of disorders that can now be diagnosed. Inherited metabolic diseases (IMD) are caused by inherited defects in the enzymes/proteins or cofactors that metabolise proteins, carbohydrates, and lipids. These disorders are the result of molecular mutations/deletions that alter metabolic pathways through reduced or absent activity of a protein. Most of these proteins are enzymes although some may act as carrier proteins or structural components. Enzymes regulate many metabolic pathways including the stepwise degradation of dietary lipids, carbohydrates, and proteins, ultimately providing energy through the complex process of oxidative phosphorylation. Others are involved in the endogenous synthesis of proteins, carbohydrates, and lipids which form building blocks within tissues or act as energy stores, predominantly in the form of adipose tissue triglycerides or liver and muscle glycogen. Yet more enzymes are involved in the synthesis /assembly of more complex macromolecules which serve as structural components or are involved in the degradation or re-cycling of cellular components.

Despite the fact that the underlying cause in a high percentage of SIDS/SUDI/SUDC cases still remains unidentified, it is recognised that a small but significant number of sudden and/or unexplained deaths in neonates, infants, and occasionally older children are a result of inherited metabolic disease IMD. Many inborn errors of metabolism can present as acute metabolic disease in the neonatal period. Most babies with inherited metabolic disorders are born apparently healthy and may show a typical asymptomatic period with clinical manifestation from the second day of life onwards. However, some disorders may present at birth or may be detected by antenatal ultrasonography or even result in death in utero. Sadly, many babies with inherited metabolic disease follow a rapid course of deterioration and may succumb before appropriate investigations can be completed or before newborn screening has been undertaken. Nevertheless, expanded newborn screening programmes are now widely implemented throughout much of the developed world (Europe, USA, Australasia) with the result that many of these inherited metabolic disorders (particularly medium-chain acyl-CoA dehydrogenase deficiency – MCADD) are identified in the neonatal period and appropriate treatment instituted. In the UK, we currently screen for 8 disorders at day 5–6 of life. These include phenylketonuria, medium-chain acyl-CoA dehydrogenase deficiency, glutaric aciduria type 1, homocystinuria, maple syrup urine disease, and isovaleric acidaemia. This is a small panel of metabolic disorders given that some states within USA claim to screen for up to fifty disorders. Consequently, in the UK a significant number of inherited metabolic diseases that are reported to present as SUDI/SIDS/SUDC remain undiagnosed in the neonatal period. Additionally, in many developing countries where the previously high infant mortality rate is being addressed through advances in public health, nutrition, and infection control, the burden of inherited metabolic disease becomes an increasingly important issue. In these countries, there is an increasing move to develop newborn screening programmes although in many developing countries these are still absent, or in their infancy.

When investigating the possibility of an underlying metabolic disorder that has resulted in an unexpected and/or unexplained death it is often helpful wherever possible to look for clues to an underlying cause by examining the pattern of deterioration in the infant, if this has been observed, as this can provide useful indicators towards a possible diagnosis (see Table 34.1).[2]

The intention of this article is to provide a brief description of the metabolic disorders that are more likely to be encountered in the context of unexplained sudden death, or death following a brief illness, in neonates, and older infants. The subsequent collection and processing of appropriate samples and types of investigations that are currently available are clearly described in Chapter 18.

Metabolic Causes of Sudden Death

Emery was the first to observe that a wide range of metabolic disorders may present as Sudden Infant Death Syndrome.[3] It may result from dramatic cardiac failure, shock, or cardiac arrest in many metabolic circumstances. Although close examination may suggest that not all these deaths were entirely unexpected, they were initially unexplained. Identification of the cause of death in such cases is a consolation to parents and offers the opportunity for future prenatal diagnosis. Although at least forty metabolic disorders are listed as causes of SIDS, there is some doubt as to the validity of some reports.[4] The most likely metabolic causes of sudden and/or unexplained death are listed below: –

1. Congenital lactic acidosis i.e. pyruvate dehydrogenase deficiency (PDH), respiratory chain disorders.
2. Inherited defects of fatty acid oxidation and ketogenesis.
3. Urea cycle disorders – most commonly ornithine transcarbamylase (OTC) deficiency.
4. Organic acidurias e.g. methylmalonic aciduria (MMA), propionic aciduria (PA) and isovaleric aciduria (IVA), glutaric aciduria type II (GAII), glutaric aciduria type I (GAI).
5. Carbohydrate disorders e.g. galactosaemia, glycogen storage disease type I (GSD I), hereditary fructose intolerance, fructose 1,6-bisphosphatase deficiency.

In practice with the exception of the fatty acid oxidation defects (FAO), the majority of these disorders do not strictly present as SIDS, but rather as an acute metabolic crisis with clear clinical symptoms, which precedes death by hours or even a few days.

Mitochondrial Respiratory Chain Disorders

Mitochondriopathies are disorders of enzymes or enzyme complexes that are directly involved in the production of chemical energy by the process of oxidative phosphorylation. These include the pyruvate dehydrogenase (PDH) complex and the respiratory chain complexes I, II, III, IV, and ATP synthase, complex V. It is estimated that the coordinated expression of around 1000 genes is required for a functioning respiratory chain. Respiratory chain disorders lead to a wide spectrum of clinical disease that can potentially involve any single or combination of organ systems. Given that almost any organ or system can be affected, the combination of seemingly unrelated symptoms with clinical disease in several tissues or organs, suggests the possibility of respiratory chain disease.[5] Cardiac disease in infants and older children is often a result of genetic defects of oxidative phosphorylation and may present as an isolated cardiomyopathy or with other multiorgan involvement. Respiratory chain disease may also lead to inter-uterine death/stillbirth or premature delivery of a sick infant with early demise before appropriate investigations can be instituted.

Fatty acid Oxidation Disorders

Inherited disorders of fatty acid oxidation are known to present as sudden unexplained death in an infant or child thought previously to be well. It is estimated that prior to newborn screening, up to 3–6% of sudden unexpected infant deaths were attributable to this group of disorders (FAO).[6–9] Defects of medium-chain acyl-CoA dehydrogenase, carnitine palmitoyltransferase type II, carnitine-acylcarnitine translocase, the high affinity carnitine transporter (mutations of the *OCTN2* gene causing primary carnitine deficiency), long-chain 3-hydroxyacyl-CoA dehydrogenase, mitochondrial trifunctional protein, very-long-chain acyl-CoA dehydrogenase, and multiple acyl-CoA dehydrogenase have all been reported as presenting initially as cases of sudden unexplained death.[6,10] However, of the fatty acid oxidation defects, medium-chain acyl-CoA dehydrogenase (MCAD) deficiency is the single most common disorder and warrants further description.

Table 34.1 Clinical patterns of deterioration / presentation associated with metabolic disorders[*]

Hypoglycaemia	Acid-Base Disorders	Cardiac Disorders	Neurological deterioration	Liver Disease	Dysmorphology
Disorders of fatty acid oxidation	Metabolic acidosis:	Disorders of fatty acid oxidation	Hyperammonaemia	Galactosaemia	Polycystic kidneys –GA II (severe)
Fructose 1,6-bisphosphatase deficiency	Organic acidaemias	Congenital disorders of glycosylation (CDG)	Organic acidaemias	α-1-antitrypsin deficiency	CPT II (severe)
Glycogen storage disease type 1 (GSD 1)	Congenital lactic acidosis	Pompe disease (GSD II)	Maple syrup urine disease	Respiratory chain disorders	Zellweger
Respiratory chain disorders	Fructose 1,6-bisphosphatase deficiency	Respiratory chain disorders	Disorders of fatty acid oxidation	Neonatal haemochromatosis	Agenesis of the corpus callosum – PDH
Organic acidaemias	3-Ketothiolase deficiency		Congenital lactic acidosis	Disorders of fatty acid oxidation	Craniofacial abnormalities – Zellweger, S-L-O,
Hereditary fructose intolerance	Respiratory alkalosis:		Peroxisomal disorders	Tyrosinaemia type 1	Respiratory chain disorders
	hyperammonaemia		Non-ketotic hyperglycinaemia (NKH)	Niemann-Pick type C	Hydrops fetalis – lysosomal storage disease
	- urea cycle defects		Molybdenum cofactor deficiency	Hereditary fructose intolerance	Cataract – Sengers disease
					Galactosaemia

[*] Adapted from J V Leonard and A A M Morris Inborn errors of metabolism around the time of birth.[2] Reprinted with permission from Elsevier.

Abbreviations:
CPT II – carnitine palmitoyltransferase type II
GA II – glutaric aciduria type II (multiple acyl-CoA dehydrogenase deficiency)
NKH – non-ketotic hyperglycinaemia
S-L-O – Smith-Lemli-Opitz syndrome
PDH – pyruvate dehydrogenase deficiency

Medium-Chain Acyl-CoA Dehydrogenase Deficiency

MCAD deficiency was first described in the early 1980s[11,12] and is the commonest fatty acid oxidation defect occurring in central Europe, affecting caucasians of northwestern European origin with an incidence as high as 1:8000 live births. The first crisis is fatal in up to 25 percent of cases, patients classically presenting with hypoketotic hypoglycaemia.[13] However, a significant percentage of genetically predisposed patients remain asymptomatic throughout life.[13,14] The disease is primarily of hepatic fatty acid oxidation. Clinically, patients may present with lethargy, emesis, encephalopathy, respiratory arrest, hepatomegaly, seizures, apnoea, and cardiac arrest.[13,15] Although hypoglycaemia with 'inappropriate' hypoketosis is usually the major presenting biochemical feature, some patients may present with hypotonia and reduced consciousness while still maintaining blood glucose concentration within the normal range. Patients presenting in crisis may often have detectable ketones in their urine. Indeed there is evidence to suggest that, at least in the well child with MCAD, medium-chain fatty acid oxidation and ketone body production and utilisation are within normal limits.[16,17] Rarely, MCAD patients may present in crisis with 'paradoxically' gross ketosis (J. Calvin, personal communication). Some patients presenting initially as SIDS have subsequently on biochemical testing been shown to have MCAD.[18] Babies can present within the first few days of life as a sudden death.[19,20] Mean age at presentation is 12 months, but presentation after the age of 5 years is rare,[13] although there are isolated reports of adult presentations following extreme metabolic stress.[21,22] The common K304E mutation accounts for 85 percent of this disease in most of Western Europe.[18] Neonatal screening programmes which now include MCAD are in place in a number of countries including Australia, some states in the USA and a number of European countries.

Other Fatty acid Oxidation Defects

Following the description of MCAD there has been considerable growth in our knowledge of previously undescribed fatty acid oxidation defects with some fifteen or so defects that directly or indirectly affect fatty acid oxidation having now been reported.[23] This group of disorders is now widely recognised as being an important cause of acute metabolic decompensation and sudden death in the neonatal period, infancy, and early childhood.[24] Cumulatively these other disorders probably account for a similar number of sudden deaths as does MCAD. Two main types of presentation are most commonly observed. The first is characterised by hypoketotic hypoglycaemia after a period of prolonged fasting. Patients may present acutely with a life-threatening illness, which may rapidly proceed to coma and death, during intercurrent infections, surgery, or other catabolic stress, having apparently been previously well or having only exhibited mild symptoms such as failure to thrive. Additionally, there may be liver disease with hyperammonaemia and cerebral oedema (Reye-like illness). Cardiac arrhythmias resulting in sudden death may be induced by accumulation of long-chain acylcarnitines, which are particularly arrhythmogenic and there may be acute cardiomyopathy with pericardial effusion.[24]

The second presentation reflects chronic impairment of muscle function with myopathy and/or cardiomyopathy, which can be either hypertrophic or dilated. Sudden death as a result of severe cardiomyopathy has been reported in patients previously thought to be well.[25]

Defects of Ketone Body Production / Utilisation

3-Hydroxy-3-methylglutaryl (HMG) CoA lyase is an enzyme required for ketogenesis as well as for the last step in leucine oxidation. Patients with deficiency of this enzyme present in infancy or early childhood with life-threatening Reye-like crisis; the picture is one of hypoketotic hypoglycaemia, metabolic acidosis, and liver disease. Analysis of urine organic acids gives a specific pattern of abnormal metabolites.

3-Ketothiolase (mitochondrial 2-methylacetoacetyl-CoA thiolase) is a ketolytic enzyme but is also an enzyme of isoleucine metabolism. Patients with a deficiency of this enzyme usually present in infancy between 6–24 months of age, but occasionally as older children, with episodes of vomiting often precipitated by intercurrent infection or occasionally by high protein intake. There is acute life-threatening ketoacidotic crisis with severe metabolic acidosis, occasionally low, but usually normal glucose and normal or moderately raised ammonia. Patients may rapidly succumb to overwhelming metabolic acidosis. Urine organic acid and blood acylcarnitine analysis will identify this disorder.

Urea Cycle Defects

Defects of the urea cycle may present in the neonatal period, infancy, and childhood, or in adolescents and adults; cumulatively they have an incidence of 1:20000. Hyperammonaemia is a potent cause of cerebral oedema in this patient group. The presentation at different age groups shows some variability but it is particularly in neonates and infants where the presentation may be of a sudden acute decompensation rapidly proceeding to coma and death. Neonates typically present on day 2 of life, following a brief asymptomatic period. There is usually disinterest in feeding, lethargy, hyperventilation, seizures, and progressive encephalopathy and coma with loss of reflexes and frequently intracranial haemorrhages resulting from coagulation defects. Respiratory alkalosis develops with marked hyperammonaemia. A misdiagnosis of sepsis is frequently made.[26,27]

Diagnosis, depending on the defect, is by amino acid analysis in plasma and urine, demonstration of elevated argininosuccinic acid in urine in the case of argininosuccinate lyase deficiency, increased orotic acid in urine in ornithine transcarbamylase (OTC) deficiency, followed by enzyme studies in leucocytes, fibroblasts, or liver and mutation studies.

Organic Acidurias

This large group of disorders result from defects of intermediary metabolism with the characteristic accumulation of carboxylic acids in urine. The majority of the important organic acidurias are caused by disorders involving the metabolism of branch-chain amino acids. Patients classically present in the neonatal period with metabolic encephalopathy resulting from 'metabolic intoxication' (see Table 34.1). There is lethargy, feeding problems, dehydration, and limb hypertonia with truncal hypotonia. Patients show multi-system failure, neurovegetative dysregulation, and coma. These disorders include isovaleric aciduria (IVA), propionic aciduria (PA), methylmalonic aciduria (MMA) and multiple carboxylase deficiency. The multiple carboxylases are biotin dependent enzymes important in the metabolism of branched-chain amino acids and disorders of these enzymes encompass biotinidase deficiency, holocarboxylase synthetase deficiency, and 3-methylcrotonylglycinuria.

GA I (glutaryl-CoA dehydrogenase deficiency) is a disorder of lysine and tryptophan metabolism. Patients are normal at birth, but usually present during infancy or early childhood with acute encephalopathic crisis and metabolic decompensation during intercurrent infection or other metabolic stress. There is often macrocephaly with fronto-temporal atrophy. The first episode may be fatal but those patients that survive are left with severe dystonic-dyskinetic movement disorder, intellect however is frequently intact. Patients presenting with this condition may be mistaken as cases of possible non-accidental injury.

Disorders of Galactose and Fructose Metabolism

Patients with classical galactosaemia resulting from galactose-1-phosphate uridyltransferase deficiency or hereditary fructose intolerance only develop clinical symptoms of disease after ingestion of lactose (milk and dairy products) or fructose/sucrose respectively. Galactose-1-phosphate and fructose-1-phosphate which accumulate in classical galactosaemia and hereditary fructose intolerance are toxic metabolites that lead to organ damage, particularly in liver, kidneys, and brain. Galactosaemia usually presents in the neonatal period on commencement of milk feeds and is frequently fatal unless detected at an early stage. Hypoglycaemia with jaundice, deranged liver function, and renal failure are the common features often with accompanying sepsis. Patients may succumb with the incorrect primary diagnosis of sepsis. Diagnosis for galactosaemia is by enzyme assay in whole blood or on a fresh Guthrie card blood spot, quantitation of galactose-1-phosphate in erythrocytes, or by mutation detection. Blood transfusion will of course invalidate the enzyme assay in blood.

Hereditary fructose intolerance may present with similar features to galactosaemia at the time of weaning with the first introduction of fructose containing feeds. Patients present with hypoglycaemia, vomiting, progressive liver dysfunction with hepatomegaly, renal tubular damage, and coma. Diagnosis is by demonstration of reducing substance in the urine (fructose) and often by demonstrating the presence of the common A149P mutation in the *aldolase B* gene. Galactosaemia and hereditary fructose intolerance show similar pathologic changes e.g. fatty change in the liver, giant cell transformation, pseudoacinar arrangement of hepatocytes, and cirrhosis.

Fructose-1,6-bisphosphatase deficiency results in severely impaired gluconeogenesis. Neonatal presentation of this disorder follows a precipitous and often lethal course. There is hypoglycaemia, hyperventilation, ketosis, lactic acidosis, apnoea, seizures, and cardiac arrest. However, infants that are rapidly treated with glucose and bicarbonate may then remain symptom-free for weeks or months before having a further attack. Episodes in older infants are often triggered by fasting and febrile episodes. There is frequently mild hepatomegaly and urine organic acids contain glycerol, glycerol-3-phosphate, and 2-ketoglutaric acid. Confirmation is by enzyme assay in liver or by mutation analysis of the *aldolase A gene.*

Glycogen Storage Disease

Glycogen storage disease (GSD) presents invariably either with pathological accumulation of glycogen (e.g. isolated hepatomegaly) and corresponding organ dysfunction (e.g. liver disease / myopathy), or with hypoglycaemia. The enzyme defect is frequently organ-specific and therefore there may be primary hepatopathic, myopathic, or mixed symptoms. The cumulative incidence of GSD is 1:20000. Patients may present in early infancy with hypotonia and severe cardiomyopathy (type II – Pompe) or with hypoglycaemic seizures, recurrent hypoglycaemia with acidosis, truncal obesity, hepatomegaly, nephromegaly, muscle atrophy and bleeding tendency (type I). Infants with type I disease may present in acute hypoglycaemic crisis with lactic acidosis which may rapidly proceed to death. Diagnosis is confirmed by biopsy / enzyme studies or mutation analysis.

References

1. Garrod AE. *Inborn Errors of Metabolism.* Oxford: Oxford University Press 1909.

2. Leonard JV, Morris AAM. Inborn errors of metabolism around the time of birth. *Lancet,* 2000; **356:** 583–7.

3. Sinclair-Smith C, Dinsdale F, Emery J. Evidence of duration and type of illness in children found unexpectedly dead. *Arch Dis Child,* 1976; **51:**424–8.

4. Saudubray J-M, Charpentier C. Clinical phenotypes: diagnosis/algorithms. In: Scriver CR, Beaudet AL, Sly WS, Valle D, eds. *The Metabolic and Molecular Basis of Inherited Disease,* 8th edn. New York: McGraw-Hill, 2000: 1327–403.

5. Munnich A, Rotig A, Cormier-Daire V, Rustin P. Clinical presentation of respiratory chain deficiency. In: Scriver CR, Beaudet AL, Sly WS, Valle D, eds. *The Metabolic and Molecular Basis of Inherited Disease,* 8th edn. New York: Graw-Hill, 2000: 2261–74.

6. Howat AJ, Bennett MJ, Variend S, Shaw L, Engel PC. Defects in the metabolism of fatty acids in Sudden Infant Death Syndrome. *Br Med J,* 1985; **290:**1771–3.

7. Rinaldo P, Yoon HR, Yu C, Raymond K, Tiozzo C, Giordano G. Sudden and unexpected neonatal death: protocol for the post-mortem diagnosis of fatty acid oxidation disorders. *Semin Perinatol,* 1999; **23:**204–10.

8. Arens R, Gozel D, Jain K, Muscati S, Heuser ET, Williams JC et al. Prevalence of medium-chain dehydrogenase deficiency in Sudden Infant Death Syndrome. *J Pediatr,* 1993; **122:**715–18.

9. Boles RG, Buck EA, Blitzer MG, et al. Retrospective biochemical screening of fatty acid oxidation disorders in post-mortem livers of 418 cases of sudden death in the first year of life. *J Pediatr,* 1998; **132**(6):924–33.

10. Chace DH, DiPerna JC, Mitchell BL, Sgroi B, Hofman LF, Naylor EW. Electrospray tandem mass spectrometry for acylcarnitines in dried post-mortem blood specimens collected at autopsy from infants with unexplained cause of death. *Clin Chem,* 2001; **47**(7): 1166–82.

11. Kølvraa S., Gregersen N., Christiensen E., Hobolth N. In vitro fibroblast studies in a patient with C6-C10-dicarboxylic aciduria: evidence of a defect in general acyl-CoA dehydrogenase. *Clin Chin Acta,* 1982; **126:**53–67.

12. Rhead WJ, Amendt BA, Fritchman KS, Felts SJ. Dicarboxylic aciduria: deficient [1-^{14} C] octanoate oxidation and medium chain acyl-CoA dehydrogenase deficiency in fibroblasts. *Science,* 1983; **221:**73–5.

13. Lafolla AK, Thompson RJ, Roe CR. Medium-chain acyl-CoA dehydrogenase deficiency: clinical course in 120 affected children. *J Pediatr,* 1994; **124:**409–15.

14. Andresen BS, Bross P, Udvari S, Kirk J, Gray RGF, Kmock S, et al. The molecular basis of medium-chain acyl-CoA dehydrogenase (MCAD) deficiency in compound heterozygous patients – is there a correlation between genotype and phenotype? *Hum Mol Genet,* 1997; **6:**695–707.

15. Wang SS, Fernhoff PM, Hannon WH, Khoury MJ. Medium chain acyl-CoA dehydrogenase deficiency human genome epidemiology review. *Genet Med,* 1999; **1**(7):332–9.

16. Heales SJR, Thompson GN, Massoud A.F, Rahman S, Halliday D, Leonard JV. Production and disposal of medium-chain fatty acids in children with medium-chain acyl-CoA dehydrogenase deficiency. *J Inher Metab Dis,* 1994; **17**(1):74–80.

17. Fletcher JM, Pitt JJ. Fasting medium chain acyl-CoA dehydrogenase-deficient children can make ketones. *Metabolism*, 2001; **50**(2):161–5.

18. Bennett MJ, Rinaldo P, Strauss AW. Inborn errors of mitochondrial fatty acid oxidation. *Crit Rev Clin Lab Sci*, 2000; **37**(1):1–44.

19. Patterson AL, Henderson MJ, Kumar R. Metabolic autopsy: lessons from an MCAD diagnosis. In: Martin SM, ed.: *Proc ACB National Meeting*, 2003; **70**:59.

20. Brackett JC, Sims HF, Steiner RD, Nunge M, Zimmerman EM, deMartinville B, et al. A novel mutation in medium chain acyl-CoA dehydrogenase causes sudden neonatal death. *J Clin Invest*, 1994; **94**(4):1477–83.

21. Ruitenbeek W, Poelis PJ, Turnbull DM, Garavaglia B, Chalmers RA, Taylor RW, Gabreels FJ. Rhabdomyolysis and acute encephalopathy in late onset medium chain acyl-CoA dehydrogenase deficiency. *J Neurol Neurosurg Psych*, 1995; **58**(2):209–14.

22. Rinaldo P, Raymond K, Barnes CA. Medium chain acyl-CoA dehydrogenase deficiency: Sudden and unexpected death of a 45-year-old woman. *J Inher Metab Dis*, 1999; **22**:104.

23. Gregerson N, Blakemore A, Winter V, Andresen BS, Kølvraa S, Bolund L, et al. Specific diagnosis of medium chain acyl-CoA dehydrogenase (MCAD) deficiency in dried blood spots by a polymerase chain reaction (PCR) assay detecting a point mutation (G985) in the MCAD gene. *Clin Chim Acta*, 1991; **203**:23–34.

24. Saudubray JM, Martin D, de Lonlay P, Touati G, Poggi-Travert F, Bonnet D, et al. Recognition and management of fatty acid oxidation defects: a series of 107 patients. *J Inher Metab Dis*, 1999; **22**:448–502.

25. Pollitt RJ, Olpin SE, Bonham JR, Cahalane SF, Naughten E. Late-presenting carnitine transport defect. *Enzyme and Protein*, 1993; **3**:175.

26. Maestri NE, Clissold DB, Brusilow S. Neonatal onset ornithine transcarbamylase deficiency: A retrospective analysis. *J Pediatr*, 1999; **134**(3):268–72.

27. Hudak ML, Jones MD, Brusilow SW. Differentiation of transient hyperammonaemia of the newborn and urea cycle enzyme defects by clinical presentation. *J Pediatr*, 1985; **107**:712–19.

35

Causes of Sudden Unexpected Death in Infancy (Other than SIDS)

Irene Scheimberg and Phillip Cox

Introduction

Sudden unexpected death in infancy (SUDI) has an incidence of 0.5 per 1000 live births[1] every year. In the UK the death is likely to be investigated through the legal (coronial/fiscal) route and a specialist autopsy will be undertaken following a detailed national protocol.[2] A specific cause of death is identified in approximately 30% of cases.[3]

Explained Natural Infant Death

A specific cause of death is found more frequently in neonates than in babies between 1 month and 1 year of age and in previously unwell babies compared to those that have been previously asymptomatic.

The most common specific causes of infant death have either an infective or a cardiac origin. Diseases of other systems may also result in sudden death in infancy, and the list of possible causes is very long.[4] Many babies present a combination of causes, particularly those with congenital conditions, some of which are only diagnosed after birth. Metabolic diseases are being diagnosed more frequently, especially when the appropriate samples are taken (See Chapter 18 and Chapter 34). Other causes include poisoning (intentional and accidental) (See Chapter 17) and unwitnessed accidents (See Chapter 36).

Infection

Bacterial infection is a common cause of death in infancy accounting for up to one-quarter of postneonatal infant deaths. Overwhelming pneumonia, septicaemia, and meningitis should be considered in cases of SUDI. Group B Streptococcus (GBS), Pneumococcus, and Meningococcus are common isolates and can lead to very rapidly progressive infection in previously healthy babies. In sepsis, disseminated intravascular coagulopathy (DIC) and acute tubular necrosis (ATN) may be identified (Figure 35.1a & b & c). In a recent study 11% of cases of sudden unexpected death in infancy (SUDI) were attributed to an infectious cause after bacteriology studies were done.[5] Infants who died of a bacterial infection were older than those whose death was unexplained. The commonest pathogen identified was *Staphylococcus aureus*, followed by *Streptococcus pneumoniae*, *ß-haemolitic Streptococcus*, and *Escherichia coli*.

Infants with bacterial pneumonia may present with non-specific symptoms of mild fever and malaise or may have minor respiratory symptoms. Inflammation may not be histologically prominent in the early stages and there may just be an eosinophilic exudate containing bacteria with scanty neutrophils. Bronchopneumonia with multiple foci in all lobes is more common than lobar pneumonia (Figure 35.2a and b). Necrotising pseudomonas pneumonia may be seen (Figure 35.3a and b).

Epiglottitis due to *Haemophilus influenzae* was once fairly common, but since the advent of the Hib immunisation it is now rare in the UK. Whooping cough (*Bordetella pertussis)* infection in unimmunised infants can be particularly severe and presents atypically without the classical cough, with a high fever, a non-specific respiratory illness, and an extremely high white-cell count. At autopsy, inflammation in the lungs may be relatively mild, but there is alveolar epithelial necrosis and there is typically profound depletion of the lymphoid tissues[6] (Figure 35.4a and b).

Primary septicaemia may result from infection with *GBS, Pneumococcus, Meningococcus, Group A Streptococcus*, and occasionally other organisms. In these cases, the origin of infection may not be found. Infants with asplenia are particularly prone to pneumococcal septicaemia. Babies with functional asplenia may be well until a fatal episode of sepsis.[7] Right atrial isomerism is accompanied by asplenia and these infants are at risk of developing fulminant sepsis.[8] Many severe infections may be associated with haemophagocytosis[9] (Figure 35.5).

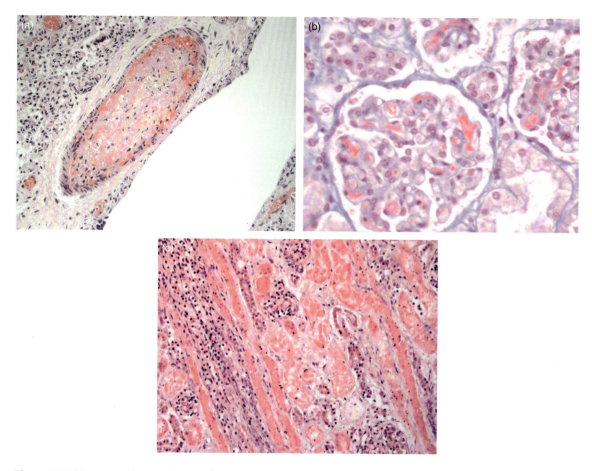

Figure 35.1 Disseminated intravascular coagulopathy (DIC) and acute tubular necrosis (ATN) in sepsis: 1a) Large thrombus in a lung blood vessel as seen in routine H&E stain. 1b) MSB (Martius Scarlet Blue) stain helps to diagnose small thrombi in renal capillaries. 1c) ATN can be diagnosed at post-mortem. Notice the tubular cells shedding into the lumen and the lack of post-mortem autolysis in surrounding tubules.

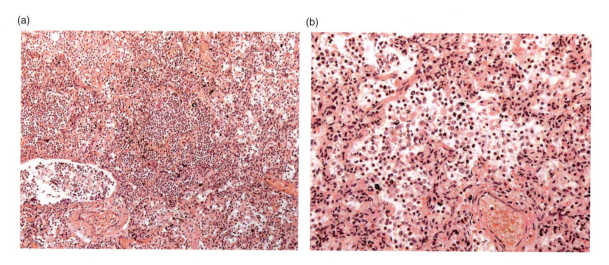

Figure 35.2a and b Low- and high-power view of bronchopneumonia showing numerous neutrophils in the alveolar lumina. On high-power view some macrophages are also present suggesting that the inflammation has been present for more than 24 hours.

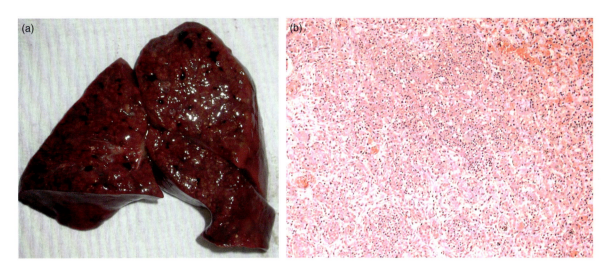

Figure 35.3 a) Gross picture of necrotising pneumonia; (note the multiple cream-coloured dots on the cut surface.) On histology alveolar wall necrosis is appreciated together with acute inflammation.

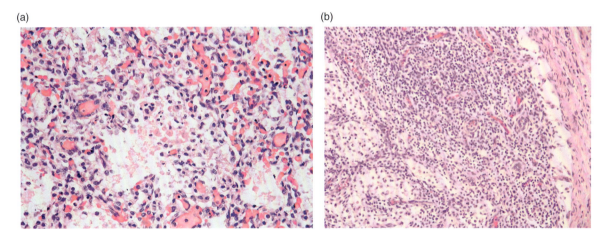

Figure 35.4 Pertussis infection. a) Lung showing alveoli with scanty inflammatory cells, apoptotic cells, and sloughing material in the lumen. b) Depleted lymph node, typical of pertussis infection in very young, non-immunised infants.

Other rare respiratory infective causes of sudden death in infants include retropharyngeal abscess;[10] and bacterial tonsillitis caused by *Clostridium perfringens* (reported in a 9-month-old baby who was found unresponsive).[11] One of the authors had a case of pseudomembranous colitis (Figure 35.6 a–d) in a 4-month-old baby.

Bacterial meningitis is an important cause of neonatal morbidity and mortality. Both neonates and older infants generally show non-specific symptoms and the typical rash of meningococcal infection (Figure 35.7) is not always present. The most common

organisms that produce bacterial meningitis in infants are *Streptococcus pneumoniae* and *Neisseria meningitidis* followed by *Haemophilus influenzae*. At post-mortem, while some cases show obvious inflammation on the surface (Figure 35.8a and b) in others the inflammatory response is poorly developed and indistinct, particularly in fulminant infection. There is frequently bilateral adrenal haemorrhage (Figure 35.8c), particularly with meningococcal but also with *Haemophilus* or pneumococcal infection. In neonates the most common organism is group B Streptococcus (*Streptococcus agalactiae*); coagulase

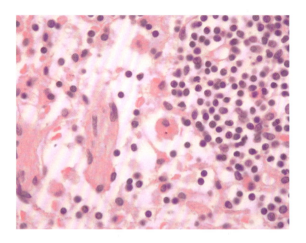

Figure 35.5 Bone marrow showing a macrophage engulfing an erythrocyte in a case of severe viral infection

negative Staphylococcus may also cause meningitis in neonates. The microorganism is isolated from blood and CSF.

Peritonitis may also occasionally present as sudden death in a child with vague symptoms. These infants usually have an underlying pathology including meconium ileus, intussusception, congenital bands, necrotising enterocolitis, volvulus, Hirschsprung's disease, etc.[12] Patients with asplenia may develop primary peritonitis due to pneumococcal infection.

Many cases of SUDI/SUID show positive bacterial cultures, particularly in samples taken at post-mortem (see Chapter 16). Frequently there is more than one organism and there is no histological evidence of infection. On the whole, mixed cultures are likely to be due to post-mortem bacterial overgrowth or contamination. In some cases, a pure growth of a single

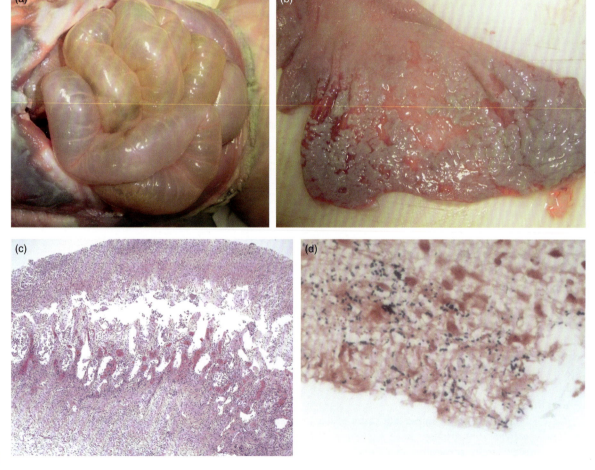

Figure 35.6 .Pseudomembranous colitis in a 4-month-old baby. a) Distended abdomen due to gas in the small intestine. b) The colon was covered by a patchy pseudomembrane. c) This is clearly appreciated in a low-power view where a pseudomembrane is present over necrotic mucosa. d) *Clostridium difficile* organisms are appreciated on gram stain.

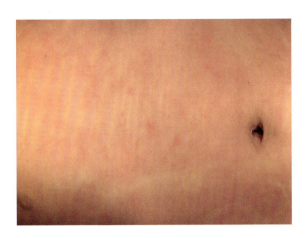

Figure 35.7 Typical rash of meningitis

pathogen is isolated. These cases require careful evaluation together with clinical colleagues, to try to determine whether death should be attributed to overwhelming infection or should be regarded as SIDS/unascertained.[13]

Although less frequent, viral infections may cause sudden death in infants, particularly viral myocarditis (Figure 35.9a and b). Myocarditis, pneumonitis, and encephalitis may all be fatal. Myocarditis may be acquired congenitally or after birth. Congenital myocarditis is most frequently due to enteroviruses, in particular type B coxsackievirus, and the organism may be detected by PCR; these babies often have myocarditis with encephalitis and it is important to sample the brain and brainstem in suspicious cases (Figure 35.10a and b). Maternal symptoms may have been minimal and the

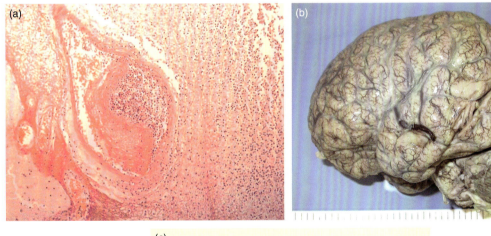

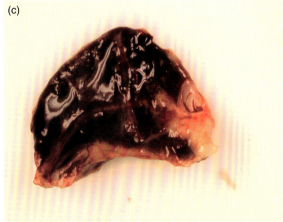

Figure 35.8 Meningococcal meningitis. a) The purulent exudate may be obvious as in this case. b) On histology the meninges show severe acute inflammation and there is an inflammatory thrombus in a bridging vein. c) Frequently there is complete haemorrhagic necrosis of the adrenals (Waterhouse-Friedrichsen syndrome).

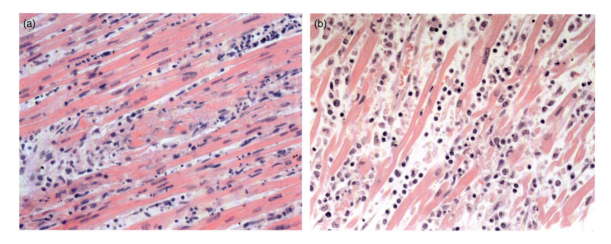

Figure 35.9 a and b. Viral myocarditis showing a lymphocytic infiltrate of the heart together with myocyte necrosis.

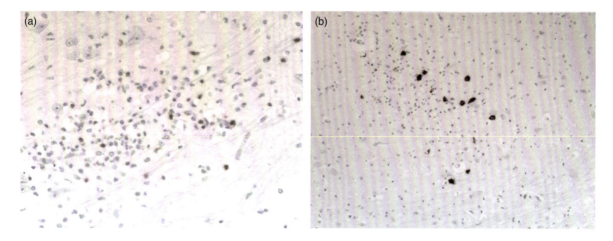

Figure 35.10 a and b. T and B lymphocytes as evidenced by CD3 and CD20 stains are seen in the brainstem of a baby with encephalomyocarditis

baby may appear non-specifically unwell, prior to its collapse in the first few weeks of life. Enteroviruses may also lead to myocarditis in later infancy, along with a host of other viruses, bacteria, and other organisms. Post-neonatal myocarditis in infants can present as sudden death. The gross findings are usually non-specific and the heart may appear normal macroscopically, therefore histology is mandatory. Both ventricles and the septum should be sampled; some authors suggest that multiple samples from each ventricle and the septum should be taken.[14] Histologically, myocardiocyte damage and an inflammatory infiltrate are seen.[15] Coxsackie and adenoviruses are the main causes, although other viruses such as cytomegalovirus (CMV) have been reported in infants[16] and parvovirus B19 has been reported in older children.

Interstitial pneumonitis is usually caused by viruses and is generally self-limiting. Viral pneumonitis, e.g. respiratory syncytial virus (RSV), is generally symptomatic, although carers, and health professionals may not appreciate the child's grave condition until it is too late. RSV may lead to apnoea in very young infants, in particular those born prematurely and with predisposing conditions such as cardiac disease.[17] Occasional overwhelming, rapidly progressive viral infections do occur, particularly with enteroviruses and adenovirus[18], and also with influenza viruses such as the H1N1 strain.[19]

Viral encephalitis is usually symptomatic, but the baby may die before reaching hospital, having been non-specifically unwell. Viral encephalitis is particularly difficult to diagnose in children with immunodeficiencies.[20] Herpes simplex is commonest after six months of age, while enteroviruses predominate in the first three months of life. Other herpes viruses, adenovirus, measles, mumps, and rubella may all also be implicated.[21] Acute encephalitis may lead to sudden collapse, through involvement of vital structures in the brainstem.

Gastroenteritis may cause death as a result of dehydration, which may not be appreciated by the family, or rarely due to septicaemia. There are always preceding symptoms of vomiting and /or diarrhoea. Hyponatraemia can result from replacement of lost fluid with water rather than electrolyte solution.

In cases of overwhelming infection, in particular viral, and pneumococcal infection, the possibility of an underlying congenital or acquired immune deficit should always be considered. Immunodeficiency syndromes should also be considered in the presence of disseminated BCGitis/BCGosis (Figure 35.11a–d).[22] Ancillary techniques will be helpful in these circumstances although the diagnosis of the type of immunodeficiency may be difficult after death.

Cardiac Disease

Cardiac disease accounts for around 10% of sudden deaths in the first year of life.[23]

Viral myocarditis has been already discussed. Eosinophilic myocarditis may occur in association with drug toxicity, infections, or hypereosinophilic syndrome (Figure 35.12).[24]

Despite advances in antenatal screening, undiagnosed congenital heart malformations remain a common cause of death in the first week of life. Affected babies are often poor feeders and parents

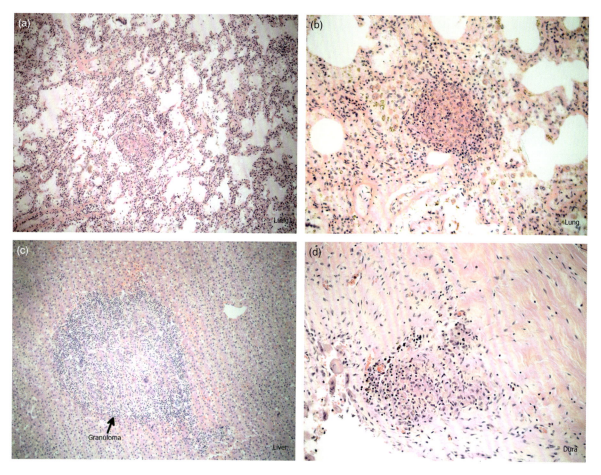

Figure 35.11 A case of BCGosis. a and b) low- and high-power view of a granuloma in the lung. There were also granulomas in the liver (c) and the duramater (d).

225

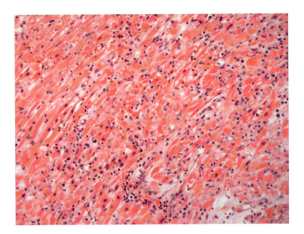

Figure 35.12 Myocardium infiltrated by lymphocyte and large number of eosinophils in a case of eosinophilic myocarditis.

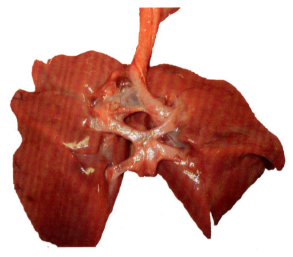

Figure 35.13 Total anomalous pulmonary venous return with confluence of the pulmonary veins in a vein draining in the inferior vena cava just above the diaphragm.

may observe that they are 'not quite right'. Death is frequently an observed collapse, rather than a 'cot death'. Cases may occasionally present later. The oldest child in the authors' experience was 19 months old when she died from undiagnosed Fallot tetralogy. Common lesions include: truncus arteriosus (single arterial trunk), transposition of the great arteries, aortic stenosis/atresia and other causes of hypoplastic left ventricle>. Total anomalous pulmonary venous return may also result in sudden collapse and death, as in a one-month-old baby examined recently by one of the authors (Figure 35.13). Anomalous origin of one or more coronary arteries is a recognised cause of sudden collapse. This may occur in association with congenital heart disease but

may be an isolated finding and grossly may mimic cardiomyopathy. Fibromuscular dysplasia of the arteries is another rare condition which may present as sudden collapse due to coronary ischaemia, or as a result of unrecognised, severe hypertension due to renal damage (Figure 35.14a and b). The vascular change affects many organs and is often focal and segmental.

Infantile cardiomyopathy may be hypertrophic or dilated and is also a cause of SUDI, again usually as an observed collapse. Many cases are due to abnormalities involving a wide range of genes affecting cardiac function. The possibility of an underlying metabolic

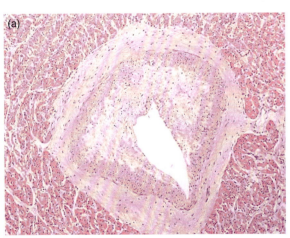

(a)

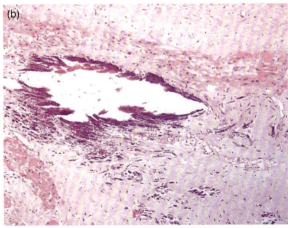

(b)

Figure 35.14 a and b. Fibromuscular dysplasia of the coronary arteries in a 10-week-old baby showing medial dysplasia with reduction of the artery lumen and dystrophic calcification in the heart.

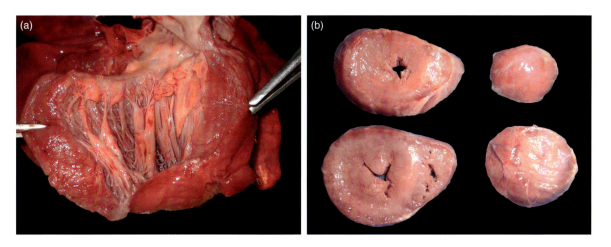

Figure 35.15 a and b. Hypertrophic cardiomyopathy in an 11-month-old baby with Noonan Syndrome

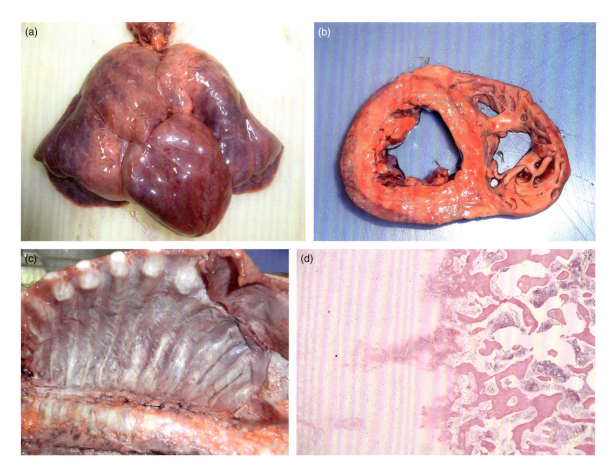

Figure 35.16 Dilated cardiomyopathy in vitamin D deficiency. a and b) The heart was enlarged and the left ventricle wall was very thin. c) A rickety rosary is seen in the inside of the rib cage; this was not seen before opening the chest. d) Histology of the rib shows the typical changes of rickets with increased hypertrophic chondrocyte layer and irregular growth plate.

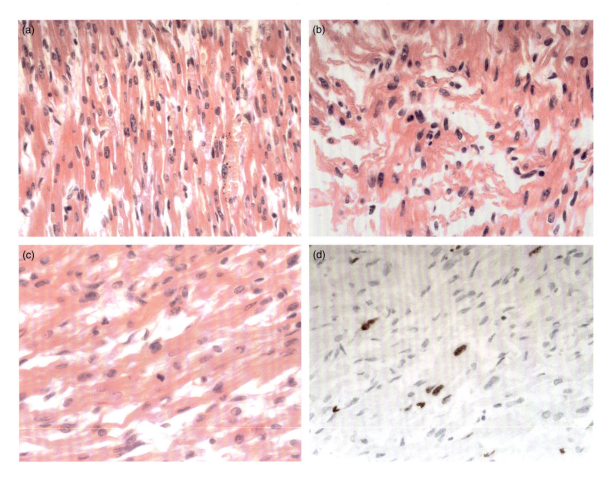

Figure 35.17 Mitogenic cardiomyopathy showing typical histological changes in a neonate: a) cigar-shaped nuclei, b) binucleated cells and c) a mitosis. d) Positive Ki67 stain reflects the mitotic activity.

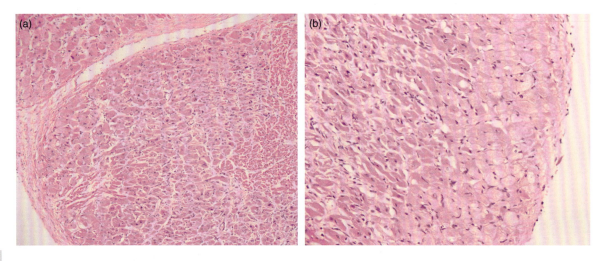

Figure 35.18 a and b. Low- and high-power view of histiocytic cardiomyopathy. The oncocytic cells are clearly differentiated from the normal myocardiocytes.

(e.g. glycogen storage disease, LCHAD) or mitochondrial disease should be considered and appropriate samples taken (see Chapter 18). Noonan syndrome typically had hypertrophic cardiomyopathy (Figure 35.15a and b). Severe vitamin D deficiency may produce dilated cardiomyopathy and if not diagnosed, may be a cause of sudden death in infancy (Figure 35.16a–d).[25] Another rare form of neonatal cardiomyopathy recently described is mitogenic cardiomyopathy (Figure 35.17 a–d).[26]

Oncocytic (histiocytoid) (Figure 35.18 a and b) cardiomyopathy may be focal, and therefore several samples of myocardium should be taken. This is thought to be an abnormality of the conduction tissue, although some cases show mutations in mitochondrial DNA.[27] Endocardial fibroelastosis (dilated cardiomyopathy with biventricular fibroelastic thickening of the endocardium) typically presents as fetal hydrops, but occasional cases may lead to SUDI/SUID (Figure 35.19). The cause of this disorder is uncertain, but metabolic disease should be considered, and there is an association with maternal autoimmune disease, in particular anti-Ro and anti-La antibodies.[28,29]

Cardiac tumours may lead to arrhythmias and severe cardiac enlargement. Multiple rhabdomyomas are the commonest cardiac tumour and raise the possibility of tuberous sclerosis. Other cardiac tumours causing SUDI/SUID are fibromas, myxomas, myofibroblastic sarcoma, and angiomyoma (Figure 35.20a and b).[30]

Long QT syndrome (LQTS) refers to a group of disorders characterised by prolongation of the QT interval in the ECG due to delayed cardiac repolarisation as a result of mutations in genes coding for cardiac ion channels and may be inherited or de novo. See also Chapters 28 and 29. LQTS was first implicated in infant death by Schwartz et al. after a retrospective study of more than 30,000 newborns.[31] It has been suggested that up to 5% of sudden infant deaths are due to LQTS mutations. Catecholaminergic polymorphic ventricular tachycardia has also been diagnosed in cases of sudden death in infancy.[32] These disorders are unlikely to be recognised in infants unless there is a family history. Diagnosis at PM is problematic as there are no gross or microscopic findings. It is therefore

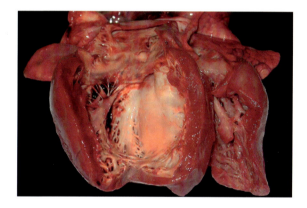

Figure 35.19 Endocardial fibroelastosis showing a pearly white fibrosed endocardium.

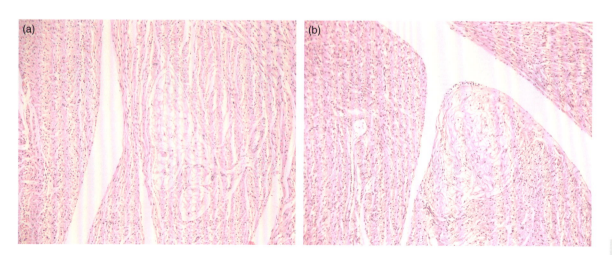

Figure 35.20 a and b. Multiple small rhabdomyomas in the heart of a child with no other features of tuberous sclerosis.

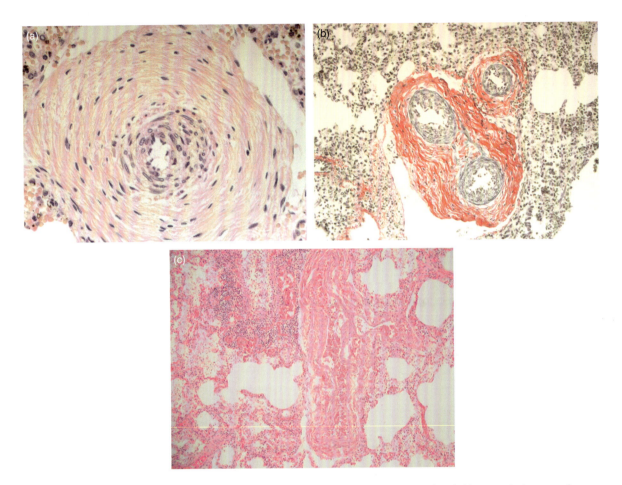

Figure 35.21 .Pulmonary arterial disease. a) pulmonary artery showing adventitial thickening and medial hypertrophy in a case of unexplained pulmonary hypertension in a 4-month-old infant; b) EVG stain confirms adventitial fibrosis and medial hypertrophy; c) thin-walled, dilated pulmonary artery in a 6-month-old with (subsequently) genetically confirmed Williams syndrome who collapsed and died suddenly.

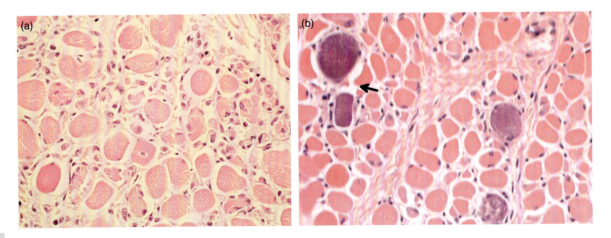

Figure 35.22 .Diaphragmatic myositis. a) active myositis in the diaphragm of a 15-month-old who collapsed and died; b) ongoing myocyte damage in the diaphragm with calcification of muscle fibres in a 9-month-old found dead in his cot.

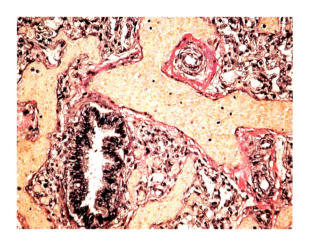

Figure 35.23 .Misalignment of blood vessels in the lung. EVG stains highlights the presence of a vein adjacent to a pulmonary artery and a bronchus.

important to store appropriate tissue for DNA testing; if suspected, and especially if confirmed, family members should be offered ECG screening.

Respiratory Tract

Infections of the respiratory tract have been discussed above. Structural malformations of the upper airways may be associated with respiratory obstruction. Disorders include choanal atresia, laryngomalacia, and tracheomalacia. Noisy breathing/stridor may be apparent and the condition may be exacerbated by concurrent respiratory infection. A careful examination of the respiratory tract is essential.[33] Infants with Pierre Robin syndrome may die suddenly and unexpectedly, although the majority have associated malformations.[34]

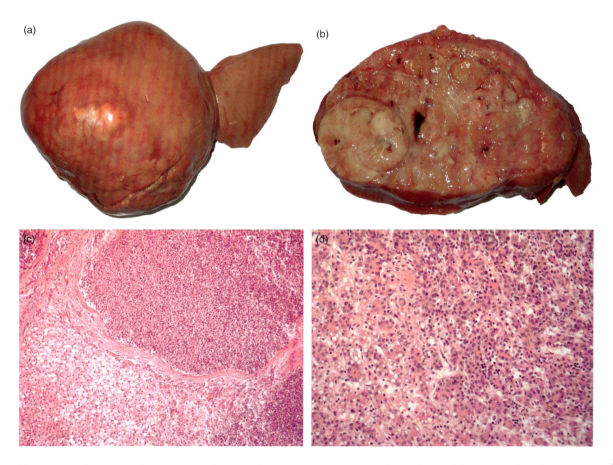

Figure 35.24 .Undiagnosed hepatoblastoma in a 6-month-old baby: a) liver with a large tumour in the inferior aspect; b) slice of liver through the tumour; c) low power view showing the interface between fetal and embryonal differentiation which can also be appreciated on high power (d).

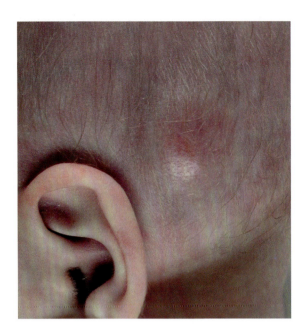

Figure 35.25 .Nodule on the scalp of a 6-week-old infant found dead in her cot, after a short illness. Histology showed juvenile myelomonocytic leukaemia. There was leukostasis in the cerebral vessels.

Pulmonary vascular disease (Figure 35.21 a–c) is difficult to diagnose in early infancy while vascular remodelling is taking place. It is typically associated with congenital heart disease but may occur in isolation, or in association with other syndromes, e.g.

Smith-Lemli-Opitz syndrome. Williams syndrome is associated with supravalvular aortic stenosis and abnormal peripheral pulmonary vessels and sudden death may result. Histological examination of the lungs may demonstrate abnormalities in the blood vessels causing sudden death[35] (Figure 35.22 a and b). In the neonatal period intractable pulmonary hypertension may be due to alveolar-capillary dysplasia[36] (Figure 35.23).

Respiratory failure may result from neuromuscular disease, including congenital myopathies, polymyositis, viral myositis, and anterior horn cell disease. These may be first diagnosed at post-mortem and disease may be confined to the diaphragm (Figure 35.22a and b).[37]

Solid Tumours and Haematological Malignancies

Various tumours may be associated with SUDI. In addition to cardiac tumours (see above), various other undiagnosed tumours have been reported in cases of sudden death. Brain tumours may occasionally present as sudden death although they tend to occur in older children. The authors have personally seen an undiagnosed hepatoblastoma in a 6-month-old baby (Figure 35.24 a–d),[38] juvenile myelomonocytic leukaemia (Figure 35.25) (unpublished) and two cases of hepatic haemangioendothelioma have been reported.[39] Other solid tumours reported as cause of sudden death in infancy are an oligondendroglioma,[40]

(a)

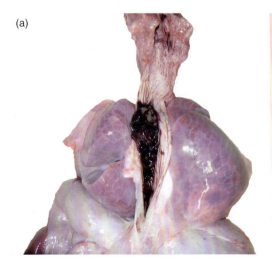

(b)

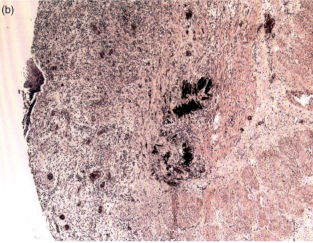

Figure 35.26 a) swallowed battery surrounded by haemorrhage stuck at the level where the oesophagus and aortic arch are adjacent to each other. b) Histology at the level of the perforation shows active chronic inflammation and calcification.

a congenital mesoblastic nephroma, a pleuropulmonary blastoma, and a malignant haemangioendothelioma.[40]

Haematological malignancies have also been described as cause of sudden death in infancy, including B cell acute lymphoblastic leukaemia and acute myelogenous leukaemia.[41]

Miscellaneous

Epileptic seizures in infants with known epilepsy may result in sudden, unobserved death. Typical features may not be apparent at post-mortem. Death is more likely in infants with underlying neurodevelopmental disease than with idiopathic epilepsy.[42] Dravet syndrome has been reported as a cause of sudden death in older children and one of the authors has encountered a case in a one-year-old.[43] Samples should be taken for anticonvulsant levels.

Children may accidentally swallow small batteries without having immediate symptoms and if the battery lodges in the upper oesophagus adjacent to the aortic arch or to a pulmonary vessel, they may exsanguinate through the erosion caused by the alkaline perforation (Figure 35.26a and b).

Conclusion

The range of possible causes of sudden unexpected death in infancy is very wide. As a result, an extensive autopsy examination needs to be undertaken by a pathologist with wide experience of paediatric disease. When providing a cause of death, it is important to correlate the findings with the known clinical circumstances.

References

1. Corbin T. Investigation into sudden infant deaths and unascertained deaths in England and Wales, 1995–2003. *Health Stat Q*, 2005; **27**:16–23.

2. *Sudden Unexpected Death in Infancy; A Multi-agency Protocol for Care and Investigation*. London: Royal College of Pathologists, Royal College of Paediatrics, and Child Health. 2004; https://www.rcpath.org and https://www.rcpch.ac.uk/ (accessed 30 October 2018).

3. Weber MA, Pryce JW, Ashworth MT, et al. Histological examination in sudden unexpected death in infancy: evidence base for histological sampling. *J Clin Pathol*, 2012; **65**(1):58–63.

4. Howatson AG. The autopsy for sudden unexpected death in infancy. *Curr Diagn Pathol*, 2006; **12**:173–83.

5. Weber MA, Klein NJ, Hartley JC, et al. Infection and sudden unexpected death in infancy: a systematic retrospective case review. *Lancet*, 2008; **371**:1848–53.

6. Sawal M, Cohen MC, Irazuzta JE, et al. Fulminant pertussis: a multi-center study with new insights into the clinico-pathological mechanisms. *Pediatr Pulmonol*, 2009; **44**(10):970–80.

7. Angelski CL, McKay E, Blackie B. A case of functional asplenia and pneumococcal sepsis. *Pediatr Emerg Care*, 2011; **27**(7):639–41.

8. Chiu SN, Shao PL, Wang JK, et al. Severe bacterial infection in patients with heterotaxy syndrome. *J Pediatr*, 2014; **164**(1):99–104.

9. Rameshkumar R, Krishnamurthy S, Ganesh RN, Mahadevan S, Narayanan P, Satheesh P, Jain P. Histopathological changes in septic acute kidney injury in critically ill children: a cohort of post-mortem renal biopsies. *Clin Exp Nephrol*, 2017; **21**(6):1075–82.

10. Coutlhard M, Issacs D. Retropharyngeal abscess. *Arch Dis Child*, 1991; **66**:1227–30.

11. Gerber JE. Acute necrotizing bacterial tonsillitis with Clostridium perfringens. *Am J Forensic Med Pathol*, 2001; **22**(2):177–9.

12. Peres LC, Cohen MC. Sudden unexpected early neonatal death due to undiagnosed Hirschsprung disease enterocolitis: a report of two cases and literature review. *Forensic Sci Med Pathol*, 2013; **9**(4): 558–63.

13. Prtak L, Al-Adnani M, Fenton P, et al. Contribution of bacteriology and virology in sudden unexpected death in infancy. *Arch Dis Child*, 2010; **95**(5):371–6.

14. Inwald D, Franklin O, Cubitt D, et al. Enterovirus myocarditis as a cause of neonatal collapse. *Arch Dis Child Fetal Neonatal Ed*, 2004; **89**:F461–2.

15. Dettmeyer R, Baasner A, Haag C, et al. Immunohistochemical and molecular-pathological diagnosis of myocarditis in cases of suspected Sudden Infant Death Syndrome (SIDS)–a multicenter study. *Leg Med (Tokyo)*, 2009; **11**(Suppl 1):S124–7.

16. Weber MA, Ashworth MT, Risdon RA, et al. Clinicopathological features of paediatric deaths due to myocarditis: an autopsy series. *Arch Dis Child*, 2008; **93**;594–8.

17. Pickens DL, Schefft GL, Storch GA, Thach BT. Characterization of prolonged apneic episodes associated with respiratory syncytial virus infection. *Pediatr Pulmonol*, 1989; **6**:195–201.

18. Dettmeyer R, Sperhake JP, Müller J, Madea B. Cytomegalovirus-induced pneumonia and myocarditis in three cases of suspected Sudden Infant Death Syndrome (SIDS): Diagnosis by immunohistochemical techniques and molecular pathologic methods. *Forens Sci Internat*, 2008; **174**:229–33.

19. Bhat N, Wright JG, Broder KR, et al. Influenza-associated deaths among children in the United States, 2003–2004. *N Engl J Med*, 2005; **353**(24):2559–67.

20. Morfopoulou S, Brown JR, Davies EG, et al. Human coronavirus OC43 associated with fatal encephalitis. *N Engl J Med*, 2016; **375**(5):497–8.

21. Modlin JF. Perinatal echovirus and group B coxsackievirus infections. *Clin Perinatol*, 1988; **15**:233–46.

22. Kourime M, Akpalu EN, Ouair H, et al. BCGitis/BCGosis in children: diagnosis, classification and exploration. *Arch Pediatr*, 2016; **23**(7):754–9.

23. Pryce JW, Weber MA, Ashworth MT, et al. Changing patterns of infant death over the last 100 years: autopsy experience from a specialist children's hospital. *J R Soc Med*, 2012; **105**(3):123–30.

24. Krous HF, Haaas E, Chadwick AE, Wagner GN. Sudden death in a neonate associated with idiopathic eosinophilic myocarditis. *Pediatr Dev Pathol*, 2005; **8**:587–92.

25. Scheimberg I, Perry L. Does low vitamin D have a role in pediatric morbidity and mortality? An observational study of vitamin D in a cohort of 52 postmortem examinations. *Pediatr Dev Pathol*, 2014; **17**(6):455–64.

26. Chang KT, Taylor GP, Meschino WS, Kantor PF, Cutz E. Mitogenic cardiomyopathy: a lethal neonatal familial dilated cardiomyopathy characterized by myocyte hyperplasia and proliferation. *Hum Pathol*, 2010; **41**(7):1002–8.

27. Andreu AL, Checcarelli N, Iwata S, Shanske S, DiMauro S. A missense mutation in the mitochondrial cytochrome b gene in a revisited case with histiocytoid cardiomyopathy. *Pediatr Res*, 2000; **48**:311–14.

28. Bennett MJ, Hale DE, Pollitt RJ, Stanley CA, Variend S. Endocardial fibroelastosis and primary carnitine deficiency due to a defect in the plasma membrane carnitine transporter. *Clin Cardiol*, 1996; **19**:243–6.

29. Nield LE, Silverman ED, Taylor GP, et al. Maternal Anti-Ro and Anti-La Antibody–Associated Endocardial Fibroelastosis. *Circulation*, 2002; **105**; 843–8.

30. Bryant VA, Booth J, Palm L, et al. Childhood neoplasms presenting at autopsy: a 20-year experience. *Pediatr Blood Cancer*, 2017; **64**(9):e26474; https://onlinelibrary.wiley.com/doi/abs/10.1002/pbc.26474 (accessed 31 October 2018).

31. Schwartz PJ, Stramba-Badiale M, Segantini A, et al. Prolongation of the QT interval and the Sudden Infant Death Syndrome. *N Engl J Med*, 1998; **338**:1709–14.

32. Tester DJ, Dura M, Carturan E, et al. A mechanism for Sudden Infant Death Syndrome (SIDS): stress-induced leak via ryanodine receptors. *Heart Rhythm*, 2007; **4**:733–9.

33. Sivan Y, Ben-Ari J, Schonfeld TM. Laryngomalacia: a cause for early near miss for SIDS. *Int J Pediatr Otorhinolaryngol*, 1991; **21**:59–64.

34. Costa MA, Tu MM, Murage KP, et al. Robin sequence: mortality, causes of death, and clinical outcomes. *Plast Reconstr Surg*, 2014; **134**(4):738–45.

35. Khairul Z, Kirsten H, Nicholson AG, Cohen MC. Abnormal Muscularization of Intra Acinar Pulmonary Arteries in 2 Cases Presenting as Sudden Infant Death (SIDS). *Pediatr Dev Pathol*, 2017; **20**(1):49–53.

36. Hung SP, Huang SH, Wu CH, et al. Misalignment of lung vessels and alveolar-capillary dysplasia: a case report with autopsy. *Pediatr Neonatol*, 2011; **52**(4): 232–6.

37. Sundararajan S, Ostojic NS, Rushton DI, Cox PM, Acland P. Diaphragmatic pathology: a cause of clinically unexplained death in the perinatal/paediatric age group. *Med Sci Law*, 2005; **45**:110–14.

38. Pryce J, Kiho L, Scheimberg I. Sudden unexpected death in infancy associated with an epithelial-type hepatoblastoma in a 6-month-old infant. *Pediatr Dev Pathol*, 2010; **13**(4): 338–40.

39. Lunetta P1, Karikoski R, Penttilä A, Sajantila A. Sudden death associated with a multifocal type II hemangioendothelioma of the liver in a 3-month-old infant. *Am J Forensic Med Pathol*, 2004; **25**(1):56–9.

40. Rajs J, Råsten-Almqvist P, Nennesmo I. Unexpected death in two young infants mimics SIDS: autopsies demonstrate tumors of medulla and heart. *Am J Forensic Med Pathol*, 1997; **18**(4):384–90.

41. Somers GR, Smith CR, Perrin DG, Wilson GJ, Taylor GP. Sudden unexpected death in infancy and childhood due to undiagnosed neoplasia: an autopsy study. *Am J Forensic Med Pathol*, 2006; **27**(1):64–9.

42. Callenbach PM, Westendorp RG, Geerts AT, et al. Mortality risk in children with epilepsy: the Dutch study of epilepsy in childhood. *Pediatrics*, 2001; **107**:1259–63.

43. Cooper MS, Mcintosh A, Crompton DE, McMahon JM, Schneider A, Farrell K, et al. Mortality in Dravet syndrome. *Epilepsy Res*, 2016; **128**:43–7.

Chapter 36

Forensic Pathology Aspects of Sudden Unexpected Death in Infancy and Childhood

Michael J. Shkrum and David A. Ramsay

Introduction

A 3-month-old previously healthy infant was breastfed and fell asleep on her mother's arm. When the mother awoke six hours later, the baby was dead. Froth was observed around her mouth, and her hands were clenched. An inquest was held. A witness testified that 'it had all the appearance of having died in a fit'. According to the local newspaper, there was neither medical evidence nor post-mortem findings to explain the infant's death. The inquest jury's verdict was: 'Died by the visitation of God of convulsion fits'.

This case was cited in an editorial entitled 'Death by 'The Visitation of God'' – published in Lancet in 1874.[1] The writer's opinion was that, 'Death by the visitation of God' was a verdict that should not be used. Regarding inquest verdicts, the editorial continued,

> their verdicts ... should, if possible, contain some statements which are comprehensible to our understanding, and therefore the less they have to do with the inscrutable and the unseen the better. If post-mortem examinations be made by properly skilled persons a failure to find a proximate cause of death will very rarely take place, and, in our judgement, no coroner should leave a stone unturned for the discovery of the same.

The investigation of sudden infant deaths has evolved beyond evoking divine intervention as an explanation. A thorough case investigation includes assessment of the death scene and an autopsy. The latter incorporates radiography, toxicology, and other ancillary studies.[2–4] The challenge for pathologists remains in distinguishing natural deaths from those occurring by unnatural means. The reality is that a cause and manner of death remain elusive in many of these cases.

The purpose of this chapter is to describe 'suspicious' autopsy findings that may be uncovered during the post-mortem investigation of infants who appear at first sight to have died suddenly and unexpectedly. Such findings either can be injury mimics due to artefacts, normal variants, trivial incidental phenomena of no relevance to the cause of death and disease, or raise the definite possibility of inflicted injuries and therefore a 'non-accidental' death. The way in which 'suspicious' findings fit the general context of similar findings in cases of non-accidental injuries will also be described.

Although this chapter is primarily concerned with post-mortem findings, the clinical, and imaging literature is a useful source of information about the characteristics of the findings under discussion. The clinical perspective is relevant to the pathologist particularly if an infant has been assessed during hospitalisation. Radiological principles will become increasingly germane for the pathologist because of the increasing use of post-mortem CT and MRI scanning to replace or supplement the autopsy. However, the clinical perspective is derived from both surviving and fatal cases, and thus will often be based on cases with less severe injuries than a pathologist will encounter.

There are many controversial issues that arise in paediatric forensic pathology and 'gold diagnostic standards' are lacking in many situations. This is particularly problematic in the literature on non-accidental or inflicted injuries. For example, problems of etiological ascertainment lie at the heart of the controversy about the so-called 'shaken baby syndrome' in which the triad of retinal haemorrhages, thin-film subdural bleeding and encephalopathy are commonly attributed to a blunt force acceleration head injury despite the lack of specific evidence of trauma (i.e., scalp bruises, and skull fractures). In these and other circumstances, the determination of the cause of suspicious injuries and death frequently rests on the opinion of the experts involved in the case and/or the judgement of a court of law.

235

Classification of Sudden Infant Deaths

Certification of sudden unexpected deaths in infancy is an ongoing issue affecting epidemiological studies and other research because of the lack of a standardised classification of these deaths and different interpretations of existing classifications.[2–4] Classifications applied to these cases should not be interpreted as causes of death because there are multiple possible etiologies.[5] They include natural disease that is undetectable by autopsy and current post-mortem testing, and mechanical asphyxial deaths.[5]

Sudden Unexpected Infant Death (SUID) applies to the death of an infant less than one year of age in which investigation, autopsy, medical history review, and appropriate laboratory testing do not identify a specific cause of death.[2] SUDI/SUID can include deceased infants who have injuries of unknown significance.[2,6]

SUID includes cases of Sudden Infant Death Syndrome (SIDS).[2–4] SIDS has been defined as the sudden death of an infant under one year of age, the death remaining unexplained after a thorough case investigation including performance of a complete autopsy, examination of the death scene, and review of the clinical history.[7]

SUID/SIDS deaths commonly occur after an infant has been put to sleep.[7] The definition of SIDS was subsequently modified by adding that the apparent onset of the fatal episode happened during sleep.[3] SUDI/SUID, rather than SIDS, can also be applied to a case where the scene and circumstances suggest that the mechanism of death could be due to asphyxia from an 'unsafe' sleep environment (Figure 36.1).[2–4]

The following information can be used by investigators to determine whether a asleep environment was 'unsafe'.[4]

- Where was the infant found?
- What type and number of bedding layers were over and under the infant?
- Were other items present either within reach of the infant or near his/her face?
- Was anyone sleeping with the infant?
- What were the original and final positions of the infant? Was the infant's death during sleep witnessed?

Asphyxia

The cause of certain sudden infant deaths has been attributed to asphyxia, but this term is a mechanism of death not a cause.[8]

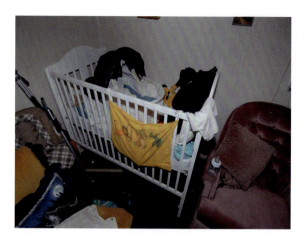

Figure 36.1 1-month-old infant found dead in a bassinet inside a crib. There was a jacket on the bassinet. The jacket may have covered the infant when she was put to sleep. The coroner described a strong tobacco odour in the residence. Both parents were heavy smokers. The carboxyhaemoglobin saturation in the infant was 18%.

The post-mortem findings associated with asphyxial deaths are non-specific; therefore, the determination of asphyxia relies on information gathered by investigators about the scene and circumstances. One of the 'signs' of asphyxia – intrathoracic petechiae – is common in SUDI/SUID/SIDS cases. They are thought to arise from airway obstruction.[7]

Asphyxia by Various Means

Sleep-related asphyxia can arise by different means.[4]

- Prone Sleeping Position, Smothering, and Overlaying:
  - Obstruction of the nose and mouth by a soft impervious sleeping surface or other items (e.g. bedding, stuffed toys) can obstruct breathing.[3]
  - Compression of the face results in areas of pallor surrounded by lividity corresponding to pressure points on the tip of the nose, around the mouth, and on the mid-forehead, cheeks, and chin (Figure 36.2).[9,10]
  - Stains by fluid or vomit from the infant's nose and mouth on the sleep surface or the bed sharer's clothing may be seen (Figure 36.3).
  - A few facial contusions or abrasions can arise if the surface is firm, but oral injuries are usually absent in infants lacking teeth.[9]

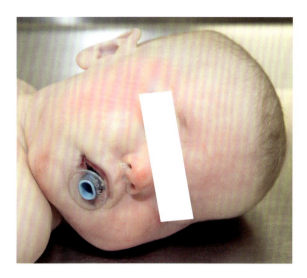

Figure 36.2 Infant found prone in a crib. Facial lividity with sparing of right cheek.

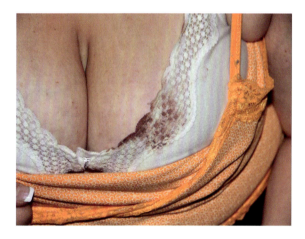

Figure 36.3 Sanguineous stain on bra of mother who fell asleep on a couch with a 15-day-old infant on her chest. There was copious bloody fluid on the infant's face and around her nostrils.

- The determination that overlaying played a role in an infant death may depend on either an admission by the bed sharer or an independent witness to the incident.
  The location of an infant under a bed sharer in the absence of ante-mortem trauma on the child's body does not necessarily mean that overlaying has occurred. The infant could have been already deceased.
- Facial and ocular petechiae are either absent or few.[9] Raised venous pressure such as from

coughing or vomiting from illness preceding the infant's death can lead to petechiae. Post-mortem petechiae from ruptured congested vessels due to lividity while the infant was prone can be observed.

- Multiple facial and intraoral injuries raise the possibility of homicidal asphyxia.[9]
- Wedging: The face, neck, or thorax of an infant is compressed between two firm structures (e.g. mattress and wall), and the infant is unable to self-extricate.
- Positional Asphyxia: This may result when an infant's face or neck position causes airway obstruction while sleeping in a car seat or stroller.
- Unsafe sleep environments pose less risk for older infants because of their ability to roll over and control their upper bodies and arms.[11]

Pulmonary Haemorrhage

Pulmonary haemorrhage arising from congestion is a common finding in infants who die from various causes including those that lead to sudden death.[6] It is usually patchy and irregularly distributed, but in some cases can be prominent. Infant position either at or after the time of discovery may play a role. A long post-mortem interval could be another factor. Resuscitation also can exacerbate intra-alveolar haemorrhage.

Pulmonary haemosiderosis resulting from healed petechiae has been considered a histological marker of previous apnoeic episodes or 'brief resolved unexplained events' (BRUE, formerly 'apparent life-threatening events' – ALTEs).[12] Studies have shown that siderophages in the lungs are not unique to SIDS cases and can arise from other identifiable causes (e.g. infections, prematurity).[13,14]

Child Abuse and Neglect

Kempe et al. described the battered-child syndrome:[15]

> The clinical manifestations of the battered-child syndrome vary widely from those cases in which trauma is very mild and is often unsuspected and unrecognised, to those who exhibit the most florid evidence of injury to the soft tissues and skeleton. . . . In these patients, specific findings of trauma such as bruises or characteristic roentgenographic changes . . . may be misinterpreted and their significance not recognised.

The abstract of this paper states: 'The syndrome should be considered in any child exhibiting evidence of fracture of any bone, subdural haematoma, failure to thrive, soft-tissue swellings or skin bruising, in any child who dies suddenly or where the degree and type of injury is at variance with the history given regarding the occurrence of the trauma'.

'Thinking dirty' about a single infant death or considering subsequent deaths in the same family as criminally suspicious has led to miscarriages of justice.[8,16,17]

The Pathologist's Role

A major challenge for a pathologist is to determine whether child abuse or neglect occurred when an infant has died suddenly with evidence of fatal and non-fatal injuries. In some cases, trauma may be unexpected based on the initial history and found only at autopsy. Although injuries may be suspicious for abuse, opinions about them are not offered in isolation but rely on a comprehensive death investigation. The pathologist considers not only external and internal post-mortem findings but also verbal, narrative, and photographic information from various investigators – coroner or medical examiner and police – about the scene, health history of the infant, and the circumstances of the death. These data are supplemented by histology and relevant ancillary post-mortem tests done on samples collected under the supervision of the case pathologist. In cases of observed or suspected trauma, specific dissections and consultations may be needed.[18] By following these steps of the 'complete' autopsy systematically, the pathologist in collaboration with the death investigation team can form an accurate opinion about the cause and manner of death.[19]

The ultimate goal of the pathologist's examination is to try to determine a cause of death and address other issues raised by investigators. A death investigation team that makes the a priori assumption that an infant death is the result of abuse may fall into 'tunnel vision' affecting the pathologist's approach to and opinions about an infant death. As a result, the pathologist's 'confirmation bias' leads to narrow or erroneous interpretations of findings to support investigators' suspicions. The result can be a 'default diagnosis' such as, 'in the absence of an adequate explanation for the injuries observed, non-accidental trauma cannot be excluded'.[8] If there is insufficient pathological evidence regarding a cause of death, then the cause can be considered 'undetermined'.[8]

A narrative and visual record of pertinent positive and negative post-mortem findings ensures that a case is reviewable by another pathologist who then is able to reach the same or different conclusions from the original case pathologist. Failures to follow proper autopsy protocol and to provide adequate documentation of post-mortem findings were issues raised after the conviction of Sally Clark for the murder of her two infant sons by suffocation.[20] The failure by the pathologist to complete each step can lead to omission of pertinent findings, mistaken interpretations, and conclusions, misdirected investigations, and unwarranted legal proceedings.

In all cases, a pathologist's opinion about trauma must be evidence-based. Any opinion is based not only on the interpretation of the findings of a complete post-mortem examination but also on peer-reviewed medical literature, particularly in a case having unusual, equivocal, or controversial findings.

Abuse or Accident?

The following investigative information raises suspicions about potential physical abuse:[21,22]

- The infant's caregivers have a history of any involvement with a child protection service agency. This includes a history of violence to children and others in the residence where the infant was found.
- There is a history of repeated trauma treated at different health facilities.
- The stated circumstances leading to the injuries are inconsistent with the physical abilities based on the infant's development. Bruises are not expected in children who are not yet crawling, cruising, or walking. In a literature search of studies that defined patterns of bruising in non-abused and abused children under the age of eighteen years, Maguire et al. found that bruising in babies who are not independently mobile was very uncommon (<1%).[22] About 17% of infants who were crawling, or cruising, had bruises. Accidental contusions increase with age and were seen in the majority of preschool and school children.
- A caregiver who has 'exclusive opportunity' to the infant at the time of the injuries provides an inconsistent explanation that may change upon further questioning. The pathologist's role is to determine whether the type, degree, and extent of

the injuries are consistent with the description of the circumstances that led to trauma.

- There is a delay in seeking treatment of injuries that would have been apparent to the caregiver. This situation may be suspected: (i) When there are healing injuries from repetitive trauma, which would either have been visible to the caregiver or have adversely affected the behaviour of the infant; (ii) If there are signs of a prolonged post-mortem interval yet the caregiver says he/she sought assistance at the time of the traumatic incident and/or as soon as the infant showed signs of acute medical distress. The proof of post-mortem signs may rely on the evidence of the emergency responders; for example, when they record severe hypothermia or when they have difficulty inserting an oral airway because of jaw rigidity resulting from established rigor mortis (the determination of time of death based on the progression of rigor mortis is only an estimate, particularly in infants because they may develop rigor more quickly owing to their relatively small muscle bulk[19]).

- There is an inappropriate response to or compliance with healthcare providers' advice by caregivers if the infant is hospitalised. This includes abandonment of the infant in the hospital.

Questions about the autopsy findings will arise during the investigation and in legal proceedings:

- Is the observation a normal variant or an abnormality arising from disease which mimics an injury?
- Was the injury ante-mortem, peri-mortem, or post-mortem?
- Could the injury have occurred during resuscitation or hospitalisation?
- How much force caused the injury?
- How old is the injury?
- What caused the injury?
- Did the injury contribute to death or disability?

Skin and Soft-Tissue Injuries

Blunt Trauma

Injuries due to blunt trauma are the most common type of trauma seen by pathologists in paediatric forensic pathology practice. Compared to penetrating injuries from either stabbing or shooting, blunt

trauma injuries can be challenging to interpret in a case of suspected physical abuse or neglect.

Bruises are the most common presenting feature of physical abuse in children, and cutaneous injuries may be the first sign at a scene or an autopsy that an infant may have been abused.[22–24]

The pathologist's documentation of external injuries may be the only complete record of the trauma sustained by an infant. Although ambulance reports, clinical notes and police records provide information about injuries described by the person who found the body (i.e. emergency responders, hospital personnel and investigators), external injuries are usually not fully or accurately described, particularly when emergency efforts are focused on resuscitation and treatment of critical internal injuries. There will be more detailed descriptions of trauma if the child has been hospitalised and assessed by child abuse specialists.

The pathologist documents location, type, appearance, number, and dimensions of any skin injuries seen during an autopsy.

Tsokos defined criteria for determination of non-accidental bruising in children:[25]

- Localisation
  - Generally, a contusion, abrasion, or laceration cannot be linked to a specific surface that caused the injury; however, the distribution or localisation of injuries on the body ('injury pattern') can be linked to certain scenarios which may or may not be consistent with the circumstances. If there is a history of a fall, then common sites of injury include the bony prominences of the forehead, tip of nose, and chin, palms, posterior elbows, knees, and anterior shins. Trauma observed around the eyes ('raccoon eyes'), outer ears, lips, and oral mucosa, external forearms, back of hands, back, posterior, or lateral thighs, buttocks, and soles are more common in child abuse.
  - Other authors have included injuries on the neck, upper arms, genitalia, and anterior thighs as suspicious for abuse.[26] Pierce et al. found that contusions, classified by them as the 'TEN-4' group (i.e. torso, ears or neck), in children less than four years old or any bruises in infants less than four months of age had a predictive value for abuse.[27] Maguire et al. opined that with the exception of patterned injuries, 'there are few bruising patterns that reach diagnostic significance. However, some patterns and

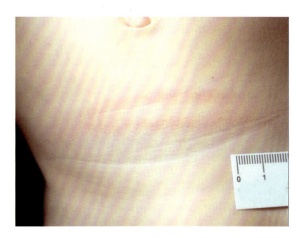

Figure 36.4 Parallel contusions on the lower abdomen of an abused infant struck by a narrow object.

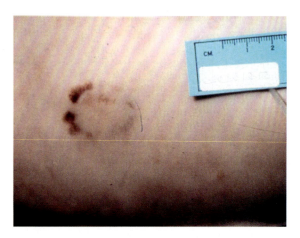

Figure 36.5 An oval array of abrasions and contusions on the torso of an infant who was bitten. Saliva swabbed from of the bite mark is a source of DNA linking the injury to an assailant.

locations of bruising are very suggestive of abuse'.[22]

- Patterned injuries
  - Less commonly, the pattern of the impacted surface or impacting object is imprinted on the skin wound and can be described as a 'patterned injury' (Figure 36.4).
  - A bite mark is an example of a patterned injury (Figure 36.5). It is characterised by two opposing round or oval abraded imprints of the teeth of the upper and lower jaws, and the canine teeth impressions in an adult are greater than 2.5 cm apart.[25]

- Repeated Injuries
  - Different coloured bruises suggest varying stages of healing, resulting from separate traumatic episodes; however, a precise age determination and linkage to a specific event are not possible.
  - Maguire et al. reviewed the medical literature of the ageing of bruises in live children less than 18 years old.[28] They could find no scientific evidence to support that the age of a bruise could be based on its colour and concluded that the dating of injuries based on the colour of bruises should be avoided in child protection proceedings. They cited one publication that described a clinical study which showed inter-observer variability on age estimates and poor inter-observer reliability on agreement of colour.[29] Red, blue, and purple bruises were more commonly seen in injuries less than 48 hours old, and yellow, brown, and green bruises were most often seen after seven days; however, the converse was also observed. Bruises caused at the same time could be of different colours. The accuracy of ageing a bruise to within 24 hours of its occurrence was less than 50%.
  - A pathologist has an advantage over a clinician in assessing the age of a bruise. Sampling of a bruise for histology can determine its stage of inflammation and healing. The periphery of a bruise, which may be fading, or of a different colour than the centre, should be sampled because this area is likely to show the most advanced inflammatory reaction. It is also good practice to sample adjacent but not contiguous grossly normal skin to ensure there are no siderophages from remote injuries that may, if found in the bruise, lead to an incorrect estimate of the bruise's age.
  - The ageing of bruises is less well-defined than for open wounds.[19,30] Extravasated red blood cells are seen initially in the bruise. Neutrophils appear and become more prominent from a half-hour to up to 24 hours after the causal event. After 24 hours, macrophages are observed, and the breakdown of haemoglobin into haemosiderin can be visualised if the section is stained

histochemically for iron. Iron-bearing macrophages (i.e., siderophages) first appear any time from 24 to 72 hours after the injury and then persist for long periods, or, after an unpredictable period, disappear. Long and overlapping intervals in the different stages of inflammation mean that the determination of an age of an injury is at best an estimate. Whether these time frames can be applied to the ageing of contusions in infants who heal more quickly is debatable. Maguire et al. cautioned quoting papers in which the data included older individuals particularly the very elderly whose bruises may evolve differently than infants.[28]

- Although the criteria used to age a contusion have their limitations, colour differences and, particularly the stages of inflammation/healing observed microscopically, provide broad estimates for the age of the lesion and thus may indicate whether a bruise occurred around the time of a fatal incident or was the result of an older event.

- Clustered injuries: A cluster of three or more injuries can be seen in the same body location. If they are on the upper arm or outer thigh of an older infant, then they may be from defensive actions by the infant.[22] Alternatively, an infant's limb may be grabbed.

In suspected cases of abuse, dissections of the deep soft tissue and muscles of the extremities and torso are done to determine if there are haematomas that are not seen on the skin. Deep soft-tissue disruption and bleeding can lead to haemorrhagic shock and fat embolism.[31]

In a clinical series of 2890 children aged less than 120 months who were evaluated for physical abuse, 137 (4.7%) had cutaneous and/non-cutaneous mimics defined as conditions or findings that clinicians thought could be due to physical abuse.[24,32] In this group, 2.4% (n=69) of the total group had cutaneous findings that mimicked physical abuse.[24] Of those who had skin findings, 70% were classified as either congenital (n=19, 28%), dermatologic (n=15, 22%), or infectious (n=14, 20%). A Mongolian spot (congenital dermal melanosis) was the most common congenital lesion that mimicked a contusion. Mongolian spots are most common on the buttocks, but they can also occur on the face, scalp and limbs (Figure 36.6).[23,33] Haemangiomas

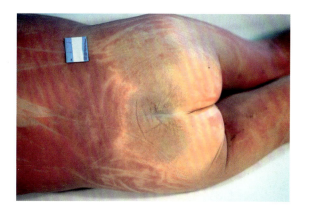

Figure 36.6 Mongolian spot in area on the natal cleft that was not affected by lividity.

and other vascular malformations can mimic bruises.[23] Microscopy can confirm the diagnosis.

Caregivers may volunteer that an infant 'bruises easily'.[26] An underlying bleeding disorder may be an issue when extensive bruising is seen at autopsy particularly if significant trauma is absent.[34] Bleeding diatheses such as von Willebrand disease, thrombocytopaenia, and platelet function disorders, coagulation factor deficiencies and fibrinogen disorders, primary and secondary bone marrow neoplasia, and marrow failure predispose to bruising.[23,33,34] In non-mobile infants, a bleeding disorder can present with contusions or petechiae during the normal handling and along pressure lines caused by clothing and infant seat fasteners.[26] Investigative information about a prior history of bleeding (e.g. excessive bleeding after circumcision, episodes of epistaxis) either in the infant or in other family members supports the caregiver's explanation.[24] Schwartz et al. found that only 7 of 2890 children evaluated for abuse had coagulopathies which mimicked abuse.[24] An underlying coagulopathy does not exclude physical abuse, if the circumstances and injuries point to it.[26,34]

Heritable non-haematological disorders such as Ehlers-Danlos syndrome and osteogenesis imperfecta are associated with bruising.[34]

Burns

Death from burns can be accidental, deliberately inflicted, or the result of neglect.

Contact burns result from the pressure of a hot object against skin (Figure 36.7).[25] The burn is typically

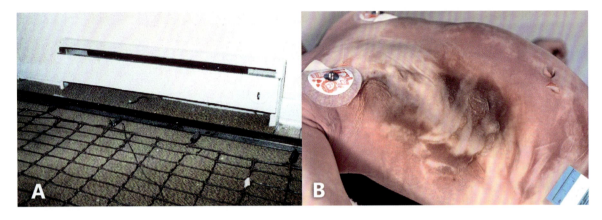

Figure 36.7 a: Infant found wedged between bed and wall over a malfunctioning electric baseboard heater. b: The infant's mother brought the lifeless infant to the hospital and explained that she had a rash. Full thickness contact burns were observed on the face, chest, and legs.

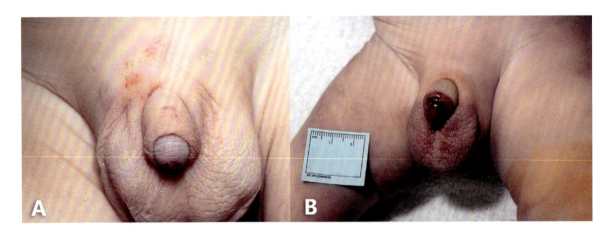

Figure 36.8 a: Multiple abrasions on the genital area of an infant who died of craniocerebral trauma. The caregiver admitted to causing these injuries. b: Erythematous penis following circumcision.

localised on the back, buttocks and outer extremities, and it can be patterned (e.g. cigarette burn). Scalding by immersion in a bathtub filled with hot water causes symmetrical burns on the buttocks and lower extremities. The edges of the burns are defined by the bathwater level. Unilateral scalds can occur when one foot is forced into hot bathwater.Chester et al. studied burns in 440 patients under the age of 16 years, four of whom had inflicted burns (two in the form of contact burns).[35] They also compared 41 burn patients who had been neglected (mean age = 4.2 years; age range = 0.5 – 14 years) to 395 patients who had been accidentally burned (mean age = 4.0 years, age range 0.25 – 15 years). Scald injuries predominated in the children in the neglected group, who also had a statistically greater chance of a delayed presentation.

Dermatoses can mimic burns or burn scars and include contact/atopic dermatitis, post-inflammatory hyperpigmentation, impetigo, tinea, and epidermolysis bullosa.[2324,33] Asian cultural practices involving applications of heat to the body (i.e., 'cupping' or 'coining') can be concerning for physical abuse.[36]

Genitalia and Anus

Anogenital injuries have been described as indicators of ongoing sexual abuse or punishment (Figure 36.8).[37] Perianal findings arising from ongoing sexual abuse include swelling, marginal haematoma, radial fissures, linear skin abrasions, thickened skin, and anal dilatation.[38] Perianal abrasions can be iatrogenic (e.g. insertion of a suppository).In deceased children in whom there was no reason to suspect abuse, McCann et al. found that widening of the anal orifice and exposure of the pectinate line and anal mucosa (which could be easily misinterpreted as fissures) were common autopsy findings (Figure 36.9).[39] Anal dilatation and venous congestion that are suspicious for abuse in living children may not be applicable to deceased infants because of lividity and decomposition.[39,40]

Skeletal Trauma

The elasticity of infant bone and its evolving anatomic structure with maturation are factors that influence fracture patterns.[41]

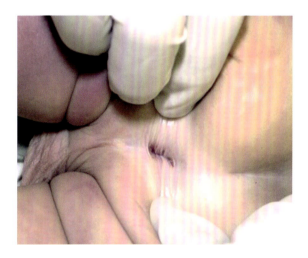

Figure 36.9 Normal anal-rectal junction.

Akbarnia et al. in a study of 74 abused infants found that 50% of their patients with fractures were younger than one year old and about 75% were under three years of age.[42] Another study of abused children found that fractures were uncommon after 2 years of age.[43]

Detection

If an infant has been hospitalised, a bone radionuclide scintiscan ('bone scan') may be done. It is more sensitive than radiography in detecting early fractures, but interpretation can be complicated by increased uptake at growth plates.[44,45]

Assessment for fractures requires a radiological skeletal survey prior to dissection.[46]

A CT scan can detect fractures of the posterior ribs, spine, skull, and pelvis not readily identified by a conventional survey.[46,47]

Information from a paediatric radiologist about definite or suspected fractures and any other abnormalities directs the pathologist's examination. A fracture can be confirmed by exposure during dissection and observation of a fracture line with associated subperiosteal and soft-tissue haemorrhage. In the case of a rib fracture, stripping of the parietal pleura will allow the internal aspect of the rib to be visualised because the external surface may be unaffected.[48] A high-resolution radiograph of a specimen removed from a suspected fracture site can assist in detection (Figure 36.10).[46 49] For example, in contrast to a healing fracture, a fresh linear incomplete or non-displaced rib fracture may not be seen in a post-mortem skeletal survey.[45,46,49,50] A periosteal bone reaction in the

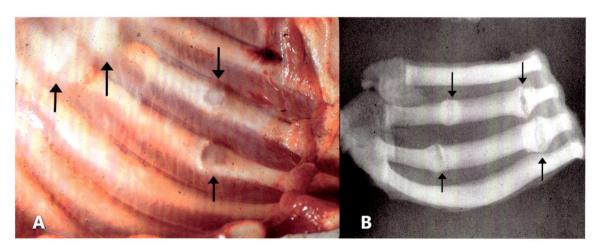

Figure 36.10 a:In-situ view of posterior rib cage with callused rib fractures (arrows). b: Excised specimen radiograph showing fractures.

absence of a fracture and cutaneous injury can be a sign of abusive injury.[45]

Ageing of Fractures

The stages of healing of a fracture proceed through haemorrhage/inflammation with resorption of necrotic bone, formation of soft callus (deposition of cartilage and non-lamellar bone) with transition to hard callus (conversion to lamellar bone) and eventual remodelling. Fractures of different relative ages imply repeated episodes of trauma.

There is little information in the literature about the precise dating of fractures in young infants by radiography and histology, because in such cases it is impossible to be certain when the causal event(s) took place.[46,50–52]

Studies of fracture healing have used data based on the healing of immobilised long-bone fractures in older children for whom the date of fracture in most cases can be reliably established.[50–52] However, these age estimates may not apply to younger children, who heal more quickly, and in whom healing is prolonged in fractures that are not immobilised (e.g. ribs).[41,50,52–54] Further, re-injury in repeated abuse can lead to different stages of healing in the same fracture.[46,50–52,54] By radiography, soft callus can be visible by 10 days; hard callus can form in 2–4 weeks.[50] Radiologic dating of non-accidental rib fractures has been described

by Sanchez et al. in sixteen infants aged 1–11 months who had been followed after injury.[52] In these cases, maximum callus thickness (at least 4 mm) was reached at 5–7 weeks post-injury.

When samples of a fracture are taken for histology, sampling of normal bone adjacent to the fracture and elsewhere is essential to ensure there is no microscopic evidence of a pre-existing bone disease that may have weakened the bone and predisposed it to injury resulting from minimal or trivial force.

Chest

Inflicted Trauma

Rib fractures caused by direct blows are typically focal and unilateral.[50] Variably healing multiple, bilateral fractures, in the absence of either metabolic disease or confirmed accidental injury, are strongly suggestive of abuse.[41,45,49] The fractures tend to be multiple and bilateral, one explanation being that they fit the span of the perpetrator's hands.[50]

Fractures from forcible chest compression by squeezing can occur at any site.[45,50] Patterned bruises on the chest suggestive of fingertip pressure may be seen (Figure 36.11). Posterior fractures are the most common, but lateral, anterolateral, anterior, and costochondral junction fractures have been described.[43,45,48,50,55,56] Fractures of the first ribs

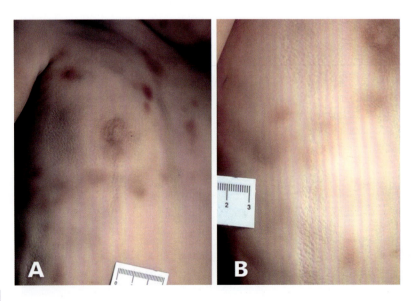

Figure 36.11 a: Multiple oval contusions on the chest of an infant who was squeezed. b: Some of the bruises show central pallor indicative of forcible fingertip compression.

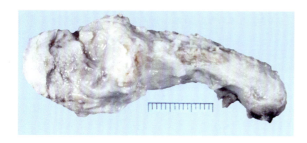

Figure 36.12 Incidental healed clavicle fracture in 5-month-old infant.

have been described as 'virtually pathognomonic' of abuse.[45,50]

A fractured sternum is caused by direct impact and is suspicious for abuse in the absence of well-documented accidental injury.[41,45,57]

Clavicle fractures are uncommon in abuse.[41,43,45,57] Mid-shaft clavicular fractures are not specific for abuse (Figure 36.12) and have been observed in resuscitated infants.[48]

A fractured scapula, due to either direct impact or twisting, is considered highly specific for inflicted trauma if there is no history of an accident.[41,45,50,57]

Cardiopulmonary Resuscitation

Attempts at cardiopulmonary resuscitation (CPR) are almost invariable when an infant is found *in extremis* and may, through chest compression, result in rib fractures. Maguire et al. searched the medical literature and, applying stringent criteria, reported in 2006 that there were six publications between 1984 and 2003 whose collective radiological and post-mortem observations indicated that CPR in children aged from birth to 14 years only rarely resulted in rib fractures.[48] Specifically, 3 of the reported 923 cases had rib fractures, including two babies aged 2 and 3 months who died suddenly, and a five-year-old drowning victim. The 2-month-old had fractures of ribs II to IV in the midclavicular line, and the 3-month-old had bilateral sternochondral fractures of ribs VIII to IX. Trained personnel attempted resuscitation in all three cases. The 3-month-old infant also had bystander CPR for 75 minutes.

Another study of 546 infant autopsies noted that contiguous anterolateral CPR-related fractures were observed ranging from the left 2nd to 6th ribs, and right 3rd to 6th ribs.[56] These fractures were either unilateral or bilateral. With the exception of infants with metabolic bone disease, posterior rib fractures

have been thought unlikely to be the result of CPR and are considered to be characteristic of abuse.[41,48,50,55] If an infant's back is on a flat surface during resuscitation, the mechanism of injury that involves levering the posterior ribs over the transverse processes does not occur readily.[48,50]

During two-handed CPR, both hands of the person administering resuscitation are wrapped around the infant's chest applying pressure to the back, and the thumbs are used to compress the sternum. A case of posterior rib fractures (right 8th and 9th) has been described in a 47-day-old infant who was found unresponsive in bed, and two-handed CPR was done by first responders.[58] In another paper, four hospitalised neonates who died of natural causes, and had two-handed CPR, were found to have posterior rib fractures.[59] In a case series of five resuscitated infants aged 1.5 to 4 months, all of whom had two-handed CPR, multiple anterolateral rib fractures were found.[60] In three cases, the fractures were bilateral. In four, there was minimal displacement. All had subtle subpleural haemorrhage.

Birth-related posterior rib fractures are rare; however, exceptions have been reported.[50] In one literature review, thirteen cases of delivery-related posterior rib fractures were found. Macrosomia, shoulder dystocia, midline unilateral posterior rib fractures, and ipsilateral clavicle fractures were common features.[61]

Long Bones

The metaphyseal corner or bucket-handle fracture has been described as pathognomonic for child abuse with the exception of birth-related trauma.[41,43,45,50] Metaphyseal fractures occur in children less than two years old. It is due to shearing force across immature bone at the end of the metaphysis.[50] Traction from manipulating a limb like a handle or flailing of an extremity when the chest is shaken is a proposed injury mechanism.[41,50] The distal femur is the most frequent site, followed by the proximal tibia, distal tibia, and proximal humerus.[50]

Diaphyseal fractures are common beyond two years of age and can be either accidental or abusive.[41,45] Transverse fractures indicate a direct blow perpendicular to the long axis of a bone. Spiral fractures are due to torsion.

A fracture of a finger or metatarsal bone is suspicious for abuse and can be caused by squeezing, forced hyperextension, or trampling.[41,45,46]

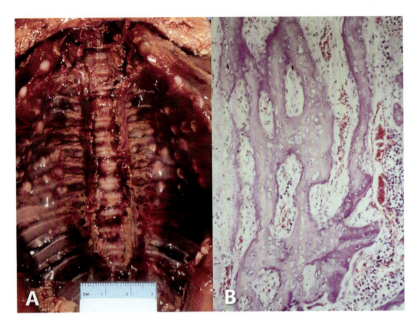

Figure 36.13 Osteogenesis imperfecta. a: Multiple rib fractures in newborn. b: Prominent non-lamellar bone (woven) in cortex.

Injury Mimics

The most common non-cutaneous mimic of child abuse in a clinical series of 2890 children less than 120 months old evaluated for physical abuse was metabolic bone disease.[32] Osteomalacia and osteo-porosis were the most common diseases followed by vitamin D deficiency and osteogenesis imperfecta (OI). These infants presented with acute or healing fractures of either the ribs or long bones.

A systematic review of the medical literature comparing fractures from chronic abuse and neglect to metabolic or genetic bone disease found that OI was the most common disease confused for abuse (Figure 36.13).[62] Individuals with OI may not always show the classic features (e.g. multiple fractures after minor trauma at an early age, blue sclera, osteopenia, wormian bones, family history of 'easy' fractures, denti-nogenesis imperfecta). Patterns of fractures of long bones and ribs including those sites highly suspicious for abuse (e.g. metaphysis, posterior rib, scapula, spinous process, sternum) did not differ between abuse and OI.

Radiological changes from either vitamin C or vitamin D deficiency can mimic metaphyseal fractures.[41]

A sample of rib to include costochondral junction for histology can detect abnormalities of the growth plate due to vitamin C and D deficiency, and OI.

Metz et al. wrote that optimal levels of vitamin D are unknown, and no level has been causally asso-ciated with fractures in normally active children.[32] They also noted that a low level of vitamin D does not mean metabolic bone disease and does not exclude the possibility that observed fractures were inflicted.

Alternatively, Cannel and Holick have controver-sially suggested that vitamin D deficiency may be the explanation for fractures in some infants who have no bruising or other evidence of trauma.[63] They described posterior rib and long bone metaphyseal fractures in two cases with very low vitamin D levels and no other evidence of trauma. Following removal from the custody of their parents, the diets of these infants were supplemented with vitamin D and no new fractures were observed in subsequent radiologic imaging. The authors cited older literature published from 1921 to 1948 to hypothesise that such fractures could occur spontaneously. They stated that radio-logic imaging was not sensitive in diagnosing rickets, and it was best determined by a bone biopsy. Further, Miller and Mirkin questioned whether classical meta-physeal lesions were true fractures based on:

- The lack of bruising, swelling, pain, and functional impairment seen typically in these apparent fractures;

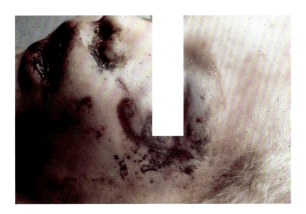

Figure 36.14 Multiple blunt trauma skin injuries including periorbital injuries in a case of child abuse.

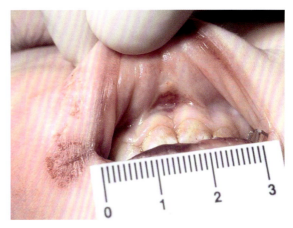

Figure 36.15 Laceration of frenulum. Impetigo, right corner of mouth.

- The fact that despite these lesions occurring in the very vascular growth plate, healing commencing with haemorrhage progressing to callus is absent on radiologic imaging;
- Absence of a healing reaction by histologic assessment when they reviewed previously published studies.[64]

From these observations, the authors hypothesised that the microscopic features, interpreted as indicating a metaphyseal fracture, could also be from processing artefacts or the result of metabolic bone disease.[64]

Facial Trauma

An abused infant can sustain blunt trauma cutaneous injuries of the face (Figure 36.14). Fractures of maxilla, mandible, and nose can occur.[65,66]

Various intraoral injuries can be seen. A torn frenulum is highly suspicious of abuse (Figure 36.15).[65,66] Forceful insertion of a finger or pressure from a soother is a possible mechanism of injury.[65] If there is a pharyngeal laceration, subcutaneous and mediastinal emphysema can occur.[65,67] Fractures or avulsions of teeth, oral contusions, lacerations, and burns are also part of the spectrum of inflicted trauma.[66]

Abrasions of the lips can occur with resuscitation and can be due to difficulty in opening a jaw in rigor during resuscitation.[68]

Other Visceral Trauma

Most extracranial visceral injuries occur beneath the diaphragm and most commonly involve the gastrointestinal tract.[69]

Intra-abdominal and Retroperitoneal Injuries

After head injuries, abdominal injuries are the second most common cause of death in an abused infant.[70] In one series, abusive abdominal injuries occurred predominantly in young children (mean age 3.73 years).[71] Accidental trauma was more common in older children (mean ages: motor vehicle collision-related cases = 9.7 years; falls = 10.39 years).

An infant's abdominal organs are susceptible to blunt trauma because the abdominal wall is less muscular and thinner. The diaphragm is more horizontal positioning the liver and spleen more anterior resulting in less protection by overlying ribs. Compression by an impact from an object may compress organs against the spine, thorax, or pelvis. A solid organ can be crushed. A hollow viscus can rupture because of sudden increased intraluminal pressure.[69,70,72] Shear stress can tear the mesentery, and the duodeno-jejunal and ileo-cecal junctions.[69,70,72]

Abusive intra-abdominal injury may be unsuspected prior to an autopsy because external evidence of trauma can be absent and clinical signs (e.g. vomiting) are too non-specific to indicate an acute abdominal crisis.[67,70–72]

Maguire et al. reviewed the medical literature on intra-abdominal trauma in children aged from birth to under 17 years and found only five 'high quality' case series or studies comparing accidental and abusive injuries.[67]

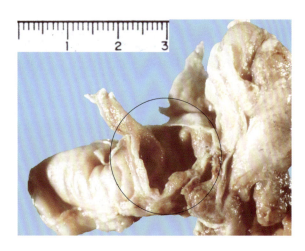

Figure 36.16 Perforated duodenum due to inflicted blunt abdominal trauma.

The following intra-abdominal and retroperitoneal injuries have been described in child abuse.[67,69,71]

- Small-bowel haematoma, perforation, or transection.
  - o The small bowel is the most frequent hollow organ injury.
  - o A duodenal injury (haematoma, perforation) under the age of four is suspicious for child abuse (Figure 36.16).[73] It may present as an isolated injury. Injuries are seen typically at the junction of the third and fourth parts of the duodenum.
  - o Caregivers may report that an infant with a small-bowel perforation fell down stairs, but one review of the medical literature, which excluded infants in walkers, found this explanation unlikely.[70] This injury has been described after a fall on a projecting surface.[72]
- Gastric perforation
- Haematoma, lacerations, or rupture of liver or spleen

Liver trauma is the most frequent solid organ injured. These organs can be injured in accidents also.

- Pancreas
- Laceration of mesentery
- Chylous ascites can arise from mesenteric injury.
- Urinary Bladder
- Kidneys
- Adrenal glands

Unilateral adrenal haemorrhage has been seen in physically abused children.[74] Associated ipsilateral rib fractures and other visceral injuries can be present. Mechanisms of injury include direct trauma, deceleration shear forces tearing adrenal vessels, and increased intra-adrenal venous pressure from impact. Microscopy reveals bleeding mainly in the medulla which contains the more fragile venous sinuses.

Rarely, intra-abdominal and retroperitoneal injuries due to resuscitation (e.g. gastric rupture, hepatic, splenic, pancreatic, and adrenal lacerations,) have been described in infants.[55,68] In a series of 362 resuscitated individuals aged 0–18 years of age, there were no significant hollow or solid organ injuries in the chest and abdomen.[75] The likelihood of injury was not increased with interventions by non-medical or untrained individuals.

Thoracic Injuries

Inflicted intrathoracic injuries are usually associated with fractures:[67,69]

- Pulmonary contusions and lacerations
- Pneumothorax
- Chylothorax

CPR – related intrathoracic trauma (e.g. cardiac rupture, pulmonary contusions, and diaphragmatic lacerations) has been described.[55,68]

Starvation

Starvation[76] of an infant can either be a deliberate act or an indicator of neglect by a caregiver. Unintentional failure to thrive can arise from prolonged breastfeeding without adequate supplementation, overdilution of formula, low-protein diets, homemade formulas, and cult diets. Most victims of fatal starvation are under one year of age. Children younger than three years are limited in their ability to independently obtain food. In the advanced stages of starvation, death may be sudden, and unexpected. Immediate causes or mechanisms of death include hypoglycaemia, ketoacidosis, arrhythmia, or infection. Manifestations of starvation include:

- Sign of decreased body weight – prominent occiput, ribs, vertebrae, scapulae, pelvis, and joints
- Wrinkled and 'semi-translucent' skin from loss of subcutaneous fat
- Signs of dehydration – sunken eyes and fontanelles

- Decubitus ulcers due to inactivity
- Diaper rash
- Focal hypopigmentation
- Alopecia or brittle hair
- Dental caries
- Loss of adipose tissue around organs.
- Muscle atrophy
- Decreased organ weights (except brain)
- Severe involution or complete atrophy of thymus
- Empty stomach and small bowel
- Dry stool in colon
- Distended gallbladder because of absence of food reducing the stimulus for bile excretion
- Hepatic steatosis
- Secondary infections

The Waterlow classification, described by Madea et al.,[76] is a method to assess starvation of an infant. The classification determined stunted growth using the height and the expected weight for height. Starved infants are not only less than 50% of the expected weight for their age group but also have impaired growth due to chronic malnutrition.

Certain diseases or anomalies can lead to dehydration and starvation and need to be excluded. They include anatomical abnormalities of the oral cavity (e.g. cleft palate) and gastrointestinal tract (e.g. pyloric stenosis), intestinal malabsorption (e.g. coeliac disease), viral gastroenteritis, malignancy, cystic fibrosis, diabetes mellitus, inborn errors of metabolism (e.g. inborn glycogen storage disease), congenital heart disease, neurological disorders (e.g. cerebral palsy), congenital adrenal hyperplasia, and immunodeficiencies

Toxicology

Toxicological analysis is part of the complete postmortem examination of an infant death. If an infant was hospitalised, then admission samples in addition to those obtained at autopsy will need to be submitted. A complete drug screen may reveal prescription or illicit drugs incompatible with a natural or non-suspicious death.

Central Nervous System and its Coverings

Preamble

This chapter does not cover in detail the various acute neuropathological conditions that may result in sudden neurological death in infants that are usually immediately obvious during the autopsy – e.g., meningitis, intracranial haemorrhage (whether extra-dural, subdural, or intracerebral) from a ruptured vascular malformations and aneurysms.[17] Similarly, infants with severe congenital, or perinatal disease in whom deaths are predictable are not covered – e.g. severe malformations or perinatal infectious and metabolic disease. The immediate and/or the proximate cause of death in these cases are usually obvious at the time of autopsy or known beforehand.

The neuropathological examination in cases of apparent SUDI/SUID should ideally include the removal and retention of the dura, brain, and the spinal cord. As part of the general autopsy, blood, and bile dot cards can be submitted for metabolic testing; cultured skin fibroblasts, frozen skeletal muscle and myocardium in appropriate preservative are three potential sources of DNA that can be analysed for evidence of, for example, heritable disorders of cardiac rhythm (e.g., channelopathies), coagulation disorders, and collagen vascular disorders. In our centre, the 'neuropathological' investigation also includes visual inspection of the optic nerves in situ and, when indicated, removal, fixation, and histologic examination of the optic nerves and the eyes.

Blocks should be taken from the following brain regions for histologic examination: dura, spinal cord (including the spinomedullary junction and representative samples from the cervical, thoracic, and lumbar segments, ensuring that nerve roots are included), brainstem (medulla, pons and midbrain), frontal region (including the periventricular white matter, at risk for hypoxic-ischaemic injury in utero, i.e. periventricular leukomalacia), mid-hippocampus, calcarine region, thalamus, and basal ganglia.

In many countries, societal concerns about organ retention have limited the extent to which a complete neuropathological examination of the central nervous system can be carried out. Again, in our centre, responding to these concerns, and in the absence of suspicious findings, the brain is placed in ice-cold formalin and fixed for a couple of hours, which makes the tissue firmer and easier to cut. The fixation is sometimes extended to 24 to 48 hours, after which time most of the brain will be released with the body (provided this has been discussed by the coroner with the family). Representative slices from regions roughly corresponding to the above-mentioned blocking areas are retained and fixed. The spinal cord, optic nerves, and eyes are not usually kept or examined microscopically in these cases.

Folkerth et al.[77] provide brain sampling recommendations for the highest cost-effective yield from the neuropathological examination of cases of sudden unexpected death in infancy and toddlers. In this series of 53 children, which included 44 live-born infants (i.e., children up to 1 year of age), critical neuropathological findings were found in nine infants (20.6%), including craniospinal trauma (3 cases), meningoencephalitis (2 cases), features suggestive of Leigh's disease (1 case), and hydrocephalus in the Dandy-Walker malformation (1 case).

Scalp

A contusion of the scalp may be visible either during the external examination or only become apparent in the form of 'sub-scalp' or 'intra-scalp' haemorrhage when the scalp is reflected. Scalp bleeding raises the possibility of a head injury resulting from an impact, whether trivial or substantial, but may be seen after the placing of venous access lines or intracranial pressure monitors during the management of the critically ill infant or after trivial injuries to patients with blood clotting disorders. Rarely, tears of emissary veins during the retraction of the scalp may result in localised, sometimes symmetrical, post-mortem scalp bleeding, which can be readily recognised when it occurs at known sites of the veins.[78]

Skull

Fractures and their Mimics

Fractures are common in definite cases of non-accidental head injury, and are almost always associated with bruising of the overlying scalp and intracranial trauma and its sequelae. The dura of the skull cap and base must always be stripped to ensure that fracture lines are not overlooked. Photographs of the exposed outer and inner calvarium and base are useful as baseline.

A skull fracture is suspected when an unfamiliar, sometimes haemorrhagic line is found in the skull in an unexpected or 'non-anatomical' location. A 'suspicious' line is unlikely to be a skull fracture if there is no haemorrhage in the overlying scalp, since an impact to the head is a prerequisite for the fracture. An exception is the occurrence of a fracture after a minor impact in patients with bone fragility (e.g. osteogenesis imperfecta).

Skull depressions and related fractures ('ping pong fractures') or linear fractures may occur during labour, either spontaneously, or after instrumentation; the lesions may be treated neurosurgically, 'reduced' using a vacuum extractor, or resolve spontaneously.[79–81] The residuum of such lesions may be found during the investigation of SUDI/SUID.

There are several developmental abnormalities of and normal lines in the skull that may mimic fractures, particularly when they are asymmetric. Examples include vascular impressions, fissures, and persistent or residual suture lines that normally disappear as the child develops (i.e., the metopic suture line, which is an extension of the sagittal suture in the frontal midline), accessory sutures (which are rare but, when they occur, are most commonly in the parietal and occipital bones because these regions of the skull have multiple ossification centres), wormian bones, and, in the neonate, overriding of the parietal and occipital bones ('moulding').[82,83] Wormian bones are accessory bones that develop within a suture, most commonly the posterior sutures. They are common in asymptomatic children[84] but are also associated with osteogenesis imperfecta, craniosynostosis, and Menkes' disease.[85,86]

It may be difficult to distinguish between fracture lines and sutures, particularly unexpected, or unilateral accessory sutures. An overlying scalp bruise and histological evidence at the lesion margins of bleeding, platelet, and thrombi deposition and, with longer survival, established organisation characterises a fracture whereas a suture line contains mesenchyme, including fibrous tissue and, depending on the infant's age, osteoprogenitor cells.[87] More generally, fractures have sharp margins and are asymmetric and linear (as opposed to the zigzag pattern of sutures); they may bifurcate, increase in diameter close to a suture line, cross the latter and, in CT scans, do not have sclerotic margins (unlike suture lines).[82,83]

Severe brain swelling, which may be found in resuscitated cases of 'delayed' SUDI/SUID, and separation of the suture margins may lead to intrasutural bleeding and therefore difficulties in distinguishing between a diastatic fracture and separation of the suture lines owing to the effects of intracranial hypertension; however, soft-tissue injury to the overlying scalp suggests a diastatic fracture.

Inflicted skull fractures, in contrast to those resulting from accidental trauma, are more likely to be bilateral, involve other than the parietal bones, cross

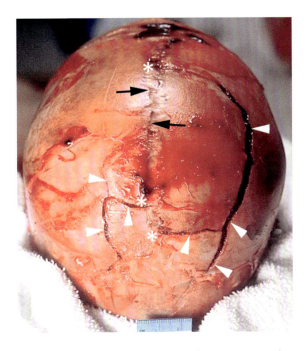

Figure 36.17 Complex fractures – view of skull vertex. Note the typical zigzag morphology of the sagittal suture (black arrows). There are also numerous fracture lines (white arrowheads), some entering the suture line (white asterisks) and one of which may have crossed the suture line in an offset. The child was said to have fallen and may have struck his head against the edge of a chair on the way down (i.e., a complex fall).

suture lines, appear comminuted or depressed, and be wider than 1 mm.[43,45]

Acute fractures can be post-mortem artefacts if the skull is inexpertly opened.

Short Falls

A caregiver may state to investigators and hospital personnel that a fall caused head injuries in an infant. The possibility that a short fall may result in a serious head injury is controversial.[88] Leaving aside the precise quantification of 'short'[89,90] and whether serious injuries resulting from a fall can be reliably distinguished from those caused by non-accidental injury,[88,89,91] the current medical literature indicates that 'short' falls rarely harm the infant, may cause an isolated scalp bruise, rarely result in simple linear fractures, and only exceptionally lead to life-threatening epidural and subdural bleeding. The interpretation of skull fractures is difficult when a 'complex fall' is claimed, i.e., a fall during which the head may have first struck a protuberance on the ground, an object on the way down and then the ground, or have followed

acceleration of the child's body (i.e., when the child is ejected from a caregiver's arm as the result of the latter tripping while walking) (Figure 36.17).

Specifically, in one series of 1,187 children who sustained skull fractures, about half the cases were due to falls. About a third of the fractures occurred from birth to six months, and another happened in infants six to twenty-four months old.[92] The estimated risk of death from a fall for infants and young children from birth to five years of age was less than 0.48 deaths per one million young children per year in one extensive review.[93] In another study of 161 children, aged 5 years and under, falling out of a bed or off a sofa from a height of less than 90 cm (36 in), there were 2 cases of skull fractures, and neither of these children had life-threatening craniocerebral trauma.[94] In a series of 556 infants up to 1 year old falling from about 2–5 feet, there were 3 skull fractures and 1 subdural haematoma.[95]

However, the association between short falls and severe acute head and brain injuries remains contentious, particularly in relation to the possibility that quite short falls on a hard surface can generate substantial force.[96]

Apparent sudden natural death in an infant with localised scalp bleeding with or without an underlying parietal fracture, and without intracranial injuries, or injuries elsewhere in the body, is potentially problematic but raises the possibility of an incidental injury or an otherwise survivable head impact that has led to a concussive cardiorespiratory arrest.[19]

Abnormalities in Skull Shape and Head/Brain Size

Abnormalities in the shape of the infant's skull are relatively common. There are various patterns, but the most common is deformational or positional flatness of the occiput (i.e. owing to the resting/sleeping position of the infant) and open sutures, which may affect as many as 20% of healthy infants. The occipital flatness may be asymmetric (plagiocephaly) or symmetric (brachycephaly). The incidence of plagiocephaly and brachycephaly has increased substantially since caregivers were encouraged to place their charges supine to reduce the risk of SIDS.[97,98]

Deformation of the skull may also indicate sporadic or syndromic/inherited premature fusion of the sutures (craniosynostosis). The pattern of deformation reflects the suture(s) involved; for example, coronal, and lambdoid craniosynostosis results in skull deformation that resembles the plagiocephalies.

Premature closure of a single suture typifies solitary craniosynostosis whereas involvement of multiple sutures is seen in syndromic/inherited forms of the disease. Facial deformation is also common in the craniosynostoses.[99,100]

The various suture lines should be inspected when skull asymmetry is observed. Appropriate samples of tissue should be frozen and stored for genetic studies in the craniosynostoses.

The plagiocephalies and craniosynostosis are unlikely causes of sudden infantile death although the latter may cause sudden death later in childhood.[100]

There are many genetic and/or environmental causes of abnormally small (microcephaly/microencephaly)[101] and large heads and/or brains (macrocephaly/macroencephaly),[102] which may be congenital, or develop in the first few years of life. Macrocephaly also results from intracranial space-occupancy (e.g., due to intracranial haemorrhage and tumours), hydrocephalus (whether isolated [i.e., aqueduct stenosis] or secondary [e.g., Dandy-Walker syndrome, following intraventricular haemorrhage of prematurity]), which may result in sudden death.

Fontanelles

The six principal fontanelles (2 midline, 4 symmetrical and bilateral) in human infants and toddlers (with their age of closure) are the posterior fontanelle (2–3 months after birth), sphenoidal fontanelles (around 6 months), mastoid fontanelles (6–18 months), and anterior fontanelle (12–24 months).[103–105]

The anterior fontanelle receives the most attention during the autopsy. It may 'bulge' because of raised intracranial pressure (i.e., resulting from tumours, brain swelling, infections) or be depressed in dehydrated infants. Early closure of fontanelles may be observed in congenital 'bulk brain growth' disorders that result in microcephaly. Innumerable conditions are associated with enlargement or delayed closure of the fontanelles, notably hydrocephalus, diseases resulting in intracranial 'space-occupancy', achondroplasia, Down's syndrome, and rickets.[104]

Dura

The infantile dura is thin and transparent so that the surface of the brain and subdural bleeding, if present, is usually visible under it.

Acute Intradural Bleeding

Mild to moderate localised dural dusky discoloration caused by intradural congestion is a common finding in

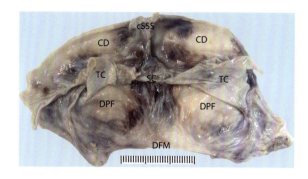

Figure 36.18 Perisinusoidal dural congestion in a 2-month-old case of SUDI/SUID. The photo shows the occipital and posterior fossa subdural surface. There is marked dusky intradural discolouration around the margins of the dural sinuses and in the posterior fossa. (CD = convexity dura, cSSS = caudal end of the superior sagittal sinus, DFM = dura at the margin of the foramen magnum, DPF = dura of posterior fossa, SC = sinus confluens, TC = tentorium cerebelli [folded].)

SUDI/SUID cases, particularly around the caudal margins of the superior sagittal sinus and adjacent to the sinus confluens and lateral sinuses (Figure 36.18). The cause is uncertain, but one explanation is agonal intradural congestion that results in capillary rupture, possibly exacerbated by post-mortem intradural settling of blood (i.e., dural livor mortis). The phenomenon is greatly exacerbated by systemic hypoxia and ischaemia.[106,107] Extension of the intradural blood into the subdural compartment also occurs, especially in critically ill infants hospitalised from birth.[106,107]

Acute Subdural Bleeding (Figure 36.19)

In most cases of significant subdural bleeding there is ample evidence for a blunt force head injury, including scalp bruises and skull fractures, and injuries elsewhere in the body.

Apparently isolated subdural bleeding may be encountered in SUDI/SUID cases without a history of head trauma or pathological evidence of an impact (i.e. scalp bruises, fractures). The subdural bleeding is usually insufficient to exert a space-occupying effect (i.e., it is 'non-surgical'). The bleeding is typically prominent at the hemispheric dorsal angles and lies thinly over the hemispheric surface, falx, and superior aspect of the tentorium.

Trauma is usually suspected because subdural bleeding commonly results from blunt force. However, there are many other causes or conditions that may predispose to or cause subdural bleeding (whether arising spontaneously or following trivial injuries) that should be excluded before trauma is

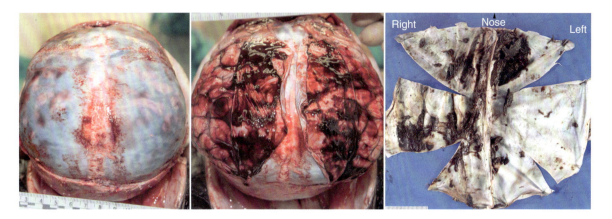

Figure 36.19 Acute subdural haemorrhage (from a 6-month-old infant with the triad). The image on the left shows the subdural bleeding visible through the convexity dura. The central image shows the cut margins of the convexity dura folded towards the midline to reveal patchy thin acute subdural bleeding. The image on the right shows the fixed dura and lightly adherent blood clot. The specimen has been flipped over so that the left is on the right and vice versa. The falx has been removed. The triangular cuts are to allow the dura to be pinned flat.

accepted as the cause.[108,109] Many of these causes can be excluded from the medical and family history and findings at the time of the autopsy (i.e., thrombotic, coagulation, infectious, and metabolic disorders). Nevertheless, it is difficult to completely exclude a coagulation disorder in a SUDI/SUID case when there has been no opportunity for extensive premortem clinical laboratory testing, especially regarding disorders of blood coagulation.[34] The role of molecular biology for this purpose is rapidly expanding but brings the added problem of determining whether and how a given molecular abnormality bears on the possibility that a clotting disorder played a role in abnormal bleeding (i.e., the usual question of cause versus coincidence).

A transient coagulopathy secondary to brain injury can occur.[26] A primary bleeding disorder can cause intracranial haemorrhage and is raised as a factor when the presentation is spontaneous or occurs after minor head trauma.[34] The type of laboratory testing is usually chosen based on the prevalence of the condition, the infant's and family history, and the perceived probability of a bleeding disorder.[24] Von Willebrand disease is the most common heritable bleeding disorder, but intracranial bleeding is very rare.[26] Although there are data for the probabilities of specific bleeding disorders causing intracranial haemorrhage, there are no specific data regarding the prevalence of bleeding disorders in infants and children with intracranial haemorrhage.[26] Other disorders (e.g. delta-storage pool disease, Ehlers-Danlos syndrome, glutaric

aciduria type 1, Menkes disease, osteogenesis imperfecta) are rarely associated with intracranial haemorrhage.[23,86,110–114]

Non-surgical subdural bleeding may be part of a triad of injuries (i.e., small 'smear-type' subdural haemorrhages, 'encephalopathy' [see Section 11.6], and optic nerve sheath/retinal bleeding). For this reason, the discovery of small subdural haematomas in an apparent case of SUDI/SUID should prompt a search for optic nerve sheath haemorrhages; the optic nerves are exposed by removing the orbital plates and dissecting the retro-orbital soft tissues (Figure 36.20). If such bleeding is present, the eyes, and optic nerves should be retained, fixed, and examined grossly and microscopically for retinal bleeding (retinal bleeding is unlikely when there is no evidence of optic nerve sheath haemorrhage). The brain, dura, and spinal cord should also be retained and fixed in such cases.

Subdural Bleeding and Non-accidental Head Injury

The triad of encephalopathy, subdural haemorrhage and retinal haemorrhage may be associated with other obvious injuries to the head and elsewhere in the body.

In other cases, there are no bruises, or fractures, i.e., there is no specific evidence of trauma. Nevertheless, the subdural bleeding is usually taken as evidence of trauma, once other causes of bleeding have been excluded. The injuries are then believed to result from a 'traceless impact' (i.e., an impact injury between the infant's head and a soft broad surface that

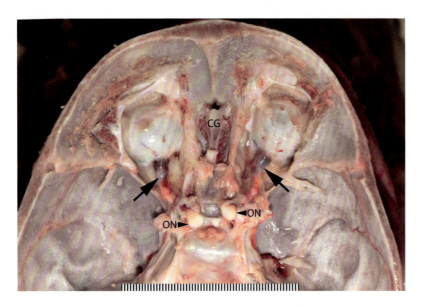

Figure 36.20 Optic nerve sheath haemorrhages: The fronto-orbital plates have been removed and the dorsal orbital soft tissues dissected to expose bilateral optic nerve sheath haemorrhages (arrows). (CG = crista galli, ON = optic nerves.)

did not injure the scalp) or a 'non-contact' blunt force acceleration head injury resulting from shaking.

In practical terms, the hypothesis that a triad case without fractures and bruises was the result of shaking or a 'traceless impact' is made once various alternative explanatory metabolic (e.g., glutaric aciduria, and urea cycle disorders – see [115]), infectious (e.g., acute bacterial meningitis may be associated with blood-stained subdural effusions) and coagulation disorders are excluded. However, the hypothesis that the triad (or subdural and ocular bleeding in cases in which there is presumed to have been insufficient time after the causal event for pathological signs of an encephalopathy to evolve) is the result of trauma is highly controversial because there is no 'gold standard' to prove that trauma occurred. A detailed analysis of this controversy is beyond the scope of this chapter but can be found, from various points of view, in the medical literature (e.g., see References [116–121]).

Old Subdural Bleeding

Faint yellow discoloration of the subdural surface and intradural haemosiderosis, particularly in the occipital and subtentorial dura may be observed in SUDI/SUID cases (Figure 36.21).[122] Subdural membranes are less common. Although these features could indicate an old head injury, they more likely are the residuum of small perinatal intradural and subdural

haemorrhages, which are relatively common and, by MRI criteria, resolve by 3 months of age.[123,124] They occur after vaginal and instrumented deliveries, and Caesarean section.

Old Optic Nerve Sheath and Retinal Bleeding

In contrast to the common finding of residual blood products in the dura in SUDI/SUID cases, a post-mortem study did not find siderosis of the optic nerve sheath in 36 such cases or, with reference to the overall study population of 53 non-trauma cases aged approximately 2 years and under (median age 9 weeks).[122] There was scant siderosis of the orbital fat and ocular muscles of many of the cases.[122] No siderosis was found in the retinae of 8 cases (the ages of each of these cases was not stated).[122] Despite these observations peripartum retinal haemorrhages are common, especially after instrumented deliveries, and tend to be bilateral, intraretinal, lie posteriorly, and rarely persist beyond 6 weeks of age.[125] (Note that retinal nerve sheath haemorrhages, whether acute or old, are not specific for inflicted injuries.[126])

Dural Sinuses

Cerebral venous and dural sinus thrombosis (CVDST) should be excluded by opening and inspecting the dural sinuses. Any suspicious areas and

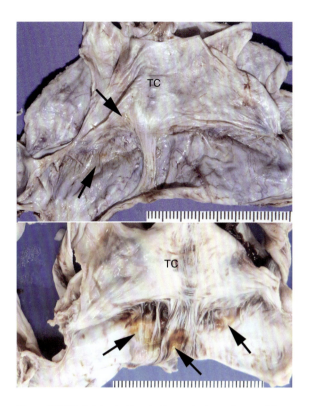

Figure 36.21 Subdural siderosis. These photographs are of the subdural surface of the posterior fossa, with the tentorium cerebelli reflected rostrally (TC), in a 4-month-old (top) and 1-month-old infant (bottom) who died of SUDI/SUID and an acute blunt force head injury respectively. The subdural haemosiderosis (arrows), both subtle (upper image) and obvious (lower image), could be the residuum of perinatal subdural bleeding.

obviously engorged firm cerebral veins should be examined microscopically.

The diagnosis of CVDST is difficult in neonates and infants,[127,128] about 50% of paediatric cases being under 1 year of age (and most of them under 3 months of age).[127] Although seizures are common, a fussy, or irritable prodrome may be the only harbinger of drowsiness, coma, and infantile sudden death. Sudden death owing to CVDST has been described in an adult[129] but is improbable in infants who do not have obvious brain changes, including brain swelling, parasagittal (sometimes subpial) and/or diencephalic haemorrhagic infarcts. The latter haemorrhagic lesions should not be confused with contusions.

A controversy surrounds the significance of CVDST in apparent cases of non-accidental head injury; specifically, is the presence of CVDST in a triad case the result of trauma (an accepted cause of dural sinus thrombosis) or the explanation for the clinical presentation and the neuropathological findings?[129–131]

Leptomeninges

Intense vascular congestion is common in SUDI/SUID and may give the gross impression of subarachnoid blood staining. It is also common to find microscopic evidence of scattered red blood cells in the subarachnoid space. Scant siderophages may be the residuum of peripartum subarachnoid bleeding.

Brain

The brain is usually grossly and histopathologically unremarkable in SUDI/SUID (although SIDS cases have various subtle histological abnormalities that may play a causal role in the mechanism of SIDS, as described elsewhere in this book). It is important, however, to recognise apparently incidental or non-specific gross and microscopic findings and not misinterpret them as recent or older traumatic lesions.

The place of post-mortem imaging in the assessment of SUDI/SUID is evolving and may eventually play a role identifying subtle brain injuries and cerebral oedema.[132]

Gross Examination

If an infant dies at the time of or soon after an event that is expected to have caused an encephalopathy (irrespective of its nature), there may be no evidence of brain injury – the brain will not be swollen and it may be grossly and histologically unremarkable or have the non-specific histological findings described below.

On the other hand, if the infant was resuscitated after being found in extremis (i.e., 'delayed death in SUDI/SUID'), there may be gross evidence of brain swelling (and microscopic features of encephalopathy, described below).[133] There is a controversy about whether this swelling, its effects and the causal hypoxia/ischaemia may lead to significant subdural bleeding and retinal haemorrhages, thus allowing 'delayed' SUDI/SUID to mimic the triad (described above in relation to non-accidental injury).[106,107,133–139]

The gross identification of brain swelling is unreliable (brain weight should not be used for this purpose) and it is uncertain when undoubted brain swelling becomes evident to the naked eye. CT scans of surviving infants may show parenchymal changes suggestive of oedema from within a couple of hours to 27 hours of the presumed causal event (assuming

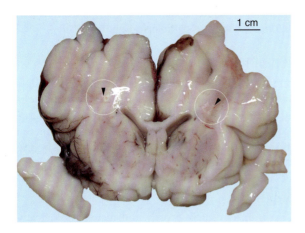

Figure 36.22 Periventricular leukomalacia. There are small bilateral foci of periventricular leukomalacia (arrows). The infant died suddenly and unexpectedly at 18 days of age (37.5 weeks corrected gestational age), 2 days after being discharged from hospital. The mother was a methadone addict. The infant had been treated with decreasing doses of morphine prior to discharge.

reliable witnesses);[140] MRI scanning is usually impractical while the infant is being stabilised in the few hours immediately following the onset of the illness.[141]

Various cyst-like or encephalomalacia-like lesions may be found in infants with a history of complications of prematurity, a complicated term delivery, and/or postnatal apnoea or seizures. The lesions, whose clinical effects on development need not be apparent in infancy, include periventricular leucomalacia (PVL – Figure 36.22) and likely variants,[142–145] subcortical lesions corresponding to radiologically described peripherally located cortical defects[146] (Figure 36.23) and organising haematomas.[147] Such lesions are unlikely to play a direct role in the death of the infant but there is one report of PVL in SUDI/SUID case.[148] Similar lesions, 'subcortical contusional tears', are seen in cases of severe and fatally injured children under 5 months of age[149–151] (Figure 36.24); although believed to be specific for traumatic head injury in young infants,[150] their resemblance to the other lesions mentioned in the previous paragraph casts some doubt on their specificity for trauma.[131]

Variations in the anatomy of the septum pellucidum include various cyst-like structures of which the cavum septum is the commonest.[152]

Unusually spacious frontal subarachnoid spaces with an impression of cerebral 'atrophy' may indicate 'benign enlargement of the subarachnoid spaces', which is usually associated with a recent rapid increase in head circumference.[153] This condition may be associated with a predisposition to 'spontaneous' subdural bleeding[154] and subarachnoid/subpial haemorrhage after a trivial head injury.[155]

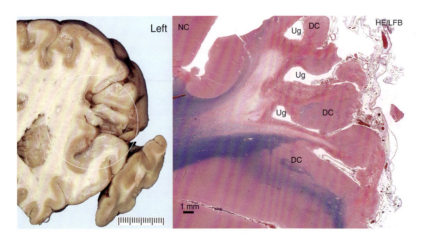

Figure 36.23 Old encephaloclastic lesion. These illustrations are from the brain of a 23-year-old man with a normal developmental history. He developed seizures three years before his death, which was attributed to 'Sudden Unexpected Death in Epilepsy' (SUDEP). He had a localised area of disruption in the left insular region (indicated by the white circle), which likely accounted for his epilepsy. The corresponding whole-mount section, stained with haematoxylin, eosin, and Luxol fast blue (HE/LFB; the latter stains myelin blue), contains areas of normal cortex (NC), disorganised cortex (DC), and dilated sulcal depths (i.e. ulegyria = Ug). The disorganised cortex includes seams of LFB-stained tissue, which are either heterotopic myelinated fibres and/or, by analogy with diencephalic 'status marmoratus', myelinated glial processes. This pattern is typical of the organisation of focal intrauterine and perinatal brain injury and likely corresponds to the fully organised form of 'peripherally located cortical defects'.

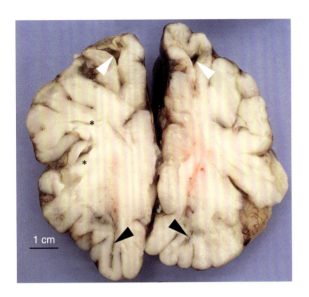

Figure 36.24 Contusional tears. This photograph is from the frontal lobes of a 3-week-old infant who became 'acutely unwell' and died shortly after. There were acute scalp bruises, multiple skull fractures, and recent subdural bleeding in and around older organising subdural membranes. There were also abundant acute optic nerve sheath/retinal haemorrhages. The black arrowheads indicate linear subcortical haemorrhages, consistent with 'contusional tears'. Symmetrical older paramedian cavities, lined by siderotic tissue, are indicated by white arrowheads. The acute scalp bruising and skull fractures prove that an impact head injury has occurred. The older subdural bleeding and paramedian siderotic cavities could be the result of an older blunt force head injury; they could also have occurred in the perinatal period. (The asterisks indicate artefactual handling tears in the brain; the redness of the white matter is the result of poor fixation, which is common in severely swollen brains.)

Microscopic Examination

The histological examination in SUDI/SUID cases may reveal numerous non-specific or incidental findings in the brain. Vascular congestion and tiny perivascular haemorrhages are common especially in the brainstem and the occipital region and are likely due to agonal effects and/or post-mortem lividity (cf. intradural bleeding). These haemorrhages should not be taken as evidence of 'diffuse traumatic vascular injury'.

There may be focal or widespread, intensely stained (i.e. duskily hyperchromatic, dense or dark) neurons or elongated hypereosinophilic neurons in the subiculum; their nuclei are often hyperchromatic and shrunken but they remain round or oval, without angulation, or fragmentation. These appearances are non-specific; they may be artefacts or very early changes resulting from blunt force or hypoxic-ischaemic injury.[19]

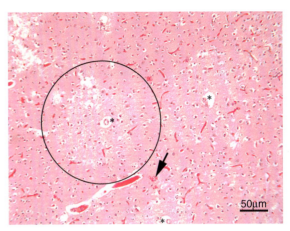

Figure 36.25 Perivascular vacuolation in brain swelling. There are two small blood vessels (asterisks) surrounded by concentric vacuoles (circle indicates this process around one of the vessels). Note the congested capillaries and secondary tiny haemorrhages (arrow), which are common non-specific phenomena (haematoxylin and eosin).

The microscopic features of the encephalopathy in cases of 'delayed' SUDI/SUID include axonal injury (see next paragraph), neuronal injury and/or microscopic evidence of cerebral oedema (i.e., in the form of microvacuoles around the blood vessels and at the interfaces between the grey matter and white matter) (Figure 36.25).[133]

β-amyloid precursor protein (βAPP) immunohistochemistry may reveal in typical cases of SIDS a focal or widespread mottled pattern of labelling with fibrillary, granular, and coarse enhancement of labelling of axons and microswellings in the denser areas (Figure 36.26). We have the impression that this pattern is more likely in infants subjected to prolonged resuscitation, which is not surprising because accumulation of βAPP in injured axons may be detectable from approximately one hour after the causal event.[156,157] This labelling pattern is non-specific and may be the early representation of injury to the axoplasmic flow of βAPP resulting from hypoxia/ischaemia, brain swelling, or trauma.

With reference to traumatic axonal injury, criteria have been proposed that may allow the early pattern of traumatic axonal injury to be distinguished from other causes, particularly in adults.[158] However, the use of βAPP patterns to distinguish traumatic from other forms of axonal injury in encephalopathic infants, particularly those with a short survival, should be avoided or employed with extreme caution.[159] Note also that traumatic axonal injury is

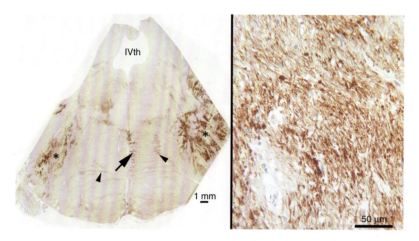

Figure 36.26 β-amyloid precursor (β APP) immunolabelling. The horizontal section of the pons (left image) shows variegated β-amyloid precursor immunolabelling of axons in the middle cerebral peduncles (asterisks), crossing fibres of the basis pontis (arrowheads), and in the midline (with interlaced or zipper-like morphology – arrow). The photomicrograph on the right shows the coarse labelling of the axons (normally there is hardly any labelling, for example in the pale areas of the whole-mount).

unusual in non-accidental injury in infants[160] although in some cases localised axonal injury in the brainstem may be apparent, prompting the suggestion that disruption of the brainstem cardiovascular centres during excessive movements of the head leads to a cardiorespiratory arrest.[160,161]

Spine

Vertebrae

Fracture with or without dislocation of the vertebrae can be inflicted.[41,57,162]

Spinal cord injuries should be suspected during the autopsy when localised bruising is found in the paravertebral soft tissues and/or there is a vertebral fracture. Heavily blood-stained CSF (draining from the spinal canal after the removal of the brain) and marked narrowing of the spinal canal, visible through the foramen magnum, suggest a high spinal cord injury as the result of atlantooccipital or atlantoaxial dislocation.

Leaving aside the dangers of generalisation, spinous process fractures from hyperflexion or hyperextension are considered highly specific for abuse.[41,45]

Ligamentous laxity, horizontally oriented, and relatively unstable facet joints, a proportionally large head, and relatively weak neck muscles predisposes the infant's spine to hyperextension or hyperflexion injury during non-physiological head movements.

Transient dislocation of the spine can occur in child abuse.[162] SCIWORA (Spinal Cord Injury Without Radiological Abnormality) describes this type of injury although SCIWORF (Spinal Cord Injury Without Radiological Fracture) may be the more apt term.[45,163] The elasticity of an infant's spine allows stretching up to 5 cm before it ruptures; however, the spinal cord, anchored to the cauda equina and brachial plexus, can tear after 0.5 to 0.6 cm of longitudinal distraction.[163]

Compression fractures may be mimicked by normal developmental variants[164] or occur asymptomatically when the bones are weakened, for example in vitamin D deficiency.[165]

Spinal Meninges and Cord

Meninges

Bleeding in the subarachnoid and subdural compartment points to a spinal injury and/or non-accidental injury[166,167] but blood may also track down from the corresponding intracranial compartments (Figure 36.27).[168,169] A lumbar puncture may result in heavily blood-stained CSF entering the subdural compartment to masquerade as a large subdural haematoma, both in CT/MRI images and in the post-mortem examination of the spinal canal.[170]

Marked congestion of the epidural surface with small haemorrhages are common artefactual findings and do not by themselves indicate spinal injury.[171,172]

Microscopic examination of the leptomeninges may reveal siderophages. Their interpretation is the same as for similar findings in the cranial leptomeninges.

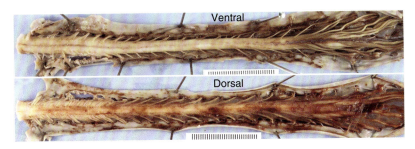

Figure 36.27 Spinal subarachnoid (SAH) and subdural bleeding (SDH). There is patchy recent SAH and SDH, which is more marked over the dependent dorsal aspect of the spinal cord.

Spinal Cord

Tonsillar herniation resulting from severe brain swelling (e.g., after resuscitation from 'near miss SUDI/ SUID') may compress, and interfere with the blood supply to the rostral spinal cord, resulting in petechial and small haemorrhages (in the spinal cord, meninges and nerve roots), cerebellar debris in the subarachnoid space (which may extend to the thecal sac), extensive βAPP immunolabelling of the nerve roots and funiculi, and grey matter necrosis. These changes alone should not be interpreted as a high cervical traumatic myelopathy.

The microscopic examination of the spinal cord is useful for distinguishing between hypoxic-ischaemic injury resulting from regional intracranial hypoperfusion associated with traumatic brain swelling (no ischaemic neurons in the spinal cord) and a cardiorespiratory arrest (necrotic neurons are often but not invariably found in the spinal cord). In severe encephalopathy, cerebral nonperfusion may supervene before histological evidence of hypoxic-ischaemic neuronal injury has had the chance to develop in the brain. However, the perfusion of the spinal cord and the evolution of neuronal necrosis resulting from a circulatory arrest may continue. Approximately 50% of fatal cases of post resuscitation hypoxic-ischaemic encephalopathy will be associated with ischaemic necrosis in the spinal cord in adults[173] although corresponding data is not available for infants.

β-APP immunolabelling of the spinal nerve roots suggests trauma but is also seen in infants dying of natural disease.[174]

References

1. Editorial. Death by 'The Visitation of God'. *Lancet*, 1874; **1**:452.

2. Corey TS, Hanzlick R, Howard J, et al. NAME Ad Hoc Committee on Sudden Unexplained Infant Death. A functional approach to sudden unexplained infant deaths. *Am J Forensic Med Pathol*, 2007; **28**:271–7.

3. Krous HF, Beckwith JB, Byard RW, et al. Sudden Infant Death Syndrome and unclassified sudden infant deaths: a definitional and diagnostic approach. *Pediatrics*, 2004; **114**:234–8.

4. Shapiro-Mendoza CK, Camperlengo L, Ludvigsen R, et al. Classification system for the Sudden Unexpected Infant Death Case Registry and its application. *Pediatrics*, 2014; **134**:e210–19.

5. Matshes EW, Lew EO. An approach to the classification of apparent asphyxial infant deaths. *Acad Forensic Pathol*, 2017; **7**:200–11.

6. Hanzlick R. Pulmonary hemorrhage in deceased infants: baseline data for further study of infant mortality. *Am J Forensic Med Pathol*, 2001; **22**:188–92.

7. Willinger M, James LS, Catz C. Defining the Sudden Infant Death Syndrome (SIDS): deliberations of an expert panel convened by the National Institute of Child Health and Human Development. *Pediatr Pathol*, 1991; **11**:677–84.

8. Goudge ST. *Inquiry into Pediatric Forensic Pathology in Ontario Report*. Toronto: Queen's Printer for Ontario, Ontario Ministry of the Attorney General, 2008.

9. Collins KA. Death by overlaying and wedging: a 15-year retrospective study. *Am J Forensic Med Pathol*, 2001; **22**:155–9.

10. Hicks LJ, Scanlon MJ, Bostwick TC, et al. Death by smothering and its investigation. *Am J Forensic Med Pathol*, 1990; **11**:291–3.

11. Leduc D. *Well Beings: A Guide to Health in Child Care*, 3rd edn (revised). Ottawa: Canadian Paediatric Society, 2015.

12. Tieder JS, Bonkowsky JL, Etzel RA, et al. Clinical practice guideline: brief resolved unexplained events (formerly apparent life-threatening events) and evaluation of lower-risk infants: executive summary.

Pediatrics, 2016; **137**(5):e20160591; http://pediatrics .aappublications.org/content/pediatrics/137/5/e20160 590.full.pdf (accessed 31 October 2018).

13. Byard RW, Stewart WA, Telfer S, et al. Assessment of pulmonary and intrathymic hemosiderin deposition in Sudden Infant Death Syndrome. *Pediatr Pathol Lab Med*, 1997; **17**:275–82.

14. Jackson CM, Gilliland MG. Frequency of pulmonary hemosiderosis in Eastern North Carolina. *Am J Forensic Med Pathol*, 2000; **21**:36–8.

15. Kempe CH, Silverman FN, Steele BF, et al. The battered-child syndrome. *JAMA*, 1962; **181**:17–24.

16. *Memorandum #63. New Protocol to be Used in the Investigation of the Sudden and Unexpected Death of Any Child Under 2 Years of Age.* Toronto: Office of the Chief Coroner of Ontario, 1995.

17. DiMaio VJM, DiMaio DJ. *Forensic Pathology.* New York: Elsevier, 1989.

18. Pinneri K, Matshes E. Recommendations for the autopsy of an infant who has died suddenly and unexpectedly. *Acad Forensic Pathol*, 2017; **7**:171–81.

19. Shkrum MJ, Ramsay DA. *Forensic Pathology of Trauma: Common Problems for the Pathologist.* Totowa, NJ: Humana Press, 2007.

20. Byard RW. Unexpected infant death: lessons from the Sally Clark case. *Med J Aust*, 2004; **181**:52–4.

21. Green FC. Child abuse and neglect: a priority problem for the private physician. *Pediatr Clin North Am*, 1975; **22**:329–39.

22. Maguire S, Mann MK, Sibert J, et al. Are there patterns of bruising in childhood which are diagnostic or suggestive of abuse? A systematic review. *Arch Dis Child*, 2005; **90**:182–6.

23. Patel B, Butterfield R. Common skin and bleeding disorders that can potentially masquerade as child abuse. *Am J Med Genet C Semin Med Genet*, 2015; **169**: 328–36.

24. Schwartz KA, Metz J, Feldman K, et al. Cutaneous findings mistaken for physical abuse: present but not pervasive. *Pediatr Dermatol*, 2014; **31**:146–55.

25. Tsokos M. Diagnostic criteria for cutaneous injuries in child abuse: classification, findings, and interpretation. *Forensic Sci Med Pathol*, 2015; **11**:235–42.

26. Anderst JD, Carpenter SL, Abshire TC. Evaluation for bleeding disorders in suspected child abuse. *Pediatrics*, 2013; **131**:e1314–22.

27. Pierce MC, Kaczor K, Aldridge S, et al. Bruising characteristics discriminating physical child abuse from accidental trauma. *Pediatrics*, 2010; **125**:67–74.

28. Maguire S, Mann MK, Sibert J, et al. Can you age bruises accurately in children? A systematic review. *Arch Dis Child*, 2005; **90**:187–9.

29. Bariciak ED, Plint AC, Gaboury I, et al. Dating of bruises in children: an assessment of physician accuracy. *Pediatrics*, 2003; **112**:804–7.

30. Vanezis P. Interpreting bruises at necropsy. *J Clin Pathol*, 2001; **54**:348–55.

31. Nichols GR, Corey TS, Davis GJ. Nonfracture-associated fatal fat embolism in a case of child abuse. *J Forensic Sci*, 1990; **35**:493–9.

32. Metz JB, Schwartz KA, Feldman KW, et al. Non-cutaneous conditions clinicians might mistake for abuse. *Arch Dis Child*, 2014; **99**:817–23.

33. Asati DP, Singh S, Sharma VK, et al. Dermatoses misdiagnosed as deliberate injuries. *Med Sci Law*, 2012; **52**:198–204.

34. Carpenter SL, Abshire TC, Anderst JD. Evaluating for suspected child abuse: conditions that predispose to bleeding. *Pediatrics*, 2013; **131**:e1357–73.

35. Chester DL, Jose RM, Aldlyami E, et al. Non-accidental burns in children – are we neglecting neglect? *Burns J Int Soc Burn Inj*, 2006; **32**:222–8.

36. Lilly E, Kundu RV. Dermatoses secondary to Asian cultural practices. *Int J Dermatol*, 2012; **51**:372–9; quiz 379–82.

37. Pollanen MS, Smith CR, Chiasson DA, et al. Fatal child abuse-maltreatment syndrome. A retrospective study in Ontario, Canada, 1990–1995. *Forensic Sci Int*, 2002; **126**:101–4.

38. Pelletti G, Tambuscio S, Montisci M, et al. Misinterpretation of anogenital findings and misdiagnosis of child sexual abuse: The role of the forensic pathologist. *J Pediatr Adolesc Gynecol*, 2016; **29**:e29–31.

39. McCann J, Reay D, Siebert J, et al. Postmortem perianal findings in children. *Am J Forensic Med Pathol*, 1996; **17**:289–98.

40. Hobbs CJ, Wright CM. Anal signs of child sexual abuse: a case-control study. *BMC Pediatr*, 2014; **14**:128.

41. Ross AH, Juarez CA. Skeletal and radiological manifestations of child abuse: Implications for study in past populations. *Clin Anat NYN*, 2016; **29**:844–53.

42. Akbarnia B, Torg JS, Kirkpatrick J, et al. Manifestations of the battered-child syndrome. *J Bone Joint Surg Am*, 1974; **56**:1159–66.

43. Merten DF, Radkowski MA, Leonidas JC. The abused child: a radiological reappraisal. *Radiology*, 1983; **146**:377–81.

44. Conway JJ, Collins M, Tanz RR, et al. The role of bone scintigraphy in detecting child abuse. *Semin Nucl Med*, 1993; **23**:321–33.

45. Brogdon BG (Byron G, Shwayder T, Elifritz J. *Child Abuse and its Mimics in Skin and Bone.* Boca Raton, FL: CRC Press, 2012.

46. Klotzbach H, Delling G, Richter E, et al. Post-mortem diagnosis and age estimation of infants' fractures. *Int J Legal Med*, 2003; **117**:82–9.

47. Sanchez TR, Grasparil AD, Chaudhari R, et al. Characteristics of rib fractures in child abuse – The role of low-dose chest computed tomography. *Pediatr Emerg Care*, 2018; **34**(2):81–3.

48. Maguire S, Mann M, John N, et al. Does cardiopulmonary resuscitation cause rib fractures in children? A systematic review. *Child Abuse Negl*, 2006; **30**:739–51.

49. Kleinman PK, Marks SC, Nimkin K, et al. Rib fractures in 31 abused infants: postmortem radiologic-histopathologic study. *Radiology*, 1996; **200**: 807–10.

50. Lonergan GJ, Baker AM, Morey MK, et al. From the archives of the AFIP. Child abuse: radiologic-pathologic correlation. *Radiogr Rev Publ Radiol Soc N Am Inc*, 2003; **23**:811–45.

51. Carty HM. Fractures caused by child abuse. *J Bone Joint Surg Br*, 1993; **75**:849–57.

52. Sanchez TR, Nguyen H, Palacios W, et al. Retrospective evaluation and dating of non-accidental rib fractures in infants. *Clin Radiol*, 2013; **68**:e467–71.

53. Chapman S. The radiological dating of injuries. *Arch Dis Child*, 1992; **67**:1063–5.

54. Prosser I, Lawson Z, Evans A, et al. A timetable for the radiologic features of fracture healing in young children. *AJR Am J Roentgenol*, 2012; **198**: 1014–20.

55. Betz P, Liebhardt E. Rib fractures in children – resuscitation or child abuse? *Int J Legal Med*, 1994; **106**:215–18.

56. Weber MA, Risdon RA, Offiah AC, et al. Rib fractures identified at post-mortem examination in sudden unexpected deaths in infancy (SUDI). *Forensic Sci Int*, 2009; **189**:75–81.

57. Kogutt MS, Swischuk LE, Fagan CJ. Patterns of injury and significance of uncommon fractures in the battered child syndrome. *Am J Roentgenol Radium Ther Nucl Med*, 1974; **121**:143–9.

58. Duval JV, Andrew TA. Two thumb method of infant CPR: Is there an increased risk for posterior rib fractures? Paper presented at National Association of Medical Examiners 41st Annual Meeting, 2007, Savannah, Georgia.

59. Clouse JR, Lantz PE. Posterior rib fractures in infants associated with cardiopulmonary resuscitation. Paper presented at American Academy of Forensic Sciences Annual Meeting, 2008, Washington, DC.

60. Matshes EW, Lew EO. Two-handed cardiopulmonary resuscitation can cause rib fractures in infants. *Am J Forensic Med Pathol*, 2010; **31**:303–7.

61. van Rijn RR, Bilo RAC, Robben SGF. Birth-related mid-posterior rib fractures in neonates: a report of three cases (and a possible fourth case) and a review of the literature. *Pediatr Radiol*, 2009; **39**:30–4.

62. Pandya NK, Baldwin K, Kamath AF, et al. Unexplained fractures: child abuse or bone disease? A systematic review. *Clin Orthop*, 2011; **469**:805–12.

63. Cannell JJ, Holick MF. Multiple unexplained fractures in infants and child physical abuse. *J Steroid Biochem Mol Biol*, 2018; **175**:18–22.

64. Miller M, Mirkin LD. Classical metaphyseal lesions thought to be pathognomonic of child abuse are often artifacts or indicative of metabolic bone disease. *Med Hypotheses*, 2018; **115**:65–71.

65. Leavitt EB, Pincus RL, Bukachevsky R. Otolaryngologic manifestations of child abuse. *Arch Otolaryngol Head Neck Surg*, 1992; **118**:629–31.

66. Phillips VM, Van Der Heyde Y. Oro-facial trauma in child abuse fatalities. *South Afr Med J Suid-Afr Tydskr Vir Geneeskd*, 2006; **96**:213–15.

67. Maguire SA, Upadhyaya M, Evans A, et al. A systematic review of abusive visceral injuries in childhood – their range and recognition. *Child Abuse Negl*, 2013; **37**:430–45.

68. Plunkett J. Resuscitation injuries complicating the interpretation of premortem trauma and natural disease in children. *J Forensic Sci*, 2006; **51**:127–30.

69. Kleinman PK, Raptopoulos VD, Brill PW. Occult nonskeletal trauma in the battered-child syndrome. *Radiology*, 1981; **141**:393–6.

70. Huntimer CM, Muret-Wagstaff S, Leland NL. Can falls on stairs result in small intestine perforations? *Pediatrics*, 2000; **106**:301–5.

71. Barnes PM, Norton CM, Dunstan FD, et al. Abdominal injury due to child abuse. *Lancet*, 2005; **366**:234–5.

72. Davison AM, Lazda EJ. Small bowel perforation and fatal peritonitis following a fall in a 21-month-old child. *Forensic Sci Med Pathol*, 2008; **4**:250–4.

73. Gaines BA, Shultz BS, Morrison K, et al. Duodenal injuries in children: beware of child abuse. *J Pediatr Surg*, 2004; **39**:600–2.

74. Nimkin K, Teeger S, Wallach MT, et al. Adrenal hemorrhage in abused children: imaging and postmortem findings. *AJR Am J Roentgenol*, 1994; **162**:661–3.

75. Matshes EW, Lew EO. Do resuscitation-related injuries kill infants and children? *Am J Forensic Med Pathol*, 2010; **31**:178–85.

76. Madea B, Ortmann J, Doberentz E. Forensic aspects of starvation. *Forensic Sci Med Pathol*, 2016; **12**: 276–98.

77. Folkerth RD Nunez J, Zhanna G, McGuone D. Neuropathologic examination in sudden unexpected deaths in infancy and childhood: recommendations for highest diagnostic yield and cost-effectiveness in forensic settings. *Acad Forensic Pathol*, 2017; **7**:182–99.

78. Mortazavi MM, Shane Tubbs R, Riech S, et al. Anatomy and pathology of the cranial emissary veins: A review with surgical implications. *Neurosurgery*, 2012; **70**:1312–18.

79. Aliabadi H, Miller J, Radnakrishnan S, et al. Spontaneous intrauterine 'ping-pong' fracture: review and case illustration. *Neuropediatrics*, 2009; **40**:73–5.

80. Heise RH, Srivatsa PJ, Karsell PR. Spontaneous intrauterine linear skull fracture: a rare complication of spontaneous vaginal delivery. *Obstet Gynecol*, 1996; **87**:851–4.

81. Loire M, Barat M, Mangyanda Kinkembo L, et al. Spontaneous ping-pong parietal fracture in a newborn. *Arch Dis Child Fetal Neonatal Ed*, 2017; **102**:F160–F161.

82. Idriz S, Patel JH, Ameli Renani S, et al. CT of normal developmental and variant anatomy of the pediatric skull: Distinguishing trauma from normality. *RadioGraphics*, 2015; **35**:1585–601.

83. Sanchez T, Stewart D, Walvick M, et al. Skull fracture vs. accessory sutures: How can we tell the difference? *Emerg Radiol*, 2010; **17**:413–18.

84. Marti B, Sirinelli D, Maurin L, et al. Wormian bones in a general paediatric population. *Diagn Interv Imaging*, 2013; **94**:428–32.

85. Bellary SS, Steinberg A, Mirzayan N, et al. Wormian bones: A review. *Clin Anat*, 2013; **26**:922–7.

86. Droms RJ, Rork JF, McLean R, et al. Menkes disease mimicking child abuse. *Pediatr Dermatol*, 2017; **34**: e132–e134.

87. Wiedijk JEF, Soerdjbalie-Maikoe V, Maat GJR, et al. An accessory skull suture mimicking a skull fracture. *Forensic Sci Int*, 2016; **260**:e11–13.

88. Plunkett J. Fatal pediatric head injuries caused by short-distance falls. *Am J Forensic Med Pathol*, 2001; **22**:1–12.

89. Reiber GD. Fatal falls in childhood. How far must children fall to sustain fatal head injury? Report of cases and review of the literature. *Am J Forensic Med Pathol*, 1993; **14**:201–7.

90. Van Ee C, Moroski-Browne B, Raymond D, et al. Evaluation and refinement of the CRABI-6 anthropomorphic test device injury criteria for skull fracture. In: *ASME 2009 International Mechanical Engineering Congress and Exposition*: vol. 2,*Biomedical and Biotechnology Engineering*. Lake Buena Vista, FL: ASME Digital Library: 2009:387–93.

91. Reece RM, Sege R. Childhood head injuries: accidental or inflicted? *Arch Pediatr Adolesc Med*, 2000; **154**:11–15.

92. Harwood-Nash DC, Hendrick EB, Hudson AR. The significance of skull fractures in children. A study of 1,187 patients. *Radiology*, 1971; **101**:151–6.

93. Chadwick DL, Bertocci G, Castillo E, et al. Annual risk of death resulting from short falls among young children: less than 1 in 1 million. *Pediatrics*, 2008; **121**:1213–24.

94. Helfer RE, Slovis TL, Black M. Injuries resulting when small children fall out of bed. *Pediatrics*, 1977; **60**: 533–5.

95. Kravitz H, Driessen G, Gomberg R, et al. Accidental falls from elevated surfaces in infants from birth to one year of age. *Pediatrics*, 1969; **44**:869–76.

96. Squier W. Shaken baby syndrome: the quest for evidence. *Dev Med Child Neurol*, 2008; **50**:10–14.

97. Huang MHS, Mouradian WE, Cohen SR, et al. The differential diagnosis of abnormal head shapes: Separating craniosynostosis from positional deformities and normal variants. *Cleft Palate Craniofac J*, 1998; **35**:204–11.

98. Rogers GF. Deformational plagiocephaly, brachycephaly, and scaphocephaly. Part II. *J Craniofac Surg*, 2011; **22**:17–23.

99. Cunningham ML, Heike CL. Evaluation of the infant with an abnormal skull shape. *Curr Opin Pediatr*, 2007; **19**:645–51.

100. Ginelliová A, Farkaš D, Iannaccone SF, et al. Sudden death associated with syndromic craniosynostosis. *Forensic Sci Med Pathol*, 2016; **12**:506–9.

101. Von der Hagen M, Pivarcsi M, Liebe J, et al. Diagnostic approach to microcephaly in childhood: A two-center study and review of the literature. *Dev Med Child Neurol*, 2014; **56**:732–41.

102. Olney AH. Macrocephaly Syndromes. *Semin Pediatr Neurol*, 2007; **14**:128–35.

103. Beasley M. Age of fontanelles/cranial sutures closure. *Centre for Academic Research and Training in Anthropogeny: Matrix of Comparitive Anthropogeny* https://carta.anthropogeny.org/moca/topics/age-closure-fontanelles-sutures (accessed 31 October 2018).

104. Kiesler J, Ricer R. The abnormal fontanelle. *Am Fam Physician*, 2003; **67**:2547–52.

105. Pindrik J, Ye X, Ji BG, et al. Anterior fontanelle closure and size in full-term children based on head computed tomography. *Clin Pediatr Phil*, 2014; **53**:1149–57.

106. Cohen MC, Scheimberg I. Evidence of occurrence of intradural and subdural hemorrhage in the perinatal and neonatal period in the context of hypoxic

Ischemic encephalopathy: an observational study from two referral institutions in the United Kingdom. *Pediatr Dev Pathol*, 2009; **12**:169–76.

107. Scheimberg I, Cohen MC, Zapata Vazquez RE, et al. Nontraumatic intradural and subdural hemorrhage and hypoxic ischemic encephalopathy in fetuses, infants, and children up to three years of age: analysis of two audits of 636 cases from two referral centers in the United Kingdom. *Pediatr Dev Pathol*, 2013; **16**:149–59.

108. Rutty GN, Squier WM. Subdural hematoma in children. In: *Essentials of Autopsy Practice: Current Methods and Modern Trends*. Berlin: Springer, 2006: 131–53.

109. Pollanen MS. Subdural hemorrhage in infancy: keep an open mind. *Forensic Sci Med Pathol*, 2011; 7:298–300.

110. De Leeuw M, Beuls E, Jorens P, et al. Delta-storage pool disease as a mimic of abusive head trauma in a 7-month-old baby: a case report. *J Forensic Leg Med*, 2013; **20**:520–1.

111. Ganesh A, Jenny C, Geyer J, et al. Retinal hemorrhages in type I osteogenesis imperfecta after minor trauma. *Ophthalmology*, 2004; **111**:1428–31.

112. Haddad MH. Hemorrhages after minor trauma (letter). *Ophthalmology*, 2005; **112**:737–8.

113. Nassogne M-C, Sharrard M, Hertz-Pannier L, et al. Massive subdural haematomas in Menkes disease mimicking shaken baby syndrome. *Childs Nerv Syst ChNS Off J Int Soc Pediatr Neurosurg*, 2002; **18**:729–31.

114. Zielonka M, Braun K, Bengel A, et al. Severe acute subdural hemorrhage in a patient with glutaric aciduria type I after minor head trauma: A case report. *J Child Neurol*, 2015; **30**:1065–9.

115. Cohen MC, Yap S, Olpin E. Inherited metabolic disease and sudden unexpected death. In: Payne-James J, Byard RW, eds. *Encyclopaedia of Forensic and Legal Medicine*, 2nd edn., Oxford: Elsevier, 2016: 85–95.

116. Christian CW. The evaluation of suspected child physical abuse. *Pediatrics*, 2015; **135** e1337–e1354.

117. Lynøe N, Elinder G, Hallberg B, et al. Insufficient evidence for 'shaken baby syndrome' – a systematic review. *Acta Paediatr*, 2017; **2**:1–7.

118. Rorke-Adams LB. The triad of retinal haemorrhage, subdural haemorrhage and encephalopathy in an infant unassociated with evidence of physical injury is not the result of shaking, but is most likely to have been caused by a natural disease: No. *J Prim Health Care*, 2011; **3**:161–3.

119. Saunders D, Raissaki M, Servaes S, et al. Throwing the baby out with the bath water – response to the Swedish Agency for Health Technology Assessment and Assessment of Social Services (SBU) report on traumatic shaking. *Pediatr Radiol*, 2017; **47**(11) 1386–9.

120. Squier W. The triad of retinal haemorrhage, subdural haemorrhage and encephalopathy in an infant unassociated with evidence of physical injury is not the result of shaking, but is most likely to have been caused by a natural disease: Yes. *J Prim Health Care*, 2011; **3**:159–61.

121. Squier W. 'Shaken baby syndrome' and forensic pathology. *Forensic Sci Med Pathol*, 2014; **10**:248–50.

122. Del Bigio MR, Phillips SM. Retroocular and subdural hemorrhage or hemosiderin deposits in pediatric autopsies. *J Neuropathol Exp Neurol*, 2017; **62**:513–69.

123. Rooks VJ, Eaton JP, Ruess L, et al. Prevalence and evolution of intracranial hemorrhage in asymptomatic term infants. *Am J Neuroradiol*, 2008; **29**:1082–9.

124. Kelly P, Hayman R, Shekerdemian LS, et al. Subdural hemorrhage and hypoxia in infants with congenital heart disease. *Pediatrics*, 2014; **134**:e773–81.

125. Watts P, Maguire S, Kwok T, et al. Newborn retinal hemorrhages: A systematic review. *J AAPOS*, 2013; **17**:70–8.

126. Leeuw MD, Beuls E, Jorens PG, et al. The optic nerve sheath hemorrhage is a non-specific finding in cases of suspected child abuse. *J Forensic Leg Med*, 2015; **36**:43–8.

127. deVeber G, Andrew M, Adams C, et al. Cerebral sinovenous thrombosis in children. *N Engl J Med*, 2001; **345**:417–23.

128. Hedlund GL. Cerebral sinovenous thrombosis in pediatric practice. *Pediatr Radiol*, 2013; **43**:173–88.

129. McLean LS; Frasier LD; Hedlund GL. Does intracranial venous thrombosis cause subdural hemorrhage in the pediatric population? *AJNR*, 2012; **33**:1281–4.

130. Krasnokutsky MV. Cerebral venous thrombosis: a potential mimic of primary traumatic brain injury in infants. *AJR Am J Roentgenol*, 2011; **197**:W503–7.

131. Squier W. The 'shaken baby' syndrome: pathology and mechanisms. *Acta Neuropathol (Berl)*, 2011; **122**:519–42.

132. Sieswerda-Hoogendoorn T, Soerdjbalie-Maikoe V, de Bakker H, et al. Postmortem CT compared to autopsy in children; concordance in a forensic setting. *Int J Legal Med*, 2014; **128**:957–65.

133. Krous HF, Haas EA, Chadwick AE, et al. Delayed death in Sudden Infant Death Syndrome: a San Diego SIDS/SUDC Research Project 15-year population-based report. *Forensic Sci Int*, 2008; **176**:209–16.

134. Geddes JF, Tasker RC, Hackshaw AK, et al. Dural haemorrhage in non-traumatic infant deaths: does it explain the bleeding in 'shaken baby syndrome'? *Neuropathol Appl Neurobiol*, 2004; **29**:14–22.

135. Smith C, Bell JE, Keeling JW, et al. Dural haemorrhage in nontraumatic infant deaths: does it explain the bleeding in 'shaken baby syndrome'? Geddes JE et al. A response. *Neuropathol Appl Neurobiol*, 2003; **29**:411–12.

136. Punt J, Bonshek RE, Jaspan T, et al. The 'unified hypothesis' of Geddes et al. is not supported by the data. *Pediatr Rehabil*, 2004; **7**:173–84.

137. Byard RW, Blumbergs P, Rutty G, et al. Lack of evidence for a causal relationship between hypoxic-ischemic encephalopathy and subdural hemorrhage in fetal life, infancy, and early childhood. *Pediatr Dev Pathol*, 2007; **10**:348–50.

138. Hurley M, Dineen R, Padfield CJH, et al. Is there a causal relationship between the hypoxia-ischaemia associated with cardiorespiratory arrest and subdural haematomas? An observational study. *Br J Radiol*, 2010; **83**:736–43.

139. Rafaat KT, Spear RM, Kuelbs C, et al. Cranial computed tomographic findings in a large group of children with drowning: diagnostic, prognostic, and forensic implications. *Pediatr Crit Care Med*, 2008; **9**:567–72.

140. Bradford R, Choudhary AK, Dias MS. Serial neuroimaging in infants with abusive head trauma: timing abusive injuries. *J Neurosurg Pediatr*, 2013; **12**:110–19.

141. Vázquez E, Delgado I, Sánchez-Montañez A, et al. Imaging abusive head trauma: why use both computed tomography and magnetic resonance imaging? *Pediatr Radiol*, 2014; **44**:589–603.

142. Blumenthal I. Periventricular leucomalacia: a review. *Eur J Pediatr*, 2004; **163**:435–42.

143. Resch B, Resch E, Maurer-Fellbaum U, et al. The whole spectrum of cystic periventricular leukomalacia of the preterm infant: results from a large consecutive case series. *Childs Nerv Syst*, 2015; **31**:1527–32.

144. Takashima S, Armstrong D, Becker L. Subcortical leukomalacia. *Arch Neurol*, 1978; **35**:470–2.

145. Takashima SAD. Cerebral white matter lesions in Sudden Infant Death Syndrome. *Pediatrics*, 1978; **62**:155–61.

146. Au-Yong ITH, Wardle SP, McConachie NS, et al. Isolated cerebral cortical tears in children: aetiology, characterisation and differentiation from non-accidental head injury. *Br J Radiol*, 2009; **82**:735–41.

147. Huang AH, Robertson RL. Spontaneous superficial parenchymal and leptomeningeal hemorrhage in term neonates. *Am J Neuroradiol*, 2004; **25**:469–75. [Erratum at AJNR (2004) 25:666]

148. Allen TB. Sudden infant death with periventricular leukomalacia. *J Forensic Sci*, 1985; **30**:1260–2.

149. Calder IM; Hill I; Scholtz CL. Primary brain trauma in non-accidental injury. *J Clin Pathol*, 1984; **37**:1095–100.

150. Jaspan T, Narborough G, Punt JAG, et al. Cerebral contusional tears as a marker of child abuse – detection by cranial sonography. *Pediatr Radiol*, 1992; **22**:237–45.

151. Lindenberg R, Freytag E. Morphology of brain lesions from blunt trauma in early infancy. *ArchPathol*, 1969; **87**:298–305.

152. Tubbs RS, Krishnamurthy S, Verma K, et al. Cavum velum interpositum, cavum septum pellucidum, and cavum vergae: a review. *Childs Nerv Syst*, 2011; **27**:1927–30.

153. Wiig US, Zahl SM, Egge A, et al. Epidemiology of benign external hydrocephalus in Norway – a population-based study. *Pediatr Neurol*, 2017; **73**:36–41.

154. Tucker J, Choudhary AK, Piatt J. Macrocephaly in infancy: benign enlargement of the subarachnoid spaces and subdural collections. *J Neurosurg Pediatr*, 2016; **18**:16–20.

155. Fingarson AK, Ryan ME, McLone SG, et al. Enlarged subarachnoid spaces and intracranial hemorrhage in children with accidental head trauma. *J Neurosurg Pediatr*, 2017; **19**:254–8.

156. Gorrie C, Oakes S, Duflou J, et al. Axonal injury in children after motor vehicle crashes: extent, distribution, and size of axonal swellings using beta-APP immunohistochemistry. *J Neurotrauma*, 2002; **19**:1171–82.

157. Hortobágyi T, Wise S, Hunt N, et al. Traumatic axonal damage in the brain can be detected using beta-APP immunohistochemistry within 35 min after head injury to human adults. *Neuropathol Appl Neurobiol*, 2007; **33**:226–37.

158. Hayashi T, Ago K, Nakamae T, et al. Two different immunostaining patterns of beta-amyloid precursor protein (APP) may distinguish traumatic from nontraumatic axonal injury. *Int J Legal Med*, 2015; **129**:1085–90.

159. Geddes JF, Whitwell HL, Graham DI. Traumatic axonal injury: practical issues for diagnosis in medicolegal cases. *Neuropathol Appl Neurobiol*, 2000; **26**:105–16.

160. Geddes JF, Vowles GH, Hackshaw AK, et al. Neuropathology of inflicted head injury in children.

II. Microscopic brain injury in infants. *Brain J Neurol*, 2001; **124**:1299–306.

161. Matschke J, Büttner A, Bergmann M, et al. Encephalopathy and death in infants with abusive head trauma is due to hypoxic-ischemic injury following local brain trauma to vital brainstem centers. *Int J Legal Med*, 2015; **129**:105–14. [Erratum in Int J Legal Med (2015) 129:115–16]

162. Swischuk LE. Spine and spinal cord trauma in the battered child syndrome. *Radiology*, 1969; **92**:733–8.

163. Kriss VM, Kriss TC. SCIWORA (spinal cord injury without radiographic abnormality) in infants and children. *Clin Pediatr (Phila)*, 1996; **35**:119–24.

164. Jaremko JL, Siminoski K, Firth GB, et al. Common normal variants of pediatric vertebral development that mimic fractures: a pictorial review from a national longitudinal bone health study. *Pediatr Radiol*, 2015; **45**:593–605.

165. Mäyränpää MK, Viljakainen HT, Toiviainen-Salo S, et al. Impaired bone health and asymptomatic vertebral compressions in fracture-prone children: a case-control study. *JBMR*, 2012; **27**(6):1413–24.

166. Choudhary AK, Ishak R, Zacharia TT, et al. Imaging of spinal injury in abusive head trauma: a retrospective study. *Pediatr Radiol*, 2014; **44**:1130–40.

167. Kemp AM, Joshi AH, Mann M, et al. What are the clinical and radiological characteristics of spinal injuries from physical abuse: a systematic review. *Arch Dis Child*, 2010; **95**:355–60.

168. Koumellis P, McConachie NS, Jaspan T. Spinal subdural haematomas in children with non-accidental head injury. *Arch Dis Child*, 2009; **94**:216–19.

169. Bortolotti C, Wang H, Fraser K, et al. Subacute spinal subdural hematoma after spontaneous resolution of cranial subdural hematoma: causal relationship or coincidence? Case report. *J Neurosurg*, 2004; **100**:372–4.

170. Adler MD, Comi AE, Walker AR. Acute hemorrhagic complication of diagnostic lumbar puncture. *Pediatr Emerg Care*, 2001; **17**:184–8.

171. Harris LS, Adelson L. 'Spinal injury' and sudden infant death. A second look. *Am J Clin Pathol*, 1969; **52**:289–95.

172. Rutty GN, Squier WM, Padfield CJ. Epidural haemorrhage of the cervical spinal cord: a post-mortem artefact? *Neuropathol Appl Neurobiol*, 2005; **31**:247–57.

173. Duggal N, Lach B. Selective vulnerability of the lumbosacral spinal cord after cardiac arrest and hypotension. *Stroke*, 2002; **33**:116–21.

174. Squier W, Scheimberg I, Smith C. Spinal nerve root β-APP staining in infants is not a reliable indicator of trauma. *Forensic Sci Int*, 2011; **212**:e31–5.

Index